AORTIC STENOSIS – ETIOLOGY, PATHOPHYSIOLOGY AND TREATMENT

Edited by **Masanori Hirota**

Aortic Stenosis – Etiology, Pathophysiology and Treatment
Edited by Masanori Hirota

Published by InTech

Janeza Trdine 9, 51000 Rijeka, Croatia

Publishing Process Manager Alenka Urbancic

Technical Editor Teodora Smiljanic

Cover Designer InTech Design Team

Additional hard copies can be obtained from orders@intechopen.com

Aortic Stenosis – Etiology, Pathophysiology and Treatment, Edited by Masanori Hirota
p. cm.
ISBN 978-953-307-660-7

For EU product safety concerns:
IN TECH d.o.o., Prolaz Marije Krucifikse Kozulić 3, 51000 Rijeka, Croatia,
info@intechopen.com or visit our website at intechopen.com.

Meet the editor

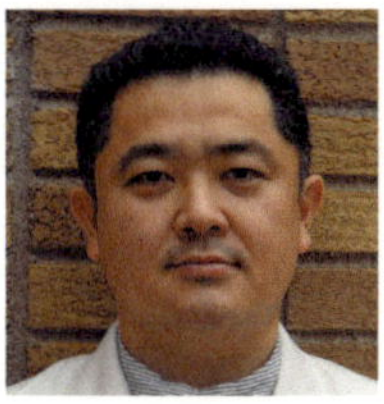

Dr. Hirota is a cardiovascular surgeon at Hayama Heart Center in Japan, one of the leading heart centers in Japan in which numerous cardiac surgeries, especially for patients with acquired heart disease, are performed, and characteristically, surgical ventricular restoration for patients with severe ischemic and non-ischemic cardiomyopathy, which has been performed for over 10 years. Dr. Hirota graduated at the Okayama University School of Medicine in 1996. He took part in a large number of cardiovascular surgeries associated with pediatric and adult heart disease, as well as vascular disease. His post-graduate research theme was on hemodynamic analysis of global ischemic hearts for heart transplantation and elucidation of endothelium-derived hyperpolarizing factor for coronary microcirculation. Dr. Hirota currently works as a cardiovascular surgeon.

Contents

Preface

At the moment, aortic stenosis (AS) is the most prevalent valvular disease in the developed countries. Pathological and molecular mechanisms of AS have been investigated in many aspects, and new therapeutic devices, such as trans-catheter aortic valve implantation, have been developed as a less invasive treatment for high-risk patients. Due to advanced prevalent age of AS, further research results and technology are required to treat elderly patients for longer life expectancy.

This book is an effort to present an up-to-date account of existing knowledge, involving recent development in this field. There are 15 chapters written by several expert researchers and clinicians, including cardiologists, cardiac surgeons, pediatricians, physiologists, pathologists and immunologists. These opinion leaders described details of established knowledge, as well as newly recognized advances associated with diagnosis, treatment and mechanism in their speciality. This book will enable close intercommunication to another field and collaboration technology for new devices. We hope that it will be an important source, not only to clinicians, but also to general practitioners, contributing to development of better therapeutic adjuncts in the future.

Masanori Hirota, MD, PhD
Department of Cardiovascular Surgery,
Hayama Heart Center, Kanagawa,
Japan

Part 1

Introduction

1

Aortic Stenosis - New Insights in Stenosis Progression and in Prevention

Parolari Alessandro, Trezzi Matteo, Merati Elisa,
Filippini Sara and Alamanni Francesco
Dept. Of Cardiovascular Sciences, University of Milano,
Centro Cardiologico Monzino IRCCS, Milano
Italy

1. Introduction

1.1 Prevalence

Aortic valve disease, in particular stenosis (AS), is the most common valvular abnormality detected in the aging population whit an AS prevalence of 3 to 5% in the population over 75 years of age (1, 2). Valvular aortic stenosis without accompanying mitral valve disease is more common in men than in women. A clear increase in prevalence of aortic sclerosis has been seen with age: 20% in patients aged 65–75 years, 35% in those aged 75–85 years, and 48% in patients older than 85 years. For the same age-groups, 1.3%, 2.4%, and 4% have frank aortic stenosis (3).

1.2 Etiology

AS is the obstruction of blood flow across the aortic valve. AS has several etiologies including rheumatic fever, congenital unicuspid or bicuspid valve, and degenerative calcific changes of the valve. Rheumatic heart disease is the main cause of valvular heart disease worldwide, but fewer than 10% of AS cases in the United States and Western Europe are rheumatic. In contrast, senile, calcific disease of the aortic valve and bicuspid valve disease are responsible for the vast majority of AS cases in those countries. Since the incidence of AS increases with age and the Western population as a whole is aging, increased numbers of patients presenting with AS are expected in the near future. Currently, the incidence of AS is estimated to be 1−2% among those over 65 years of age and 4% among octagenarians.
Rheumatic AS is rarely an isolated disease and usually occurs in conjunction with mitral valve stenosis. Rheumatic AS is characterized by diffuse fibrous leaflet thickening of the tricuspid valve with fusion of the commissures with scarring and eventual calcification of the cusps. A congenital malformation of the valve may also result in stenosis and is the most common cause in young adults. Bicuspid aortic valve is the most common cause of aortic stenosis in patients under age 65. About 2% of people are born with aortic valves that have only two cusps (bicuspid valves). Although bicuspid valves usually do not impede blood flow when the patients are young, they do not open as widely as normal valves with three cusps. Therefore, blood flow across the bicuspid valves is more turbulent, causing increased wear and tear on the valve leaflets. Over time, excessive wear and tear leads to calcification,

scarring, and reduced mobility of the valve leaflets. About 10% of bicuspid valves become significantly narrowed, resulting in the symptoms and heart problems of aortic stenosis.
The most common cause for AS in adults is senile degenerative AS, with the calcification of a normal trileaflet or a congenital bicuspid valve (4). Even if it was considered to be the result of years of mechanical stress on an otherwise normal valve, the evolving concept is that the degenerative process leads to proliferative and inflammatory changes. Calcific aortic-valve disease refers to progressive aortic leaflet thickening and calcification, beginning with the early lesion of aortic-valve sclerosis leading to advanced leaflet disease of aortic-valve stenosis, characterized by restricted leaflet motion and outflow obstruction. The pathobiology of the aortic-valve lesion involves an atheromatous, osteogenic, inflammatory process sharing some histologic similarities with coronary atherosclerosis (5)

1.3 Pathophysiology

Valvular aortic stenosis results in chronic left ventricular pressure overloading. At any stage of life, however, the natural history of aortic stenosis largely reflects the functional integrity of the mitral valve. As long as adequate mitral valve function is maintained, the pulmonary bed is protected from the systolic pressure overloading imposed by aortic stenosis. Compensatory concentric left ventricular hypertrophy allows the pressure-overloaded ventricle to maintain stroke volume with modest increases in diastolic pressure, and patients remain asymptomatic for many years. In early stages the development of concentric hypertrophy appears to be an appropriate and beneficial adaptation to compensate for high intracavitary pressures. Unfortunately, this adaptation often carries adverse consequences. The hypertrophied heart may have reduced coronary blood flow and also exhibit a limited coronary vasodilator reserve, even in the absence of epicardial coronary artery disease, that`s why one of the symptoms is angina. In later stages of severe AS, cardiac output declines, and the pulmonary artery pressure rises, leading to pulmonary hypertension. The first symptom of this condition is increasing shortness of breath and the last consequence is heart failure. The onset of any of the classic symptoms of left ventricular outflow obstruction—angina, syncope, or heart failure—in a patient with valvular aortic stenosis indicates advanced valve disease and should be carefully and promptly evaluated. Syncope most commonly is due to the reduced cerebral perfusion that occurs during exertion secondary to the decrease in arterial pressure consequent to peripheral vasodilation in the presence of a fixed cardiac output. For years the cause of the calcification of the aortic valve was thought to be the passive accumulation of calcium in the valve leaflets, causing nodular deposits and an eventual stenosis. Clinical studies have demonstrated that the risk factors for this process include hypercholesterolemia, diabetes, smoking, hypertension, male sex, and elevated high sensitivity C-reactive protein (6), suggesting that calcification of the aortic valve results from an inflammatory process triggered by these factors of atherosclerotic risk and that drug therapies to retard this process may be a useful strategy in the future. Hyperuricemia has been identified as another risk factor for development of aortic valvular disease. Calcific AS is also observed in a number of other conditions, including Paget disease of bone and end-stage renal disease. Ochronosis with alkaptonuria is another rare cause of AS, which also can cause a rare greenish discoloration of the aortic valve. Recent experimental models have shown that there is a relationship between hypercholesterolemia and the development of aortic valvular disease (7). Studies of human tissue also suggest that the development of aortic valvular calcification represents an active cellular biology. O'Brien et al. have described the early valvular lesion (aortic sclerosis) as an entity very similar to the early lesion of the atherosclerotic plaque (8). These lesions show similarities to the atherosclerotic process, with a predominance of 'atherogenic' lipoproteins, especially LDL and lipoprotein(a), evidence of LDL oxidation, inflammatory cellular infiltrates and the development of calcification. The presence of lipids stimulates the production of many factors such as modified TGF-b1, tumor necrosis factor and cytokines in the aortic valve leaflets (9). In particular early valvular sclerotic lesions demonstrate a chronic inflammatory cell infiltrate (macrophages and T lymphocytes), lipid accumulation (apolipoprotein [apo] B, apo(A) and apo(E) and α-actin–expressing cells in the lesion and adjacent fibrosa; end-stage calcified valves contain mature lamellar bone with expression of specific bon markers important in the development of osteoblast bone formation (10). In addition, angiotensin-converting enzyme (ACE) and angiotensin II type 1 (AT1) and type 2 (AT2) receptors are present in stenotic aortic valves, implicating this signaling pathway in the disease process (11). These observations are analogous to the cellular findings in vascular atherosclerosis and corroborate epidemiological studies that showed similar associations of clinical risk factors with both atherosclerosis and aortic valve disease (12). The mechanism for valvular calcification is similar to skeletal bone formation and that calcification occurs in areas of neoangiogenesis, which is stimulated by an active inflammatory process and the release of vascular endothelial growth factor (VEGF). VEGF is well known to play a key role in angiogenesis in pathological inflammatory diseases.(13) Deckers et al (14) have suggested that VEGF regulates bone remodeling by attracting endothelial cells and by stimulating osteoblast differentiation. Our findings indicate that VEGF is localized to cells in inflammatory regions of the valve fibrosa, specifically the macrophages and myofibroblasts. Rajamannan recently demonstrated that an osteoblast phenotype is associated with nonrheumatic, degenerative calcific aortic stenosis. The current data, including the production of osteopontin and osteocalcin proteins (both osteoblast cell products) and proliferating myofibroblast cells synthesizing bone matrix proteins, indicate that a similar osteoblast-like process that occurs in degenerative calcific aortic stenosis develops in the calcification process in rheumatic valves (10). Although calcification in rheumatic valves has been described in the literature for years, the cellular mechanisms responsible for the calcification have not been previously described. These new observations support the hypothesis that mineralization of rheumatic cardiac valve tissue is similar to skeletal bone formation that is associated with neoangiogenesis and show that studying this disease process will provide important information on the treatment of valvular heart disease (15). In contrast to mitral valve degeneration, Caira et al. found that the Lrp5/Wnt3 signaling markers are present in the calcified aortic valve greater than the degenerative mitral valve. These data provide the evidence of a mechanistic pathway for the initiation of bone differentiation in degenerative valve lesions, which is expressed in the mitral valve as a cartilage phenotype and in the calcified aortic valve as a bone phenotype. These results indicate that there is a continuum of an earlier stage of osteoblast bone differentiation in the mitral valves as compared with the calcified aortic valves. In normal adult skeleton formation, the initiation of bone formation occurs with the development of a cartilaginous template, which eventually mineralizes and forms calcified bone. Therefore, the mitral valve expresses an early cartilage formation, and the aortic valve demonstrates the mineralized osteoblast phenotype,which follows the spectrum of normal skeletal bone formation. The calcified aortic valves express an osteoblast phenotype: "bone" in the aortic valve that is responsible for the stenosis present in symptomatic aortic stenosis requiring surgical valve replacement. This study demonstrates that hypercholesterolemia may play a role in the initiating event of calcification. This is the first study to demonstrate the presence of chondrocytes in mitral valves, and osteoblasts in aortic valves implicating this pathologic mechanism in the development of mitral regurgitation in myxomatous mitral valves and stenosis in calcific aortic valves (16). In bicuspid aortic valve, the calcification and progressive stenosis typically occur faster than in tricuspid aortic valves, Rajamannan demonstred that the eNOS protein expression was decreased in the BAV vs. the tricuspid aortic valves. This data provides further evidence of the potential functional importance of eNOS enzymatic activity in the developmental level for the formation of the congenital heart abnormality in addition to the actual role in the calcification process. More, bone sialoprotein, osteocalcin, and osteopontin are increased and are markers of extracellular matrix synthesis in the valve whereas Notch1 is decreased in the valve. The protein and RNA expression also demonstrated a decrease in overall Notch1 in these disease tissues, indicating that the loss of normal Notch1 is necessary for valve calcification similar to the implications of the loss of function mutation in the genetic study. Overall, the loss of Notch1 function and the increase in Lrp5 signaling demonstrate the role of these important regulators of bone metabolism in these diseased tissues. Than, the mechanism of BAVD results in a decrease in Notch1 function and an increase in Lrp5 expression which activates bone formation within the valve myofibroblast (17).

2. Clinical presentation

The diagnosis of the aortic stenosis is usually made on physical examination with detection of the classical systolic outflow murmur. The severity of aortic stenosis can be determined reliably by echocardiography, based on the extent of the valvular calcification, the peak flow velocity across the valve, the mean gradient and the valvular area computed by the continuity equation. Evaluation of serial echocardiograms in patients with aortic stenosis make it possible to obtain valuable information over a period of time to determine the progression of the disease and the timing of surgery (9).

2.1 Signs and symptoms

The classical symptoms of AS are angina, dispnea, syncope, and heart failure, which represent also the dramatic inflection in the natural history of this disease.

In adults with AS, the obstruction develops gradually. Many patients with aortic stenosis will remain asymptomatic for decades. The diagnosis of aortic stenosis is usually made in the asymptomatic patient on the basis of a systolic murmur on auscultation and confirmed by echocardiography. The development of symptoms therefore is a critical point in the natural history of patients with AS, infact the risk of sudden death in asymptomatic patient with initial manifestation of severe aortic stenosis is very low (<1% per year), but it is high once any symptom is present, so that valve surgery is appropriate with even mild symptoms.

Most prospectively followed patients present with more subtle symptoms, typically decreased exercise tolerance, or dyspnea on exertion. It is not uncommon for patients to decrease their activity level below their symptom threshold—a careful history comparing

current and last year's activity levels is needed to recognize that these patients, in fact, are symptomatic.
In asymptomatic patients, the risks of valve surgery are weighed against the risk of an adverse outcome without surgical intervention. Aortic valve repair is not an option, so that the long-term durability and risks of a prosthetic valve also must be considered. (18)

2.2 Diagnosis

The physical examination, electrocardiogram, chest radiograph, echocardiography, and cardiac catheterization are important for the diagnosis.
The physical examination demonstrates a weak and slowly rising pulse ("parvus and tardus"). Systolic ejection murmur is best heard at the base of the heart and is harsh in quality, but does not correlate with the severity of stenosis.
The electrocardiogram demonstrated findings consistent with the presence of left ventricular hypertrophy and show an overload pattern.
The chest radiograph has a normal appearance in the vast majority of patients. Left ventricular hypertrophy may be present and is demonstrated in the rounding of the left ventricular free wall. Severe calcification of the aortic valve can frequently be seen in adult patients with severe or critical aortic stenosis.
Echocardiography is the most commonly used noninvasive diagnostic method for assessing the significance of aortic stenosis. Two-dimensional echocardiography can determine valvular motion and the presence or absence of valve thickening and calcification. However, Doppler echocardiography is necessary to assess the hemodynamic severity of the stenosis. Echocardiography is the clinical standard for evaluation of adults with suspected or known valvular AS. Anatomic images show the etiology of AS, level of obstruction, valve calcification, leaflet motion, and aortic root anatomy (19).
It is important to determine the severity of aortic stenosis based upon hemodynamic measurements. The echocardiographic criteria were established to define the grading of stenosis by ACC/AHA 2006 (20) and includes the following:
Valve area

1. mild aortic stenosis: area > 1.5 cm2
2. moderate aortic stenosis: area 1 to 1.5 cm2
3. severe aortic stenosis: area < 1.0 cm2.

Aortic velocity allows classification of stenosis as

1. mild (less than 3.0 m/s)
2. moderate (3 to 4 m/s)
3. severe (>4 m/s).

but in the revision and the update of ACC/AHA guidelines (2006) the grading of aortic stenosis in evaluated also by the transvalvular gradiente as following.

1. mild (mean gradient less than 25 mm Hg)
2. moderate (mean gradient 25 to 40 mm Hg)
3. severe (mean gradient greater than 40 mm Hg)

When stenosis is severe and ejection fraction (EF) is normal, the mean transvalvular pressure gradient is normally greater than 40 mm Hg. However, when cardiac output is low, severe stenosis can be present with a lower transvalvular gradient and velocity. So to grade the severity of the stenosis also the Ef must to be evaluated. Doppler echocardiography is also used to determine diastolic dysfunction by the presence of

abnormal left ventricular relaxation. Moderate to severe diastolic dysfunction does not increase early mortality but may increase late mortality after AVR. Stress echocardiography is used in patients with normal left ventricular function (LVF) to demonstrate the presence of diastolic dysfunction (i.e., signs of elevated left ventricular filling pressure) as the cause of symptom development during exercise.
Doppler echocardiography has replaced cardiac catheterization in most centers for evaluation of the hemodynamic severity of aortic stenosis (21). Cardiac catheterization is reserved for hemodynamic evaluation in patients in whom reliable echocardiographic data cannot be obtained or when the clinical and echocardiographic data are divergent. Catheterization is also necessary in most patients undergoing aortic valve replacement (usually men with age > 40, post menopausal women, history of coronary artery disease and suspected myocardial ischemia or LV systolic dysfunction) to determine if there is associated coronary artery disease that can be treated at the time of operation (9).

3. Predictors of Aortic Stenosis

3.1 C reactive protein

The dynamic and inflammatory nature of calcific aortic stenosis has been well appreciated in recent years, and many pathobiologic features of calcific aortic valve disease exhibit striking similarity to coronary atherosclerosis. C-reactive protein (CRP), which has been an useful predictive biomarker of the inflammatory process and prognosis of atherosclerosis, is increased in subsets of patients with calcific aortic stenosis, and this has led to the hope that CRP could be used as well to identify those patients likely to progress or develop severe calcific aortic stenosis (22).
Recent data suggest that oxidative stress and high-sensitivity CRP plasma levels as a marker of systemic inflammation could be involved in the pathogenesis of rheumatic valve disease. Therefore, the role of inflammation in rheumatic valve disease progression should be considered. Indeed, the persistence of high levels of high-sensitivity CRP has been shown in patients with chronic rheumatic valve disease, particularly in patients with multivalvular disease, who showed significantly higher plasma levels of CRP (23).
If inflammation is the fundamental process of early aortic valve disease, with calcification predominating in the later stages, one might anticipate that markers of inflammation, such as CRP, would reflect early aortic valve disease activity and perhaps be less useful as a marker in later stages. The available data do not support such a concept. CRP has been localized in the valve tissue of aortic stenosis in both native valves and bioprosthetic aortic valves, with a positive correlation between serum CRP values and valve CRP expression (24). C-reactive protein values are increased in patients with severe symptomatic aortic stenosis awaiting valve surgery compared with matched controls and decline after aortic valve replacement. On the other hand, Navaro et al show that there is no relationship between elevated CRP levels and the presence of calcific aortic-valve disease or of incident aortic stenosis. C-reactive protein appears to be a poor predictor of subclinical calcific aortic-valve disease. They observed that older age, male gender, hypertension, coronary artery disease, and renal insufficiency, but not CRP values, are associated with the presence of increasing calcific aortic valve abnormality and that CRP values are not related to the progression from a normal aortic valve to aortic sclerosis or stenosis, nor progression from aortic sclerosis to aortic stenosis. African-American ethnicity was significantly protective

from developing calcific aortic valve disease. How do we make sense of these apparent discrepancies that CRP appears not to reflect the early inflammation phase of calcific aortic valve disease but does reflect the later calcific stages of the disease? The first methodologic consideration is that the single CRP value at study entry may have been too distant from the time that calcific aortic stenosis was developing during the follow-up period to reflect the inflammatory change that would later occur. It is also possible that the inflammatory process in early calcific aortic valve disease was not substantial enough to lead to an elevated serum value. It is also clear from the previously noted associations between CRP and severe aortic stenosis that CRP may be a more active, direct participant in the later stages of the disease progression and not simply a biomarker passively reflecting the early inflammatory stages of disease. CRP provides valuable prognostic information concerning adverse cardiovascular events in coronary disease as well, but it does not reflect the presence or severity of subclinical anatomic coronary artery disease (25). The study by Novaro et al. does add important new understanding concerning the genetic determinants of calcific aortic valve disease. Genetic characteristics of calcium metabolism may be central to the development of valvular calcification, and the observation that African Americans are protected from development of calcific aortic valve disease, may be related to a genetic predisposition toward less calcification of vascular and valve tissue and lower incidence of osteoporosis. It would be of enormous value to identify a biomarker to predict patients likely to develop aortic sclerosis and those likely to progress to aortic stenosis. Only a few studies have examined the relationship between CRP and aortic stenosis. Galante et al. (6) published the initial study demonstrating elevated CRP levels in association with calcific aortic stenosis. In a surgical series, CRP levels were higher in severe aortic stenosis patients compared to patients with pure aortic regurgitation (26). In those who underwent aortic valve replacement for aortic stenosis, CRP levels decreased from before to 6 months after valve replacement. Recently, CRP has been localized in valve tissue of both calcific aortic-valve stenosis and degenerative aortic-valve bioprostheses , with a positive correlation between serum CRP levels and valvular CRP expression. Thus, from the available human studies, it is apparent that CRP levels are elevated in aortic stenosis patients with severe disease awaiting surgery, do not correlate with stenosis severity, and decrease after valve replacement, supporting the histologic evidence that the aortic valve is a site of active inflammation. (5)

3.2 Others predictors

Whereas cardiovascular risk factors and CRP levels failed to predict incident aortic stenosis, only 4 demographic variables (increasing age, male gender, white ethnicity, and shorter height) were associated with an increased risk of incident aortic stenosis. Increasing age is a well-recognized risk factor related to aortic stenosis. Gender appears to have an impact on the risk of both aortic stenosis and the degree of aortic valve calcification , with men showing a greater predilection of both (5).

Genetic factors can also be important in the development of valvular calcification. In a recent case–control study, 100 patients with similar demographic characteristics were compared, with and without aortic stenosis, and significant differences between the two groups were observed in the genotype of the vitamin D receptors (27). Another study identified polymorphisms of the apolipoproteins AI, B and E as predisposing factors for development of calcification and valvular stenosis (28). Finally, a unique study by Garg et al.

demonstrated the unique signaling pathway Notch as important in the development of calcific aortic stenosis and also congenital heart abnormalities. These important studies indicate that genetic predisposition and risk factors may play a role in the development of disease (9). In a recent study Kamalesh et al. revealed that diabetes accelerate progression of calcification in subjects who have moderately severe aortic stenosis. Therefore, for this patients may need intensive follow-up for their aortic stenosis rather than non diabetic subjects (29). The finding that the multifunctional glycophosphoprotein osteopontin (OPN) is involved in both cell-mediated inflammation and biomineralization has generated considerable interest in the role of OPN in ectopic calcification and calcific aortic valve disease as shown by Yu et al. (30). Although other serum markers, such as C-reactive protein and B-type natriuretic peptide have previously been shown to be associated with aortic calcification and stenosis, OPN is the only molecule that is implicated in both inflammation and biomineralization processes, which lead to aortic valve calcification and subsequent stenosis. Also Ferrari and Grau demonstrates a direct correlation of NT-pro-BNP, BNP, and osteopontin and the presence of calcific AS, while fetuin A showed an inverse correlation. Plasma ADMA and homocysteine levels were comparable in the calcific AS patients and healthy individuals. A new study analyzed osteopontin level and its phosphorilation status in CAVD and demostred that phospho-threonina levels of purified OPN are higher in healthy controls when compared to CAVD patients. This study showed that phospho-OPN prevent calcium deposition, whereas the dephosphorylated protein mimicking the patient's plasma OPN, lose its protective role allowing calcium depositation on the cellular surface. This data suggest the role of circulating OPN and its phosphorilation status as biomarker and inhibitory factor for the pathogenesis of calcific CAVD. (31)

4. Treatment

There are different choises of treatment, based on clinical symptoms, echocardiographical criterias and evaluation of risk factors.

The development of symptoms in patients with severe aortic stenosis is associated with a 50% mortality within a period of 5 years. Thus, symptomatic severe aortic stenosis is a clear class I recommendation for surgical intervention (21). At present, there is no medical treatment recommended for asymptomatic patients with aortic stenosis, and only clinical monitoring is recommended (5).

However, recent epidemiologic studies evaluating the independent risk factors for calcific aortic stenosis have demonstrated that the risk factors for aortic stenosis are similar to those of coronary artery disease, which include hypertension, elevated low-density lipoprotein, smoking, diabetes, and male gender (32). These atherosclerotic risk factors provide the evidence for the potential of medical therapy for this disease process. (19)

4.1 Initial treatment

The management of patients with aortic stenosis depends upon the severity of aortic stenosis and the presence or absence of symptoms. In patients with only mild stenosis and no symptoms, management is continued observation. Serial echocardiography should be performed every 3 years in patients with mild aortic stenosis and every 1–2 years in those with moderate stenosis. Prompt echocardiography should be performed anytime there is new symptom onset. Infective endocarditis prophylaxis should be followed. Patients with moderate-to-severe aortic stenosis should avoid athletics, which require high dynamic and static muscular demands. There are no proven medical treatments to slow or prevent disease progression. However, aggressive lipid lowering therapy may be of benefit, especially in patients with less-severe valve calcification, and will ameliorate progression of vascular atherosclerosis that frequently coexists and increases their comorbidity. Patients with symptoms and severe aortic stenosis should be considered for operation with aortic valve replacement. Delays to surgery have been associated with poorer outcome following operation Over the past two decades, the risk of operation has decreased substantially. Isolated aortic valve replacement in a patient less than 70 years old should be able to be performed with a risk of less than 1%. The risk should be less than 2–3% among septuagenarians and even less than 5% in octogenarians in the absence of significant comorbidities. Therefore, age is not a contraindication to surgery. Concomitant coronary artery bypass grafting should be performed for coronary atherosclerosis when epicardial lesions are >50%.

Since statins lower levels of high-sensitivity C-reactive protein as well as cholesterol, different studies hypothesized that people with elevated high-sensitivity C-reactive protein levels might benefit from statin treatment. (33) The treatment of the asymptomatic patient with severe aortic stenosis is more controversial. When there is left ventricular dysfunction, valve replacement is indicated even in asymptomatic patients. In these patients, the critical increase in afterload has started to overwhelm the compensatory mechanisms of left ventricular hypertrophy and the outcome is poor without surgical intervention. Importantly, aortic valve replacement can also now be done with a low operative mortality and there is enhanced durability of the new prostheses. Thus, surgery is reasonable to consider in asymptomatic patients when there is critical aortic stenosis and the expected operative mortality is <1.0%. Aortic valve replacement may also be considered for adults with severe asymptomatic aortic stenosis if there is evidence or high likelihood of rapid progression or when there may be delayed rapid access to medical care if symptoms arose. Progression of aortic stenosis may be considered rapid when the Doppler peak velocity increases by >0.3 m/s per year or when the valve area decreases by >0.1 cm2 per year .

4.2 Future directions in medical treatment

As greater understanding of the cellular mechanisms, pathogenesis and progression of aortic valvular disease evolves, new pharmacological strategies are being proposed that are targeted more directly to mechanisms of the disease, both for preventing its progression and ultimately for achieving its regression. The two pharmacological agents that have been studied experimentally and that demonstrate the most potential benefit are the HMG-CoA reductase inhibitors (statins) and the ACE inhibitors (19,20,22,33). The clinical implementation of these pharmacological treatments will require a strict validation of the experimental and retrospective studies to date (34–38), in order to establish a clear cause–effect benefit in any pharmacological treatment system.

Conventionally ACE-Is are contraindicated in patients with severe AS. However, we may safely administer ACE-Is to patients with mild AS because hemodynamic effects of stenotic aortic valve are well compensated in such patients. The renin-angiotensin system contributes to the inflammatory nature of the aortic valve lesion. Angiotensin converting enzyme (ACE), as well as angiotensin II and the angiotensin II type-1 receptor, have been identified in aortic sclerotic lesions , which stimulate monocyte infiltration and macrophage uptake of modified LDL (34). Calcification, the hallmark characteristic of aortic valve stenosis, is also clearly a feature of the active inflammatory process, occurring in valve

regions of lipid disposition, especially oxidized lipids, with additional stimulus provided by macrophage- and T lymphocyte-produced cytokines. Early in the disease process, active microscopic areas of calcification are seen co-localizing in areas of lipoprotein accumulation and inflammatory cell infiltration; as the disease progresses, active bone formation is seen.
ACE inhibitors are thought to interfere with the renin-angiotensin system and exert beneficial actions on vascular tissues beyond their blood pressure–lowering effects.
Regarding statins, there are a number of experimental models testing the effects of a cholesterol diet on the aortic valve in mice model. Sarphie (39) demonstrated the first histochemical effects of cholesterol on the development of valvular heart disease. Studies by Rajamannan and Charest et al have also shown that endothelial nitric oxide enzyme activity plays a role in the early valve lesions. Elevated cholesterol decreases the enzyme expression and induces early mineralization in the aortic valve. Therefore, these early studies provide the evidence that aortic valve disease has similar initiating mechanism of oxidative stress that is found in vascular atherosclerosis. The next critical step toward understanding of aortic valve calcification is to determine the signaling mechanisms involved in the development of this disease (40). The studies from Mohler (41) and Rajamannan (40) have shown that the aortic valve calcifies secondary to a bone phenotype. Recent studies from Rajamannan and Shao et al. have demonstrated that the mechanism by which calcification develops is activation of the LDL receptor 5 (Lrp5)/Wnt pathway in the vascular and valvular interstitial cells (40). These studies confirm that the presence of bone formation is the phenotypic expression of calcification in the aortic valve (10). Over time, the valve leaflet synthesizes bone matrix, which eventually calcifies and forms bone. If the aortic valve has an actual biology that is initiated by elevated cholesterol, then in the future, medical therapy such as statins or angiotensin-converting enzyme inhibitors may slow the progression of this disease.
Also Nagy et al. studied the role of proinflammatory signaling through the leukotriene (LT) pathway in aortic stenosis and demonstred that the messenger RNA levels of the LT-forming enzyme 5-lipoxygenase increased in thickened and calcified tissue compared with normal areas of the same valves. Moreover they showed that leukotriene C4 (LTC4) increased intracellular calcium, enhanced reactive oxygen species production, reduced the mitochondrial membrane potential, and led to morphological cell cytoplasm changes and calcification. This data suggest the up-regulation of the pathway LT and the potentially detrimental LT-induced effects on valvular myofibroblasts as possible role in the development of aortic stenosi and induce to considerate innovative therapeutic interventions(42).
The first landmark randomized, prospective trial published in this field, Scottish Aortic Stenosis and Lipid Lowering Trial, Impact on Regression (SALTIRE), (43) demonstrated, however, that high-dose atorvastatin does not slow the progression of this disease. SALTIRE initiated atorvastatin in patients who had more advanced aortic stenosis as defined by the mean aortic valve area of 1.03 cm2, with heavy burden of calcification as measured by aortic valve calcium scores. Newby et al recently acknowledged that the timing of therapy for aortic valve stenosis may play the key role in the future treatment of this disease. The important issue may be treating this disease earlier in its process to slow the progression of bone formation in the aortic valve (44). The potential benefit of statin therapy, however, is controversial and widely debated, as recent randomized studies done in patients with moderate to severe degrees of aortic stenosis failed to consistently show substantial benefits of this class of drugs. Antonini et al. provides evidence for a positive effect of statins in

reducing the progression of rheumatic AS and in a large series of patients with long-term follow-up, statins were effective in slowing the progression of aortic valve disease in aortic sclerosis and mild AS, but not in moderate AS. These results suggest that statin therapy should be taken into consideration in the early stages of this common disease (23). The RAAVE (Rosuvastatin Affecting Aortic Valve Endothelium) study suggests that earlier treatment with statins is more efficacious in the prevention of progression of aortic valve stenosis than late treatment, similar to the effects of statins in the regression of vascular atherosclerosis (45). Importantly, results of the randomized trials will provide further evidence to define the treatment of this complex disease process, in which timing of therapy and characteristics of the valve lesion will need to be taken into account in the future treatment approaches. In the RAAVE trial, the rate of progression of aortic stenosis in those with hypercholesterolemia treated with rosuvastatin is slower than in those with lower lipid levels who are not treated. This is the first study to provide positive clinical evidence for the potential of targeted therapy in patients with asymptomatic aortic stenosis (45). Finally Parolari et al. (46) performed a meta-analysis of studies was performed comparing statin therapy with placebo or no treatment on outcomes and on aortic stenosis progression echocardiographic parameters. This meta-analysis identified 10 studies with a total of 3822 participants (2214 non-statin-treated and 1608 statin-treated). No significant differences were found in all-cause mortality, cardiovascular mortality or in the need for aortic valve surgery. Lower-quality (retrospective or non-randomised) studies showed that, in statin-treated patients, the annual increase in peak aortic jet velocity and the annual decrease in aortic valve area were lower, but this was not confirmed by the analysis in high-quality (prospective or randomised) studies. Statins did not significantly affect the progression over time of peak and mean aortic gradient. Taken together, this evidences suggest that the progression of calcific aortic stenosis is a complex process; the multitude of the mechanisms involved in AS indicates that drug therapy should address the earliest stages of the disease, as it is now evident that pharmacological treatment administered in more advanced stages of the disease may be ineffective (47). At the end, all studies of statins have had the "wrong target" trying to treat patients with severely calcified valves. In our opinion we should treat patients at earlier stages of the disease, since statins side-effects are considered marginal and moreover statins have been proven beneficial to delay atherosclerosis progression and CAD, than quite often accompany AS.

4.3 Surgical treatment

Aortic valve replacement is indicated in patients who have severe aortic stenosis in the absence of other major comorbidities. Patients who undergo aortic valve replacement have an improvement in symptoms and increased survival after valve replacement surgery. Currently, there is no indication for surgical valve replacement in patients who have asymptomatic critical aortic stenosis unless they have left ventricular dysfunction or abnormal hemodynamic response to exercise. Patients who have moderately depressed ventricular function do as well as those with normal ventricular function. Depressed ventricular function may be due to afterload mismatch or an intrinsic depression of contractility. Both the safety and prognosis of aortic valve replacement relate to distinguishing between these two causes of reduced ventricular function. Patients with true afterload mismatch do well after aortic valve replacement despite very low ejection fractions. Depressed contractility from myocardial disease does not respond as well to aortic valve replacement (19)

Aortic valve replacement in patients without symptoms is controversial, infact asymptomatic patients with AS have outcomes similar to age-matched normal adults. While the short-term prognosis in such patients is excellent without surgery, there is still a small but definite risk of sudden death. Obviously there is also a small but definite risk of morbidity and mortality related to aortic valve replacement and to complications resulting from the presence of a prosthetic valve.

4.4 Aortic valve replacement

When planning AVR, the chief issues related to surgical decision making involve the type of valve prosthesis to be inserted, the timing of surgery, and issues related to concomitant procedures. The ideal prosthesis for AVR is characterized by excellent hemodynamics, minimal residual transvalvular pressure gradient, and laminar flow through the prosthesis. In addition, the valvular prosthesis should be durable, easy to implant, quiet, biocompatible, and resistant to thromboembolism. The two major categories of valvular prostheses, which account for the vast majority of implanted aortic valves, include mechanical and bioprosthetic valves. Regarding the decision between bioprosthetic and mechanical valves, the primary advantage of mechanical valves is their durability and
reliable performance. Conversely, the primary disadvantage of mechanical valves relates to the need for lifelong warfarin anticoagulation and attendant lifestyle limitations and thromboembolic (TE) and bleeding risks. When anticoagulation is managed appropriately, the risk of TE with mechanical valves is similar to that for bioprosthetic valves. Bileaflet mechanical valves are the standard in current practice. Conversely, the primary advantage of bioprosthetic valves is that systemic anticoagulation with warfarin is not required. As a result, patients receiving tissue valves have a lower rate of anticoagulation-related bleeding complications. However, their limited durability (freedom from structural valve deterioration and need for reoperation) and suboptimal hemodynamics, due to a generally smaller effective orifice area size-for-size as compared to mechanical valves, have historically been the drawbacks of bioprosthetic valves. As a result, use of bioprosthetic valves has generally been recommended for patients older than 65 years of age or with reduced life expectancy. These tendencies are nowadays changing in light of improved tissue engineering, the increased lifespan of new generation tissue valves and the relative low risk of reoperation for isolate valve re-replacement. Moreover, the increasing trend to use transcatheter aortic valve implantation (TAVI) and the possibility to replace a previously implanted biological prosthesis with the method of valve in valve, the implantatation of a trancatheter valve into the old and degenerated prothesis, without a new open heart operation, moves the needle of the balance toward greater use of biological prosthesis, even if the duration of TAVi in young patient is not still known.

The most important problem in the use of mechanical prosthesis is anticoagulation for all the life. Anticoagulation for the long-term treatment has been accomplished by vitamin K antagonists for the last half century. Although effective under optimal conditions, the imminent risk of a recurrent adverse event of INR the risk of bleeding due to the narrow therapeutic window, numerous food- and drug interactions, and the need for regular monitoring complicate the long-term use of these drugs and render treatment with these agents complicated. But new anticoagulants which selectively block key factors in the coagulation cascade are being developed (48). Dabigatran is the first available oral direct thrombin inhibitor anticoagulant, it specifically and reversibly inhibits thrombin, the key enzyme in the coagulation cascade. Its oral bioavailability is low, but shows reduced

interindividual variability. Studies show a predictable pk/pd profile that allows for fixed-dose regimens. The anticoagulant effect correlates adequately with the plasma concentrations of the drug, demonstrating effective anticoagulation combined with a low risk of bleeding. Rivaroxaban will probably be the first available oral factor Xa (FXa) direct inhibitor anticoagulant drug. It produces a reversible and predictable inhibition of FXa activity with potential to inhibit clot-bound FXa. Its pharmacokinetic characteristics include rapid absorption, high oral availability, high plasma protein binding and a half-life of aprox 8 hours. (49)
The development of new anticoagulant, safer , with less risk of bleeding, and which allow to the patient the possibility of a fixe assumption, without monitoring INR every week, could change the choice criteria between biological and mechanical prosthesis.

4.5 Aortic balloon valvotomy

Percutaneous balloon aortic valvotomy (BAV) is a procedure in which 1 or more balloons are placed across a stenotic valve and inflated to decrease the severity of AS. Although BAV is useful in children with congenital AS, the calcified lesion of acquired AS in the adult does not respond well to BAV. After a modest acute reduction in stenosis severity, restenosis recurs usually within 6 months. Immediate hemodynamic results include a moderate reduction in the transvalvular pressure gradient, but the postvalvotomy valve area rarely exceeds 1.0 cm2. Despite the modest change in valve area, an early symptomatic improvement is usually seen. However, serious acute complications occur with a frequency greater than 10% (50, 51).

5. The future

Prolonged life expectancy has resulted in an aging population and, consequently, in an increased number of patients with degenerative calcific aortic stenosis (52). AS has increased markedly in developed countries and AS, caused by valve calcification in the elderly, will continue to increase as the aging of society accelerates. For symptomatic patients with severe aortic valve stenosis, open heart surgery for aortic valve replacement (AVR) with use of cardioplegia under cardiopulmonary bypass remains the gold standard. Although surgery is still the gold standard treatment, it is considered high risk in elderly patients because of high complication rates, which leads to substantial hesitation in submitting such patients to surgery. The surgical approach is associated with substantial operative mortality rates in high-risk patients. Consequently, almost one-third of patients with severe aortic stenosis are not offered surgery owing to a combination of reasons such as advanced age, impaired left ventricular function, re-do procedure, or multiple comorbidities (50). Moreover, as longevity within the general population is increasing, the proportion of aortic stenosis patients with contraindications for surgery is also expected to increase. Decision-making is particularly complex in the elderly who represent a heterogeneous population, resulting in a wide range of operative risk, as well as life expectancy, according to individual cardiac and non-cardiac patient characteristics. The two most striking characteristics of patients who were denied surgery were older age and LV dysfunction. Age and LV dysfunction are associated with an increased operative risk and a poor late outcome after surgery, which may explain the reluctancy to operate on such patients. Age is a strong predictor of operative risk and poor late survival in cardiovascular surgery, in particular, in the case of AS. Four percent of the elderly population has significant aortic stenosis and the size of the population older than 65 years will grow 50% between 2000 and 2030. In very old patients with many comorbidities, the outcome of AVR is less favourable than in average poulation, and many of those patients may be inoperable or carry an unacceptably high perioperative risk. Some patients with aortic valve disease defer surgery in light of mild symptoms, whereas others are deemed too ill to undergo cardiac surgery. The latter currently have been treated expectantly or by balloon aortic valvuloplasty (BAV), but this technique offers poor magnitude and durability of the physiologic improvement in aortic valve orifice area. In most patients, balloon valvotomy reduces severe AS to moderately severe AS. The gradient typically is reduced by 50% and averages approximately 35 mm Hg after the procedure. Unfortunately, in 50% of patients, restenosis occurs within 6 months. Overall, balloon valvotomy has not reduced the high mortality seen in patients who do not undergo surgery for symptomatic AS. Recent technological advances, however, now indicate that catheter techniques similar to those used for BAV can be used for percutaneous aortic valve replacement, avoiding open cardiac access or the use of cardiopulmonary bypass. As with any medical procedure, the risk/benefit ratio of TAVI must be carefully considered. The benefits provided by this novel procedure must be weighed eventually against what is considered today the "gold standard" that is surgical AVR. Bearing in mind, however, the excellent track record of surgical AVR, it seems prudent to initially target those patients who are at high surgical risk due to severe comorbidities. Thus, the patients currently enrolled in these studies are chosen based on a risk score, such as the EuroSCORE or STS score. The other set of patients who may be considered at present are those with a deteriorated aortic bioprosthesis and deemed at high risk for surgical reoperation, and this "valve-in-valve" concept has already been reported. With technological advancements, it is expected that the ease of implantation will improve and complications will decrease. In order to consider lower risk and younger patients as candidates for this new technology, additional long-term durability data will be required before advocating this procedure as a possible substitute to surgical AVR. Risk algorithms have been used to assess operative risk, anticipate outcomes, and provide for comparability of patients among diverse centers and countries. Unfortunately, these tools are inherently imprecise and frequently exclude comorbidities encountered in this population. Therefore, the comparison of transcatheter procedural outcomes to anticipated results based upon predictive risk scoring remains somewhat subjective. The presence of CAD has been clearly demonstrated to increase procedural risk with conventional aortic valve replacement. However, its overall influence on outcomes of transcatheter therapy for aortic stenosis has not been clearly delineated. This is especially true given the fact that TAVI is generally considered a stand-alone procedure, with variable degrees of concomitant coronary artery disease tolerated without intervention. It has been shown that patients with CAD as indicated by previous CABG or PCI had significantly higher 30-day and overall mortality with transcatheter valve implantation.

6. Risk stratification

The Euro Heart Survey has shown that, in current practice, there is general agreement between the decision to operate and the existing guidelines in asymptomatic patients. However, in patients with severe symptoms, intervention is underused for reasons that are often unjustified. This stresses the importance of the widespread use of careful risk stratification. In the absence of evidence from randomized clinical trials, the decision to intervene in a patient with VHD relies on an individual risk-benefit analysis, suggesting that improvement of prognosis compared with natural history outweighs the risk of intervention and its potential late consequences, in particular, prosthesis-related complications. Factors predicting operative mortality have been identified from large series of patients undergoing cardiac surgery or, more specifically, heart valve surgery. They are related to heart disease, the patient's age, comorbidity, and the type of surgery. The easiest way to integrate the weight of the different predictable factors is to combine them in multivariate scores, enabling operative mortality to be estimated.

6.1 Euroscore

It is a risk model which allows the calculation of the risk of death after a heart operation. The model asks for 17 items of information about the patient, the state of the heart and the proposed operation, and uses logistic regression to calculate the risk of death. First published in 1999, the model has been adopted worldwide, becoming the most widely used risk index for cardiac surgery, and its use is believed to have contributed substantially to the improvement in the results of heart surgery seen at the beginning of the millennium. It is now aging and a new model (EuroSCORE 2010) is being prepared. Briefly, comprehensive data were obtained for over 19,000 consecutive patients undergoing open heart surgery in 128 centers in eight European countries. The database thus generated was subjected to multiple logistic regression analysis to determine which risk factors were associated with operative mortality. Weights were allocated to each risk factor on the basis of the odds ratios and a risk model was constructed in which the percentage predicted mortality for a patient could be calculated by adding the weighted values of risk factors which are present. The additive EuroSCORE model, by virtue of its nature, tends to underestimate risk in very high-risk patients. Some very high-risk patients may be better assessed, for individual risk prediction, by using the full logistic EuroSCORE model. EuroSCORE was initially designed to be a user-friendly system, in the hope of encouraging as many units as possible to embark on programs of risk-adjusted quality monitoring. In this setting, although derived from a logistic regression methodology, only the simple additive version of the score was originally published. This score could be easily calculated at the bedside and could therefore be used widely in Europe even in hospitals with little information technology. Using the same risk factors, the logistic regression version of the score (the 'logistic EuroSCORE') can be calculated. Many risk factors have been associated with cardiac surgical mortality and morbidity. The EuroSCORE was derived from data obtained from patients operated on in 1995, and the details were first published in 1999. The system is now 10 years old, and is based on data that are even older. Yet, since the introduction of EuroSCORE, there has been a quantum improvement in cardiac surgical survival which mainly occurred during the first two to three years of the new millennium. Evidence from countries with national databases has suggested that mortality in some of these countries has approximately halved, despite a gradual worsening of the risk profile of patients. In the United Kingdom, for example, mortality has fallen to approximately 55% of logistic EuroSCORE prediction, giving a UK RAMR (risk adjusted mortality ratio obtained dividing the actual mortality by the predicted mortality) of around 0.55. In a consecutive series of patients with severe AS undergoing AVR, Kalavrouziotis and coworkers found that the logistic EuroSCORE was not an accurate risk assessment tool in all categories of risk but especially in high-risk patients. Therefore, this predictive model should not be used to determine procedural risk in patients with severe AS. Furthermore, the utilization of the logistic EuroSCORE in the assessment of operability in patients with severe AS may not be appropriate.

6.2 STS (Society of Thoracic Surgeons) risk score

More than 20 years ago, the STS was one of the first specialty organizations to recognize the importance of developing a prospectively maintained clinical data registry. The resulting STS National Adult Cardiac Surgery Database (STS NCD) has achieved widespread acceptance by the provider community as well as interested third parties, including health policy researchers, government regulators, accrediting agencies, and payers. The Society of Thoracic Surgeons' risk models predict the risk of operative mortality and morbidity after adult cardiac surgery on the basis of patient demographic and clinical variables. The models are primarily used to adjust for case mix when comparing outcomes across institutions with different patient populations. The STS currently has three risk models: CABG, Valve, and Valve + CABG. The models apply to seven specific surgical procedure classifications:

CABG model

1. Isolated Coronary Artery Bypass (CABG Only)

Valve model

2. Isolated Aortic Valve Replacement (AV Replace)
3. Isolated Mitral Valve Replacement (MV Replace)
4. Isolated Mitral Valve Repair (MV Repair)

Valve + CABG model

5. Aortic Valve Replacement + CABG (AV Replace + CABG)
6. Mitral Valve Replacement + CABG (MV Replace + CABG)
7. Mitral Valve Repair + CABG (MV Repair + CABG)

New STS models, developed using STS data from 2002 to 2006, account for endpoints as for operative mortality, permanent stroke, renal failure, prolonged ventilation (> 24 hours), deep sternal wound infection, reoperation for any reason, a major morbidity or mortality composite endpoint, prolonged postoperative length of stay, and short postoperative length of stay. Recently, the STS risk algorithm was reported to be the most sensitive score in defining the risk of patients undergoing isolated AVR. Predictive value of many of the currently available scoring systems is insufficient to allow a reliable risk assessment in patients undergoing isolated aortic valve replacement. The overestimation is most prominent in high-risk patients. Risk stratification using the STS score was accurate in predicting the risk of mortality in high-risk patients. Nevertheless, even this most recently built score systematically overestimates procedural risk. From the clinician's standpoint there is a need for an objective risk assessment tool.

6.3 Do we need new or better tailored risk models?

Risk stratification models for operative mortality have gained widespread acceptance in cardiac surgery. These models, however, are not 100% accurate. A number of factors can influence their performance. Generally speaking, available risk models for cardiac surgery can be divided into three categories: (1) **general cardiac surgery models -** that is, coronary artery bypass surgery, valve surgery or other related cardiac surgery; (2) **general valve surgery models**; and (3) **specific aortic valve surgery risk models**. Risk models can serve multiple purposes if used correctly. Firstly, risk models can be used for benchmarking; they may allow for control of procedural complexity when analyzing hospital and surgeon performance. Secondly, risk models can help educate patients and improve informed patient consent. Risk models can also be incorporated into guidelines to help identify high risk patients who may benefit from additional work-up or alternative treatment strategies. If risk models can accurately identify high risk patients with expected longer lengths of stay in hospital, they may be useful for administrative logistic and budget planning. Differences in epidemiology of disease, risk profiles, surgical strategies, decision making, selection bias, and referral bias can all influence the applicability and performance of a model. Regarding EuroScore performance in valve surgery Parolari suggested that EuroSCORE might not be the appropriate tool for risk prediction in isolated valve operations or those combined with other cardiac procedures. The area under the curve (AUC) derived from the meta-analysis he performed provided estimates of 0.72 to 0.74, which are in a range of a performance considered less than satisfactory for a risk stratification algorithm. EuroSCORE discrimination is also substantially lower with respect to the performance of the Society of Thoracic Surgery (STS) algorithm, which is about 0.8 for isolated valve operations and about 0.75 for valves plus CABG. The explanation for this is that the STS score is updated almost annually, and, for this reason, it may better follow the changes occurring in valve patient population with relative ease, whereas the EuroSCORE is now undergoing its first revision since its introduction. The discriminatory power and precision in risk prediction of the EuroSCORE in valve surgery has recently become increasingly important for two reasons. The first is that in the most centers, valve procedures—either isolated or combined - actually represent more than 50% of the total caseload; therefore, accurate risk estimation in this patient population—mainly elderly and very elderly people—has become much more important. The second reason is strictly related to the recent evolution in technical options in aortic valve operations that has led to a steady increase in the adoption of transcathether aortic valve procedures in patients at the highest risk or in very elderly people.

7. References

[1] US National Library of Medicine/National Institute of Health MedlinePlus: *Aortic Stenosis.*

[2] Rossebø AB et al. (2008). *Intensive Lipid Lowering with Simvastatin and Ezetimibe in Aortic Stenosis.* N Engl J Med 10.1056

[3] Carabello BA, Paulus WJ. (2009) *Review. Aortic stenosis.* The lancet vol 373,march 14, 2009

[4] Roberts WC, Ko JM. (2005). *Frequency by decades of unicuspid, bicuspid, and tricuspid aortic valves in adults having isolated aortic valve replacement for aortic stenosis, with or without associated aortic regurgitation.* Circulation 2005;111:920–5.

[5] Novaro GM, Katz R, Aviles RJ, Gottdiener JS, Cushman M, Psaty BM, Otto CM, Griffin BP.(2007). *Clinical Factors, But Not C-Reactive Protein, Predict Progression of Calcific Aortic-Valve Disease The Cardiovascular Health Study.* Journal of the American College of Cardiology Vol. 50, No. 20, 2007

[6] Galante A, Pietroiusti A, Vellini M, et al. (2001). *C-reactive protein is increased in patients with degenerative aortic valvular stenosis.* J Am Coll Cardiol 2001;38:1078–1082.

[7] Rajamannan NM, Edwards WD, Spelsberg TC. (2003). *Hypercholesterolemic aortic valve disease.* N Engl J Med 2003; 349:717–718.

[8] O'Brien KD, Reichenbach DD, Marcovina SM, et al. (1996). *Apolipoproteins B, (a), and E accumulate in the morphologically early lesion of 'degenerative' valvular aortic stenosis.* Arterioscler Thromb Vasc Biol 1996; 16:523–532.
[9] Mouraa LM, Magantib K, Puthumanab JJ, Rocha-Gonc F¸ Alvesc and Rajamannan NM. (2007). *New understanding about calcific aortic stenosis and opportunities for pharmacologic intervention.* Current Opinion in Cardiology 2007, 22:572–577
[10] Rajamannan NM, Subramaniam M, Rickard D et al. (2003). *Human aortic valve calcification is associated with an osteoblast phenotype.* Circulation.2003;107:2181–2184.
[11] O'Brien KD, Shavelle DM, Caulfield MT et al. (2002). *Association of angiotensin-converting enzyme with low-density lipoprotein in aortic valvular lesions and in human plasma.* Circulation. 2002;106:2224–2230.
[12] Rajamannan NM, Otto CM, MD (2004). *Targeted Therapy to Prevent Progression of Calcific Aortic Stenosis.* Circulation September 7, 2004
[13] Moulton KS, Vakili K, Zurakowski D, Soliman M, Butterfield C, Sylvin E, Lo KM, Gillies S, Javaherian K, Folkman J. (2003). *Inhibition of plaque neovascularization reduces macrophage accumulation and progression of advanced atherosclerosis.* Proc Natl Acad Sci U *S A*. 2003;100:4736–4741.
[14] Deckers MM, van Bezooijen RL, van der Horst G, Hoogendam J, van Der Bent C, Papapoulos SE, Lowik CW. (2002). *Bone morphogenetic proteins stimulate angiogenesis through osteoblast-derived vascular endothelial growth factor A.* Endocrinology. 2002;143:1545–1553.
[15] Rajamannan NM, Nealis TB, Subramaniam M, Pandya S, Stock SR, Ignatiev CI, Sebo TJ, Rosengart TK, Edwards WD, McCarthy PM, Bonow RO, Spelsberg TC. (2005). *Calcified Rheumatic Valve Neoangiogenesis Is Associated With Vascular Endothelial Growth Factor Expression and Osteoblast-Like Bone Formation.* Circulation. 2005;111:3296-3301.
[16] Caira FC, Stock SR, Gleason TG, McGee EC, Huang J, Bonow RO, Spelsberg TC, McCarthy PM, Rahimtoola SH, Rajamannan NM. (2006). *Human Degenerative Valve Disease Is Associated With Up-Regulation of Low-Density Lipoprotein Receptor-Related Protein 5 Receptor-Mediated Bone Formation.* J Am Coll Cardiol 2006;47:1707–12
[17] Rajamannan NM. (2011). *Bicuspid aortic valve disease: the role of oxidative stress in Lrp5 bone formation.* Cardiovascular Pathology (2011) in press.
[18] Otto CM. (2006) *Valvular Aortic Stenosis. Disease Severity and Timing of Intervention.* Journal of the American College of Cardiology Vol. 47, No. 11, 2006
[19] Rajamannan NM. (2005) *Calcific Aortic Stenosis: Medical and Surgical Management in the Elderly.* Current Treatment Options in Cardiovascular Medicine 2005, 7:437–442
[20] ACC/AHA 2006 *Guidelines for the Management of Patients With Valvular Heart Disease*
[21] Bonow RO, Carabello BA, Kanu C, et al. *ACC/AHA 2006 guidelines for the management of patients with valvular heart disease: a report of the American College of Cardiology/American Heart Association Task Force on Practice Guidelines.* Circulation 2006; 114:e84–e231.
[22] Stone PH. (2007). *C-Reactive Protein to Identify Early Risk for Development of Calcific Aortic Stenosis Right Marker? Wrong Time?* Journal of the American College of Cardiology Vol. 50, No. 20, 2007
[23] Antonini-Canterin F, Leiballi E, Enache R,. Popescu BA, Rosca M, Cervesato E, Piazza R, Ginghina C˘, Nicolosi GL. (2009). *Hydroxymethylglutaryl Coenzyme-A Reductase Inhibitors Delay the Progression of Rheumatic Aortic Valve Stenosis A Long-Term*

Echocardiographic Study. Journal of the American College of Cardiology Vol. 53, No. 20, 2009

[24] Rajamannan NM, Subramaniam M, Springett M et al. (2002). *Atorvastatin inhibits hypercholesterolemia-induced cellular proliferation and bone matrix production in the rabbit aortic valve.* Circulation 2002;105: 2660–5.

[25] Gunduz H, Akdemir R, Binak E et al. (2003). *Can serum lipids and CRP levels predict the "severity" of aortic valve stenosis?* Acta Cardiol 2003;58:321- 6.

[26] Gerber IL, Stewart RAH, Hammett CJK et al. (2003). *Effect of aortic valve replacement on C-reactive protein in nonrheumatic aortic stenosis.* Am J Cardiol 2003;92:1129 -32.

[27] Ortlepp JR, Hoffmann R, Ohme F et al. (2001). *The vitamin D receptor genotype predisposes to the development of calcific aortic valve stenosis.* Heart 2001; 85:635–638.

[28] Avakian SD, Annicchino-Bizzacchi JM, Grinberg M et al. (2001). *Apolipoproteins AI, B, and E polymorphisms in severe aortic valve stenosis.* Clin Genet 2001; 60:381–384.

[29] Kamalesh et al. (2009) *Does diabetes accelerate progression of calcific aortic stenosis?* European Journal of Echocardiography, 30 aprile 2009

[30] Yu PJ, Skolnick A, Ferrari G, Heretis K, Mignatti P, Pintucci G, Rosenzweig B, Diaz-Cartelle J, Kronzon I, Perk G, Pass HI, Galloway AC, Grossi EA, Grau JB. (2009). *Correlation between plasma osteopontin levels and aortic valve calcification: potential insights into the pathogenesis of aortic valve calcification and stenosis.* J Thorac Cardiovasc Surg. 2009 Jul;138(1):196-9

[31] Grau J.B., Sainger R., Poggio P., Seefried W.F., Field B., Koka E., Ferrari G.. (2011). *Dephosphorilation of circulating human Osteopontin correlates with severe valvular calcification in patiemts wuth Calcific Aortic Valve Degeneration.* In press. Per concessione dell'autore.

[32] Stewart BF, Siscovick D, Lind BK et al. *(1997). Clinical factors associated with calcific aortic valve disease. Cardiovascular Health Study.* J Am Coll Cardiol 1997, 29:630–634.

[33] Ridker PM, Danielson E, Fonseca FAH, Genest J, Gotto AM, Kastelein JJP, Koeni W, Libby P, Lorenzatti AJ, MacFadye JG, Nordestgaard BG, Shepherd J, Willerson JT, and Glynn RJ for the JUPITER Study Group. (2008). *Rosuvastatin to Prevent Vascular Events in Men and Women with Elevated C-Reactive Protein* N Engl J Med 2008;359:2195-207.

[34] O'Brien KD. (2006). *Pathogenesis of calcific aortic valve disease: a disease process comes of age (and a good deal more)*. Arterioscler Thromb Vasc Biol 2006;26:1721- 8.

[35] Helske S, Lindstedt KA, Laine M et al. (2004). *Induction of local angiotensin II-producing systems in stenotic aortic valves.* J Am Coll Cardiol 2004;44:1859–66.

[36] Rosenhek R, Rader F, Loho N et al.*(2004). Statins but not angiotensin-converting enzyme inhibitors delay progression of aortic stenosis.* Circulation 2004; 110:1291–1295.

[37] Lonn E. *Angiotensin-converting enzyme inhibitors and angiotensin receptor blockers in atherosclerosis.(2002).* Curr Atheroscler Rep. 2002;4: 363–372.

[38] O'Brien KD, Zhao XQ, Shavelle DM et al. (2004). *Hemodynamic effects of the angiotensin-converting enzyme inhibitor, ramipril, in patients with mild to moderate aortic stenosis and preserved left ventricular function.* J Investig Med. 2004;52:185–191.

[39] Sarphie TG. (1986). *A cytochemical study of the surface properties of aortic and mitral valve endothelium from hypercholesterolemic rabbits.* Exp Mol Pathol. 1986; 281–296.

[40] Rajamannan NM, Subramaniam M, Caira F, Stock SR, Spelsberg TC. (2005). *Atorvastatin inhibits hypercholesterolemia-induced calcification in the aortic valves via the Lrp5 receptor pathway.* Circulation. 2005;112(Suppl I):I-229–I-234.

[41] Mohler ER III, Gannon F, Reynolds C, Zimmerman R, Keane MG, Kaplan FS. (2001). *Bone formation and inflammation in cardiac valves.* Circulation. 2001;103: 1522–1528.

[42] Nagy E, Andersson DC, Caidahl K, Eriksson MJ, Eriksson P, Franco-Cereceda A, Hansson GK and Bäck M. (2011). *Upregulation of the 5-Lipoxygenase Pathway in Human Aortic Valves Correlates With Severity of Stenosis and Leads to Leukotriene-Induced Effects on Valvular Myofibroblasts.* Circulation. 2011;123:1316-1325

[43] Cowell SJ, Newby DE, Prescott RJ, Bloomfield P, Reid J, Northridge DB, Boon NA. (2005). *A randomized trial of intensive lipid-lowering therapy in calcific aortic stenosis.* N Engl J Med. 2005;352:2389–2397.

[44] Newby DE, Cowell SJ, Boon NA.(2006). *Emerging medical treatments for aortic stenosis: statins, angiotensin converting enzyme inhibitors, or both?* Heart, 2006 Jun;92(6):729-34

[45] Moura LM, Ramos SF, Zamorano JL, Barros IM, Azevedo LF, Rocha-Gonçalves F, Rajamannan NM. (2007). *Rosuvastatin Affecting Aortic Valve Endothelium to Slow the Progression of Aortic Stenosis.* J Am Coll Cardiol 2007;49:554–61

[46] Parolari A, Tremoli E, Cavallotti L, Trezzi M, Kassem S, Loardi C, Veglia F, Ferrari G, Pacini D, Alamanni F. (2011). *Do statins improve outcomes and delay the progression of non-rheumatic calcific aortic stenosis?* Heart. 2011 Apr;97(7):523-9.

[47] Parolari A, Loardi C, Mussoni L, Cavallotti L, Camera M, Biglioli P, Tremoli E, Alamanni F.(2009). *Nonrheumatic calcific aortic stenosis: an overview from basic science to pharmacological prevention.* Eur J Cardiothorac Surg. 2009 Mar;35(3):493-504

[48] Steffel J, Braulwald E. (2011). *Noval anticoagulants: focus on stroke prevention and treatment of venous thrombo-embolism.* Eur Heart J. 2011 Mar 18

[49] Ordovas Baines JP, Climent Grana E, Jover Botella A, Valero Garcia I. (2009). *Pharmacokinetics and pharmacodynamics of the new oral anticoagulants dabigatran and rivaroxiban.* Farm Hosp. 2009 May-June; 33(3):125-33

[50] Iung B, Cachier A, Baron G, Messika-Zeitoun D, Delahaye F, Tornos P et al. (2005). *Decision making in elderly patients with severe aortic stenosis: why are so many denied surgery?* Eur Heart J 2005; 26:2714–2720.

[51] Cribier A, Eltchaninoff H, Tron C, Bauer F, Agatiello C, Sebagh L et al. (2004). *Early experience with percutaneous transcatheter implantation of heart valve prosthesis for the treatment of end-stage inoperable patients with calcific aortic stenosis.* J Am Coll Cardiol 2004; 43:698–703.

[52] Iung B, Baron G, Butchart EG, Delahaye F, Gohlke-Ba¨rwolf C, Levang OW et al. (2003). *A prospective survey of patients with valvular heart disease in Europe: the Euro Heart Survey on valvular disease.* Eur Heart J 2003; 24:1231– 1243.

Part 2

Etiology and Pathophysiology

2

Aortic Stenosis: Geriatric Considerations

Petar Risteski, Andreas Zierer, Nestoras Papadopoulos,
Sven Martens, Anton Moritz and Mirko Doss
Department of Thoracic and Cardiovascular Surgery, Johann Wolfgang Goethe University
Germany

1. Introduction

In developed countries, the most frequent heart valve disease is aortic stenosis (AS) (Lung et al., 2003). Approximately, 25% of the population aged over 65 years have aortic valve thickening and some 3% of people older than 75 years have severe AS (Lindroos et al., 1993; Stewart et al., 1997). Its prevalence further increases with age and since life expectancy continues to extend, it is expected that the population of elderly patients with AS will grow in future.

Aortic valve replacement (AVR) is the gold standard treatment of severe and symptomatic AS. The current American College of Cardiology and American Heart Association as well as the European Heart Association Guidelines do not restrict operative treatment in relation to the age of the patient (Bonow et al., 2006; Vahanian, 2007).

Most of the large studies now report of more than 20% of patients undergoing surgery for AS being over the age of 80 years (Charlson et al., 2006). Still, in every day clinical practise, advanced age is considered one of the main reasons to decline surgery.

In the Euro Heart Survey on valvular heart disease (Lung et al, 2003), despite presence of severe and symptomatic AS, aortic valve surgery was refused in as many as 33% of elderly patients (defined as age over 75 years). Advanced age and left ventricular dysfunction were the most striking characteristics of the patients being refused, while comorbidities played a less important role.

The decision to operate an elderly with AS must be carefully considered, and made then when the benefits of the operation, as compared to conventional treatment, outweigh the risk of the intervention.

2. Natural history of aortic stenosis and conventional treatment

Drs. Ross and Braunwald were the first to show that aortic stenosis develops latent over many years, with a near-to-normal survival until the symptoms develop (Ross & Braunwald, 1968). Once the symptoms of angina, dyspnea or syncope develop, the survival declines abruptly. Around 75% of symptomatic patients will expire within 3 years after the onset of symptoms, without valve replacement. The worst prognosis had the patients with global heart failure associated with severe AS, with a median survival of less than one year.

Some other more contemporary studies looked at the survival of patients after being medically or surgically treated for AS. Bouma and coworkers identified three predictive factors for poor outcome of non-operated patients with aortic stenosis (Bouma et al., 1999). Advanced heart failure (New York Heart Association Class III or IV), associated mitral regurgitation as well as severe left ventricular systolic dysfunction identified patients as high-risk for mortality, with a three-year survival of only 20%. Their study showed a 3-year survival rate of 80% in the group of patients treated operatively versus only 49% in the group of patients treated medically. Still, 41% of these patients with severe symptomatic AVS were treated medically.

A similar survival pattern was observed in the study by Varadarajan and coworkers (Varadarajan et al., 2006). In their hands, surgically treated patients showed improved 1-year, 2-year and 5-year survival rates of 87, 78 and 68%, respectively, as compared with 52, 40 and 22%, respectively, in those managed medically.

With this issue in hand, Pierard and coworkers from Brussels, Belgium have looked at the determinants and their prognostic impact of operative refusal or denial in octogenarians with severe AS (Pierard et al., 2011). Advanced age, a lower transaortic pressure gradient, a larger aortic valve area and presence of diabetes were identified as independent predictors of AVR refusal or denial, which occurred in 40% of all patients with severe and symptomatic AS, and had a profound impact on long-term prognosis, leading in a twofold excess mortality of patients treated without surgery (Pierard et al, 2011).

Nowadays, there is no reason to put into question the decision to perform the operation on an elderly patient with severe AS, since optimal medical treatment remains ineffective when AS becomes symptomatic.

3. Operative treatment of elderly with AVS

Advanced age at the time of the operation has a strong influence upon the perioperative mortality and morbidity. Bridgewater and co-workers, on behalf of the European Association of Cardio-Thoracic Surgery, reported recently that early mortality following isolated AV surgery averaged 1.2% for patients under the age of 56 years, and progresses to 3.7% for patients between 71-75 years, further to 4.1% for patients between 76-80 years of age, and finally to 6.1% for patients older than 80 years (Bridgewater et al, 2010). The same authors also conclude, based on a survey on 40111 operated patients in developed countries that patients older than 80 years stay, on the average, more than 3 days longer than those under 61.

This, however, represents a significant improvement of early results in contemporary aortic valve surgery as compared to outcomes reported two or three decades ago. In a paper published in Circulation in 1994, from the group from Rennes, France, Dr. Logeais and coworkers report of higher early postoperative mortality risk, averaging 6.2% for patients age 60-70 years, and 11.2% for patients older than 70 years of age (Logeais et al, 1994). A better understanding of the role of the preoperative respiratory preparation, improved myocardial protection of otherwise severely hypertrophic myocardium, as well as normothermic cardiopulmonary bypass may be attributed to the improved early postoperative results in the recent studies as compared to those several decades ago.

Another approach to improve early and long-term survival of elderly patients undergoing AV surgery is to have them undergo surgery in due time. Surgery in octagenarians, as reported by Pipper and coworkers (Pipper, 2009) should not be postponed until chronic myocardial decompensation finally convinces patients, relatives and cardiologists that AV surgery is inevitable, as the preoperative chronic decompensation strongly increases operative mortality and morbidity and negatively impacts long-term survival.

The surgical community worked over the last two decades vigorously to reduce the trauma of the conventional aortic valve operation. Minimally invasive approaches like partial upper sternotomy have replaced the conventional complete median sternotomy when performing AVR in many centres. Aiming for smaller incision, without compromising the quality of the operation and the effectiveness of myocardial protection, improved early outcomes have been reached.

We reported the safety and reliability of AVR via a partial upper sternotomy in 2003 (Dogan et al, 2003). In a prospective randomised trial, we showed that minimally invasive AVR can be performed with only slightly longer operative times, good cosmetic results and improved rib cage stability as well as significantly less blood loss. Furthermore, limited surgical access affected negatively neither the patients' neurological outcome nor the efficacy of myocardial protection.

More recently, the implantation technique for AVR has been also modified, without compromise in hemodynamic performance of the valve substitute, all in order to reduce implantation times, and therefore the myocardium ischemia as well as cardiopulmonary bypass times. We recently reported on the initial clinical experiences with the sutureless, nitinol-stented 3f Enable (Medtronic Inc., Minnesota, USA) aortic valve prosthesis in 32 patients. Implantation time could be significantly reduced down to 9±5 minutes (Martens et al., 2009). The first report of multicenter experience with this particular valve substitute and implantation technique in 140 patients was published in the European Journal of Cardiothoracic Surgery in 2011 (Martens et al., 2011). Reproducibility as well as feasibility and safety with the ATS 3f Enable Bioprosthesis were demonstrated. Valve implantation resulted in excellent hemodynamics and significant clinical improvement. Further comparative studies are underway to prove the clinical benefit using this less-time-consuming implantation technique versus the conventional one.

In the last few years, intensive interest has been put toward the development and perfection of a catheter-delivered valve substitutes for use in patients with aortic stenosis in whom surgical therapy has been rejected (Walther et al, 2007a). Two delivery routes have been used to deploy the valve substitute in such patients.

The transapical route (TAP-AVI – transapical aortic valve implantation), is the one used by the surgeons. By avoiding the sternotomy incision, the cardiopulmonary bypass, aortic crossclamping as well as the cardioplegic cardiac arrest during the procedure, one aims at reduction of perioperative risk in an otherwise high-risk population of patients. The vast majority of patients targeted for this therapy are elderly with multiple severe comorbidities rendering them as high-risk or not suitable for conventional AVR. The mean age of the patients being reported on in the initial multicenter experience was 81 years (Walther et al., 2007b).

We went further on and compared our experience with TAP-AVI versus minimally invasive AVR through partial upper sternotomy in matched population of elderly patients (Zierer et al., JTCVS 2008). Mean age in our collectives were 85 years for the TAP-AVI group and 82 years for the ministernotomy group.

Patient age, preoperative comorbidities and perioperative risk, expressed as logistic EuroSCORE (38%±14% for the TAP-AVI group and 35%±9% for the ministernotomy group) were matched between the groups. Although the TAP-AVI approach was associated with faster postoperative recovery, early and late morbidity and mortality were comparable with those of the surgery group, suggesting that patient age and comorbidities are independent predictors of adverse outcome after AVR, regardless of the surgical approach.

4. Long-term survival of elderly patients after AVR: the issue of left ventricular hypertrophy

The long-term survival after the surgery, although superior to the medical treatment, is still not satisfactory. Reported survival rates in all age groups range between 50% and 66% (David et al, 2001; Hammermeister et al, 2000) and further decrease to 18% at 15 years in patients older than 75 years of age (Jamieson et al., 1994). Several studies have related these poor results after AV surgery with the incomplete regression of the left ventricular hypertrophy (Levy, 1991; Rossi et al, 2000).

Left ventricular hypertrophy (LVH), a known complication of aortic stenosis, has been strongly associated with increased risk of sudden death, congestive heart failure, and overall cardiovascular mortality. Incomplete regression of the LVH in patients undergoing AVR has been linked to the obstructive nature of the valve sewing ring and stent, or to patient-prosthesis mismatch, which are being held responsible for persistently elevated transvalvular gradients.

In the late 1980s, stentless valves were introduced with the goal of maximizing the effective orifice area for flow by eliminating the valvular stent and sewing ring, therefore facilitating faster and more complete regression of LVH. Over the next decade, several groups have published their initial results; many of them indicating faster and more complete regression of left ventricular mass after stentless as compared with the stented AVR (Jin et al., 1996, Thomson et al., 1998). However, these advantages have been obtained in the setting of nonrandomized trials. Our team had therefore set forth to determine, if we could measure these early and mid-term postoperative improvements in older patients receiving a stentless versus a stented bioprosthetic aortic valve, in a prospective randomized setting (Risteski et al., 2009).

Between September 1999 and January 2001, 40 patients with severe symptomatic aortic stenosis, over the age of 75 years, were randomly assigned to receive either the stented Perimount (n=20) or the stentless Prima Plus (n=20) bioprosthesis.

The aortic valve was approached through a hockey stick aortotomy. After complete resection of the native aortic valve and debridement of the aortic annulus, accurate sizing was carried out using the respective Carpentier-Edwards sizers for the Prima Plus stentless and the Perimount stented valves.

The Prima Plus stentless valves were implanted in the subcoronary position. The commissures were positioned 120° apart, with the muscular shelf corresponding to the right coronary sinus. Care was taken to suture the base of the valve subannularly, to ensure that the coaptation line of the leaflets was at the height of the native annulus. Single interrupted unpledgeted 4-0 braided polyester sutures were used for the proximal end, and the rims of the valve commissures were sutured to the native aorta using 4-0 polypropylene running sutures. For the Carpentier-Edwards Perimount stented valve implantation, interrupted mattressed pledgeted 2-0 braided polyester sutures were placed circumferentially from below the annulus. The valves were implanted in the supra-annular position, with the valvular stent positioned so as not to interfere with the coronary ostia.

Clinical outcomes, left ventricular mass regression, effective orifice area, ejection fraction and mean gradients were evaluated at discharge, six months, one year and five years after surgery.

Left ventricular mass index (LVMI) was calculated using the formula postulated by Devereux and Reichek, as follows:

$$LVMI\ (g/m^2) = (1.05 \times [(EDD + PWTd + IVSTd)^3 - EDD^3] - 13.6) / BSA$$

where the EDD is the LV end-diastolic diameter (cm), the PWTd is the LV postero-lateral diastolic wall thickness (cm), the IVSTd is the interventricular septum diastolic thickness (cm), and the BSA is the body surface area of the patient (Devereux & Reichek, 1997).

At five years, there were 5/20 (25%) deaths in the stentless group and 6/20 (30%) deaths in the stented group (all non-valve-related). There was one case of endocarditis in each group, early postoperatively. All patients displayed continuous clinical improvement after the operation; at five years, all of the survivors were in New York Heart Association class I or II. Mean transvalvular gradients (Fig. 1a) have remained consistently low throughout the follow-up with neither clinical nor statistical relevance in the differences between the groups at any of the given time points. Also noted was the lack of significant difference in the follow-up values of the effective orifice areas (Fig. 1b) of both prostheses, although a tendency toward increase of the same in both groups was obvious early in follow-up (at 12 months with regards to 6 months) only to disappear at the 5-year follow-up examination.

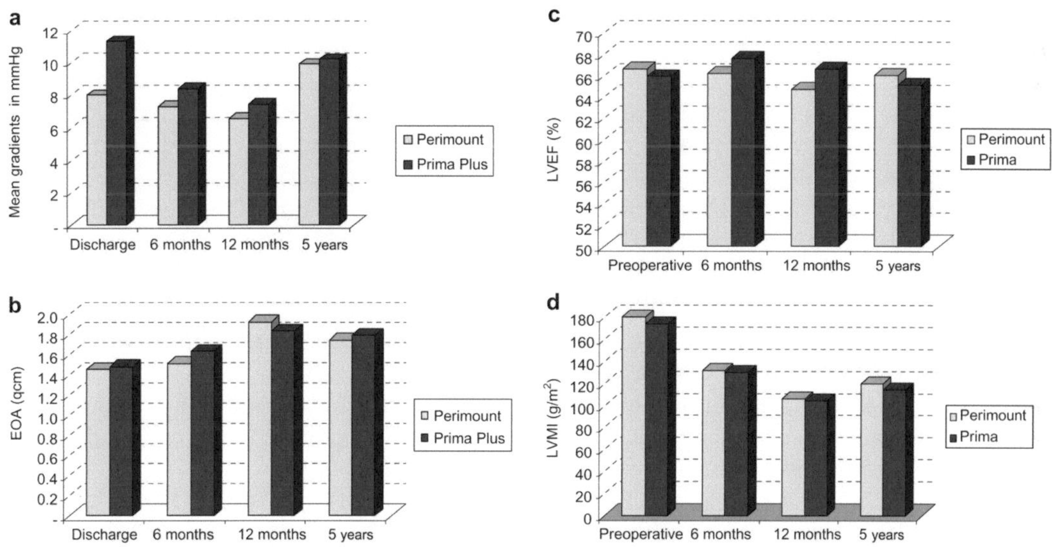

Fig. 1. Hemodynamic results after AVR with Edwards Perimount Stented Valve vs. Prima Plus stentless valve in elderly. (a) Mean transvalvular gradients. (b) Mean effective orifice area (c) Left ventricular ejection fraction (d) Left ventricular mass index.

The left ventricular ejection fraction (Fig. 1c) did not change over the time of follow-up. At 6 and 12 months, as well as at 5 years it did not differ between the groups. The left ventricular mass index (LVMI, Fig. 1d) did display a continuous rate of decrease in the first years after the surgery; however, this tendency was lost after the first year as the mean LVMI at 5 years was almost the same to that at 12 months. Finally, the index failed to reach the normal range in both groups. At all time points, the difference between the groups did not reach statistical significance.

At five years, stentless valves were not superior to the stented valves, with regards to hemodynamic performance, regression of left ventricular mass and clinical outcome. Survival of the patients was not related to the nature of the biologic valve.

Overall, the complexity of stentless valve implantation with its prolonged cross-clamping times might not be justifiable under these circumstances, if as we found, the same results can be achieved with a standard stented bioprosthesis. Our results are in concordance with some other prospective randomized studies that emerged in the meantime (Ali et al., 2007, Perez de Arenaza et al., 2005).

5. Conclusion

There is no scientific reason to put into question the decision to perform the operation on an elderly patient with severe AS, since optimal medical treatment remains ineffective when AS becomes symptomatic. Elderly patient may benefit from one of the available minimally invasive techniques for aortic valve replacement. The regression of the left ventricular hypertrophy as well as the long-term survival after aortic valve replacement is not influence by the nature of the valvular substitute, failing to justify a rather more complex implantation of stentless valve substitute in an elderly patient.

6. References

Ali A, Halstead JC, Cafferty F, Sharples L, Rose F, Lee E, Rusk R, Dunning J, Argano V & Tsui S. (2007) Early clinical and hemodynamic outcomes after stented and stentless aortic valve replacement: results from a randomised controlled trial. Ann Thorac Surg 83:2162–2168.

Bonow RO, Carabello BA, Kanu C, de Leon AC Jr, Faxon DP, Freed MD, Gaasch WH, Lytle BW, Nishimura RA, O'Gara PT, O'Rourke RA, Otto CM, Shah PM, Shanewise JS, Smith SC Jr, Jacobs AK, Adams CD, Anderson JL, Antman EM, Faxon DP, Fuster V, Halperin JL, Hiratzka LF, Hunt SA, Lytle BW, Nishimura R, Page RL & Riegel B. (2006) ACC/AHA 2006 guidelines for the management of patients with valvular heart disease. J Am Coll Cardiol. 48(3):e1-148.

Bouma BJ, van Den Brink RB, van Der Meulen JH, Verheul HA, Cheriex EC, Hamer HP, Dekker E, Lie KI & Tijssen JG. (1999). To operate or not elderly patients with aortic stenosis: the decision and its consequences. Heart 82:143-8.

Bridgewater B, Gummert J, Walton PKH & Kinsman R. (2010) *Forth EACTS adult cardiac surgical database report 2010.* Dendrite Clinical Systems Ltd, ISBN 1-903968-26-7, United Kingdom.

Charlson E, Lagedza ATR & Hamel MB (2006) Decision-making and outcomes in severe symptomatic aortic stenosis. J Heart Valve Dis 15:312-321

David TE, Ivanov J, Armstrong S, Feindel CM & Cohen G. (2001) Late results of heart valve replacement with the Hancock II bioprosthesis. J Thorac Cardiovasc Surg 121:268–277.

Devereux RB & Reichek N. (1977) Echocardiographic determination of left ventricular mass in man: anatomic validation of the method. Circulation 55:613–618.

Dogan S, Dzemali O, Wimmer-Greinecker G, Derra P, Doss M, Khan MF, Aybek T, Kleine P & Moritz A. (2003) Minimally invasive versus conventional aortic valve replacement: a prospective randomized trial. J Heart Valve Dis 12:76-80.

Hammermeister K, Sethi GK, Henderson WG, Grover FL, Oprian C & Rahimtoola SH. (2000) Outcomes 15 years after valve replacement with a mechanical versus bioprosthetic valve: final report of the Veterans Affairs randomised trial. J Am Coll Cardiol 36:1152–1158.

Jamieson WR, Burr LH, Tyers GF & Munro AI. (1994) Carpentier-Edwards standard and supraannular porcine bioprosthesis: 10 year comparision of structural valve deterioration. J Heart Valve Dis 3:59–65.

Jin XY, Zhang ZM, Gibson DG, Yacoub MH & Pepper JR. (1996) Effects of valve substitute on changes in left ventricular function and hypertrophy after aortic valve replacement. Ann Thorac Surg 62:683–690.

Levy D. (1991) Clinical significance of left ventricular hypertrophy: insights from the Framingham Study. J Cardiovasc Pharmacol 17(Suppl 2):S1–S2.

Lindroos M, Kapari M, Heikkala J & Tilvis R. (1993) Prevalence of aortic valve abnormalities in the elderly: an echocardiographic study of a random population sample. J Am Coll Cardiol 21:1220-5.

Logeais Y, Langanay T, Roussin R, Leguerrier A, Rioux C, Chaperon J, de Place C, Mabo P, Pony JC & Daubert JC. (1994) Surgery for aortic stenosis in elderly patients. A Study of surgical risks and predictive factors. Circulation 90:2891-2898

Iung B, Baron G, Butchart EG, Delahaye F, Gohlke-Bärwolf C, Levang OW, Tornos P, Vanoverschelde JL, Vermeer F, Boersma E, Ravaud P &Vahanian A. (2003) A prospective survey of patients with valvular heart disease in Europe: the Euro Heart Survey on valvular heart disease. Eur Heart J 24:1231-43.

Martens S, Ploss A, Sirat S, Miskovic A, Moritz A & Doss M. (2009) Sutureless aortic valve replacement with the 3f Enable aortic bioprosthesis. Ann Thorac Surg 87:1914-17.

Martens S, Sadowski J, Eckstein FS, Bartus K, Kapelak B, Sievers HH, Schlensak C & Carrel T. (2011) Clinical experience with the ATS 3f Enable(®) Sutureless Bioprosthesis. Eur J Cardiothorac Surg doi:10.1016/j.ejcts.2010.12.068

Perez de Arenaza D, Lees B, Flather M, Nugara F, Husebye T, Jasinski M, Cisowski M, Khan M, Henein M, Gaer J, Guvendik L, Bochenek A, Wos S, Lie M, Van Nooten G, Pennell D & Pepper J. (2005) ASSERT (Aortic Stentless versus Stented valve assessed by Echocardiography Randomized Trial) Investigators. Randomised comparison of stentless versus stented valves for aortic stenosis: effects on left ventricular mass. Circulation 112:2696–2702

Piérard S, Seldrum S, de Meester C, Pasquet A, Gerber B, Vancraeynest D, El Khoury G, Noirhomme P, Robert A & Vanoverschelde JL. (2011) Incidence, determinants and prognostic impact of operative refusal or denial in octogenarians with severe aortic stenosis. Ann Thorac Surg 91:1107-12

Piper C, Hering D, Kleikamp G, Körfer R & Horstkotte D. (2009) Valve replacement in octogenarians: arguments for an earlier surgical intervention. J Heart Valve Dis. 18(3):239-44

Risteski P, Martens S, Rouhollahpour A, Wimmer-Greinecker G, Moritz A & Doss M. (2009) Prospective randomized evaluation of stentless vs. stented aortic biologic prosthetic valves in the elderly at five years. Interact CardioVasc Thorac Surg 8:449-453.

Ross J, Jr., Braunwald E. (1968) Aortic stenosis. Circulation 38 Suppl V:V-61-7.

Rossi A, Tomaino M, Golia G, Anselmi M, Fuca G & Zardini P. (2000) Echocardiographic prediction of clinical outcome in medically treated patients with aortic stenosis. Am Heart J 140:766–771.

Stewart BF, Siscovick D, Lind BK, Gardin JM, Gottdiener JS, Smith VE, Kitzman DW & Otto CM. (1997) Clinical factors associated with calcific aortic valve disease: Cardiovascular Health Study. J Am Coll Cardiol 29:630-4

Thomson HL, O'Brian MF, Almeida AA, Tesar PJ, Davison MB & Burstow DJ. (1998) Haemodynamics and left ventricular mass regression: a comparision of the stentless, stented and mechanical sortic valve replacement. Eur J Cardiothorac Surg 13:572–575

Vahanian A, Baumgartner H, Bax J, Butchart E, Dion R, Filippatos G, Flachskampf F, Hall R, Iung B, Kasprzak J, Nataf P, Tornos P, Torracca L & Wenink A. (2007) Guidelines on the management of valvular heart disease. Eur Heart J 28:230-68.

Varadarajan P, Nikhil K, Bensal RC & Pai RG. (2006) Survival in elderly patients with severe aortic stenosis is dramatically improved by aortic valve replacement: results from a cohort of 277 patients aged ≥80 years. Eur J Cardiothorac Surg 30:722-727

Walther T, Falk V, Borger MA, Dewey T, Wimmer-Greinecker G, Schuler G, Mack M & Mohr FW. (2007) Minimally invasive transapical beating heart aortic valve implantation—proof of concept. Eur J Cardiothorac Surg 31:9–15.

Walther T, Simon P, Dewey T, Wimmer-Greinecker G, Falk V, Kasimir MT, Doss M, Borger MA, Schuler G, Glogar D, Fehske W, Wolner E, Mohr FW & Mack M. (2007) Transapical minimally invasive aortic valve implantation: multicenter experience. Circulation 116(11 Suppl):I240-5.

Zierer A, Wimmer-Greinecker G, Martens S, Moritz A & Doss M. (2009) Is transapical aortic valve implantation really less invasive than minimally invasive aortic valve replacement? J Thorac Cardiovasc Surg. 138:1067-72.

3

Pathophysiologic Mechanisms of Age – Related Aortic Valve Calcification

Alexandros Alexopoulos[1], Nikolaos Michelakakis[2] and Helen Papadaki[1]
[1]*Department of Anatomy, School of Medicine, University of Patras*
[2]*Department of Cardiology, General Hospital of Athens "G. Gennimatas"*
Greece

1. Introduction

Tricuspid aortic valve is a flexible membrane that opens and closes 100,000 times a day (Fig. 1) [1].

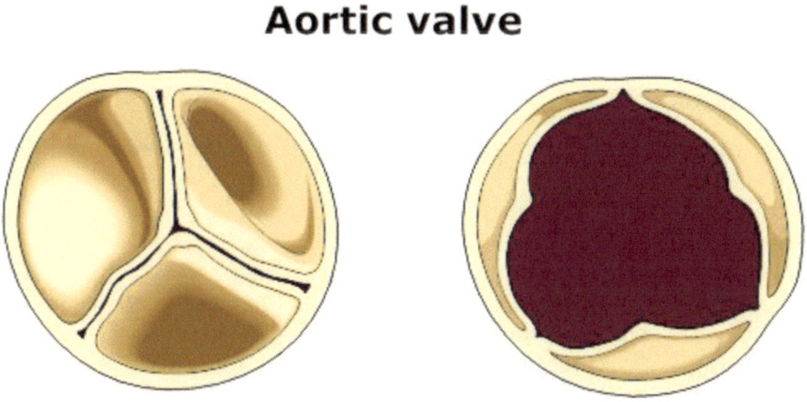

Fig. 1. Normal tricuspid aortic valve in closed and open position.

Aortic stenosis is the most common valvular lesion in Europe and North America [2]. As incidence of acute rheumatic fever has declined, calcific aortic stenosis (CAS) has become the most common indication for surgical valve replacement in the United States (Fig. 2) [3].
Regarding population aged>65 years, its incidence is 2-7% [2]. Interestingly, aortic sclerosis (aortic valve calcification without hemodynamic compromise) is present in more than 25% of patients older than age 65 years [5].
Recent studies provide evidence that atherosclerosis and CAS share common features in relation to risk factors and histopathologic lesions [3]. Moreover, histopathologic evidence suggests that early lesions in CAS are not just a result secondary to aging, but an active cellular process. Recent research implies that the classical "response to injury hypothesis", initially described in atherosclerosis, seems to represent the cornerstone of pathophysiology [4].

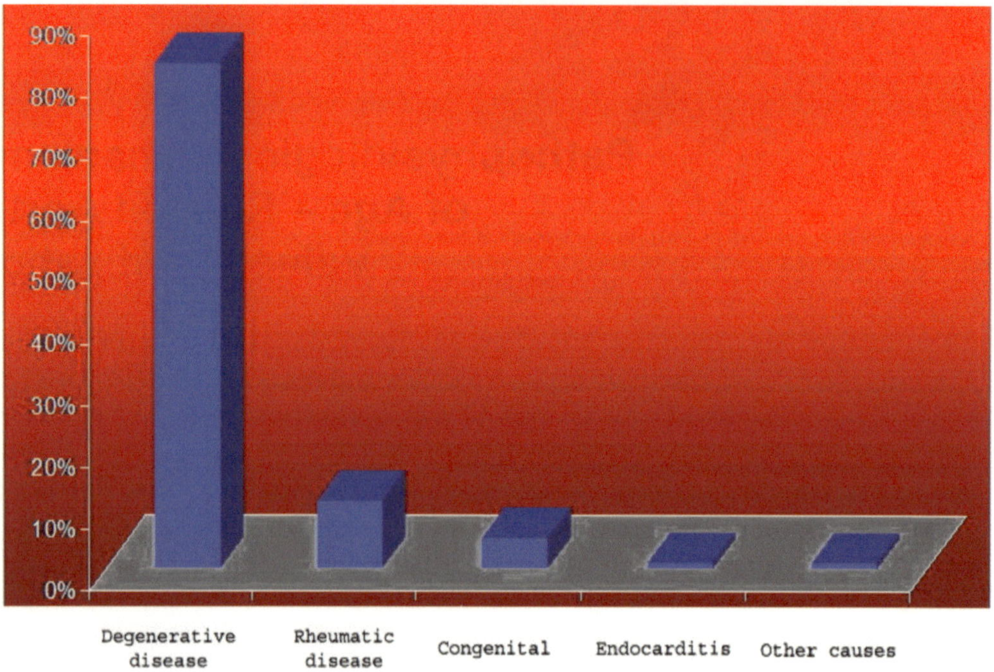

Fig. 2. Causes of aortic valve stenosis.

2. Anatomy - histology

Aortic valve is normally tricuspid, although in 1% of the population it is found to be congenitally bicuspid.

The internal collagen framework of the leaflets is arranged in three layers: fibrosa, spongiosa and ventricularis.

Fibrosa with its dense connective tissue provides strength, spongiosa with its loose matrix of glycoproteins provides a cushion for the mechanical forces, and ventricularis provides elasticity for changes of shape during opening and closing [6].

All three layers of aortic valve are avascular and are innervated by adrenergic and cholinergic neural networks [6].

In aortic sclerosis and stenosis, calcified nodules are initially observed at the base of the cusps and their presence is gradually extended towards the orifice. All three cusps are usually affected but one or more may be dominant. Heavy calcification is associated with hemodynamic impairment leading ultimately to need for valve replacement [7].

3. Calcific aortic stenosis (CAS) and atherosclerosis

3.1 Risk factors

Several studies suggest that traditional risk factors for atherosclerosis such as male gender, hypertension, dyslipidemia and renal failure are implicated in pathogenesis of CAS (Fig. 3) [2, 3, 8].

In addition, as we will discuss later, histologic lesions of CAS and atherosclerosis share common features. Inflammatory infiltration, lipid accumulation, cellular apoptosis and profileration and remodeling of extracellular matrix are present in both situations. Genetic

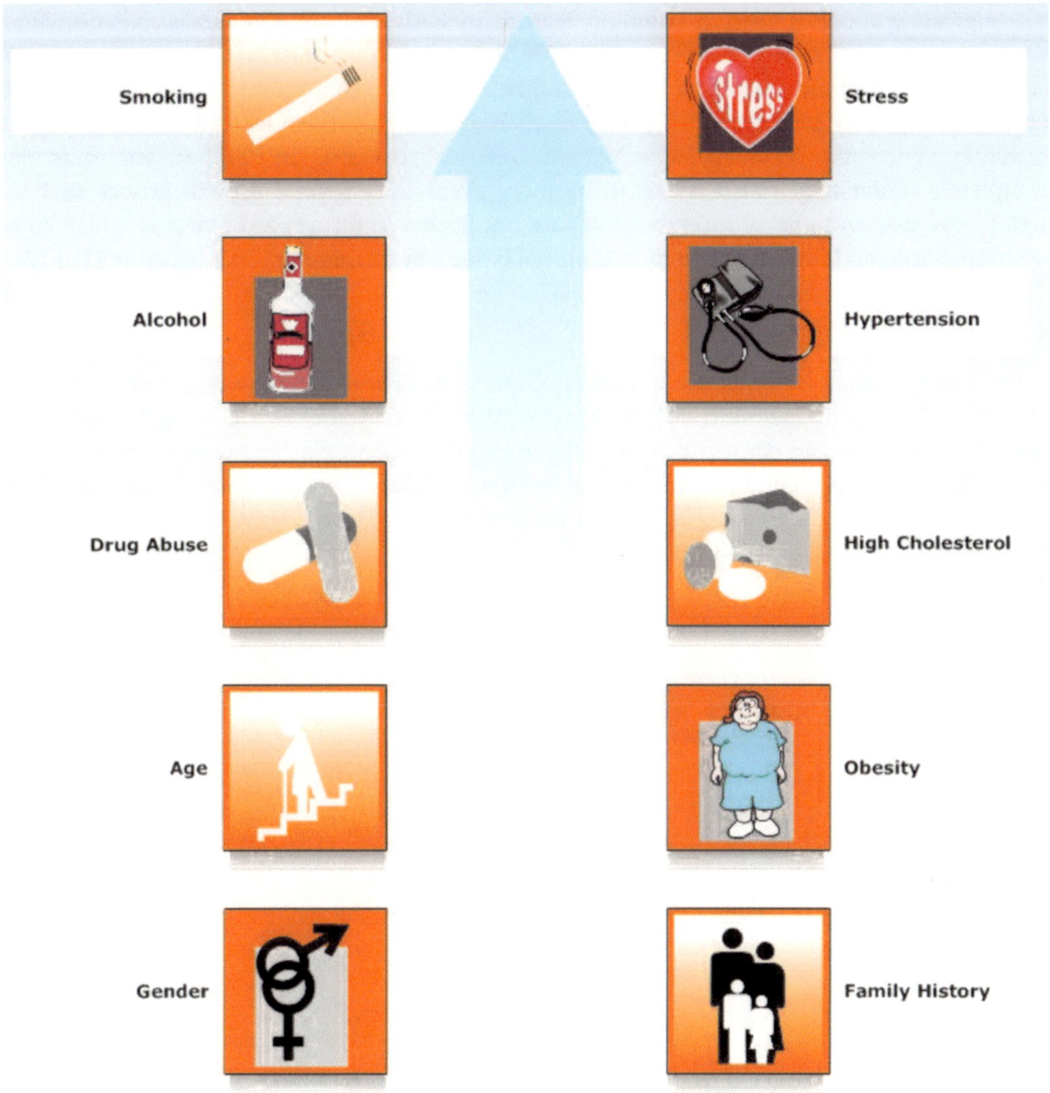

Fig. 3. Risk factors for calcific aortic stenosis.

polymorphisms and activation of certain pathways such as renin-angiotensin system seem to play vital role and elucidation of their participation in pathophysiology of CAS comprises major challenge [2, 6].

3.2 Similarities in histopathology

CAS and atherosclerosis present characteristic lesions with fibromyxomatous degeneration, inflammatory infiltration and lipid accumulation. Mechanical forces play significant role in progression of lesions [9].

However, pattern of disease is more diffuse in CAS in relation to atherosclerosis where lesions are characterized by necrotic core and fibrous cap. In addition, calcification is more prominent in aortic cusps and is observed even in early stages of pathophysiologic process [6].

Neoangiosis comprises, also, a common feature in CAS and atherosclerosis. Nevertheless, there are some differences. Normal valves are avascular in contrast to artery wall which is supplied by vasa vasorum. New vessels in atherosclerotic lesions are, actually, branches of vasa vasorum and present some defective characteristics as their wall is thin and friable resulting very often in intraplaque hemorrhage. Angiogenesis in calcified valves is not completely understood but it seems to be more organized. Several growth factors such as VEGF (vascular endothelial growth factor) are implicated in formation of vessels which have developed interendothelial junctions and partial basement membrane - like structures [10-12].

4. Pathophysiology of Calcific aortic stenosis (CAS)

Several factors lead to activation of endothelium with subsequent expression of significant factors such as cytokines and adhesion molecules. Subendothelial accumulation of lipids and inflammatory cells comprise the early lesions which trigger a "response to injury". This phase includes remodeling of extracellular matrix and transformation of quiescent valvular interstititial cells to activated interstitial cells (VICs) that consequently gain osteoblastic phenotype (Fig. 4).

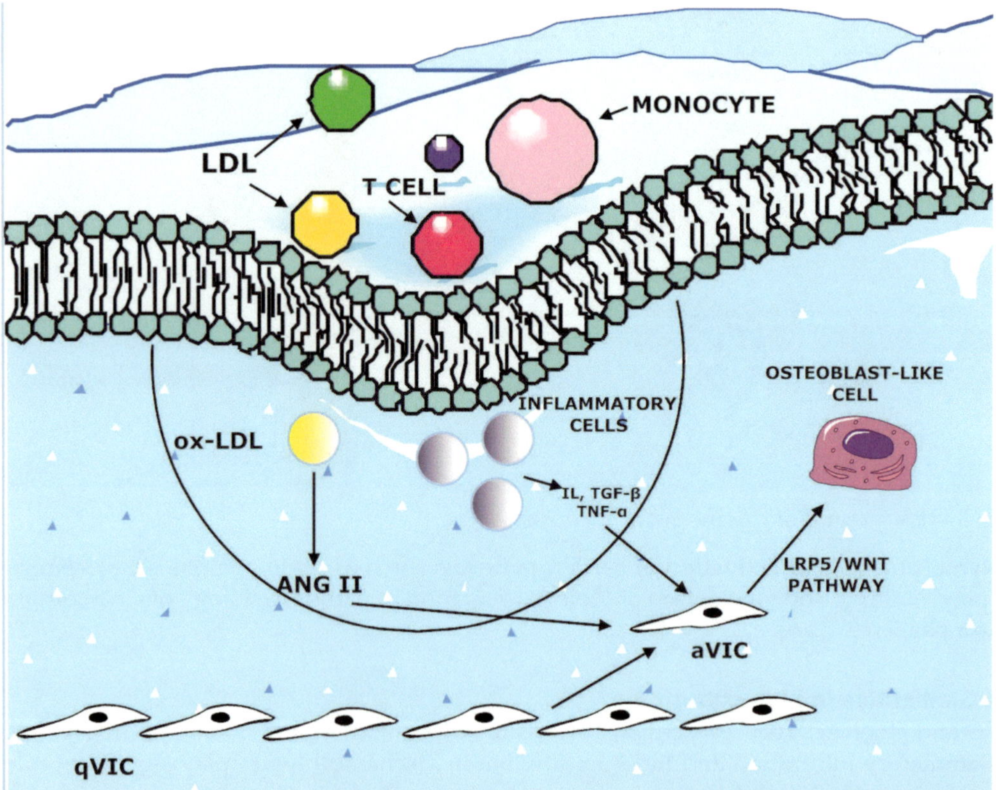

Fig. 4. Schematic illustration of pathophysiology of calcific aortic stenosis (ox-LDL: oxidized LDL, ang II: angiotensin II, qVIC: quiescent valvular interstitial cell, aVIC: activated valvular interstitial cell).

Expression of bone regulatory factors is related to formation of calcified nodules, lesions which represent later stages of aortic stenosis [8].
We will discuss further in detail all aspects of pathophysiologic process.

4.1 Endothelium

Abnormal activation of aortic valve endothelium was observed initially in experimental hypercholesterolemia rabbits [3].
Recent research has shown increased E-selectin plasma levels in patients with severe CAS which normalize after aortic valve surgery [13,14]. In addition, high levels of endothelial microparticles have been found in these patients. Endothelial microparticles are small vesicles that consist of a plasma membrane surrounding a small amount of cytosol. The membrane of the endothelial microparticle contains specific receptors and cell surface molecules which enable the identification of the endothelial origin of the microparticle. Inflammatory infiltration in calcified aortic valves has been related to circulating levels of endothelial microparticles [13, 15]. Several endothelial markers such as CD31, CD34, von Willebrand factor, and CEACAM1 (carcinoembryonic antigen-related cell adhesion molecule) were markedly expressed in tissue samples of human aortic valves that were from patients undergoing valve replacement for severe calcific, non-rheumatic aortic stenosis [13].
Remarkably, decreased availability of nitric oxide and prostacyclin was noticed in these specimen. These molecules are considered to be major modulators of inflammatory processes [1].

4.2 Valvular Interstitial Cells (VICs)

Valve integrity is determined by extracellular matrix. Moreover, quality and quantity of extracellular matrix components are depended on function of VICs [16].
Not surprisingly, age - related reduction of this cellular population is accompanied by fibrous degeneration [17].
VICs are elongated, spindle - like cells and most of them are located in fibrosa. They display morphological and functional characteristics of fibroblasts, smooth muscle cells and myofibroblasts [17].
Five distinct phenotypes of VICs have been recognized:

1. Embryonic progenitor endothelial/mesenchymal VICs
2. Quiescent VICs
3. Activated VICs
4. Adult progenitor VICs
5. Osteoblastic VICs

These cells present plasticity and are capable of changing their phenotype under certain circumstances (Fig. 5) [18].
VICs preserve stability and integrity of the valves and are involved in synthesis and remodeling of extracellular matrix [17].
Calcified nodules consist of nonviable myofibroblasts and crystals of hydroxyapatite. Viable osteoblast-like cells surround these structures expressing bone regulatory proteins. Alkaline phosphatase constitutes unquestionable proof of bone formation in areas of tissue injury [1].

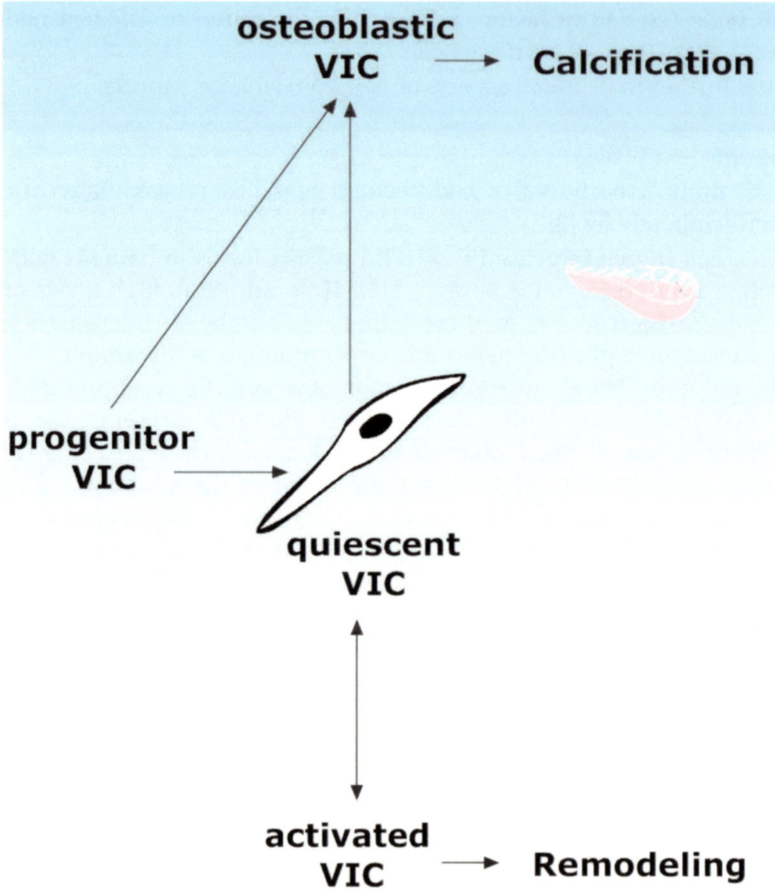

Fig. 5. Subtypes of Valvular Interstitial Cells.

VICs resemble to vascular smooth muscle cells (VSMCs) but their embryology is different. VSMCs derive from cardiac neural crest and lateral mesoderm-derived mesenchyme [6]. Myocardin-related transcription factor-B is the master regulator of differentiation of VSMCs that originate from the neural crest [19]. On the other hand, endothelial to mesenchymal transformation (EMT) phenomenon is considered to be responsible for the origin of VICs. The process seems to be regulated by TGF-β (transforming growth factor-β), NOTCH1, and Wnt/β-catenin signals [20].

4.3 Mechanical forces

Aortic valve cusps are subjected to unceasing influence of severe mechanical forces during lifetime. It is believed that the attachment area of the aortic leaflets to the aortic root encounters the strongest mechanical influence, which may provoke endothelial dysfunction. As we aforementioned, activation of endothelium is related to expression of adhesion molecules and cytokines that initiate several pathophysiologic processes [3].
Leucocyte infiltration and lipid accumulation take place initiating tissue injury with reactive fibro-proliferative changes. Alteration of valve morphology leads to further increase of local shear stress and ultimately a vicious circle is set up [13].

Preliminary studies suggested the 'wear and tear' theory in order to underline significance of mechanical stress in pathogenesis of aortic stenosis [4].
However, mechanical stress does not necessarily hold primary role in pathogenesis. Genetically predisposed individuals in atherosclerosis and aortic valve sclerosis are very prone to mechanical forces that trigger effortlessly key molecular signaling pathways in both diseases [13].

4.4 Genetic influence

4.4.1 Inhibitory proteins

Activation of signaling pathways is depended on expression of inhibitory proteins. Recent evidence has shown that BMP (bone morphogenetic protein), a major bone regulator, is inhibited by several proteins such as noggin, chordin, follistatin, gremlin and Smad proteins. Relative deficiency of these factors could be responsible for aortic valve ossification [1].

4.4.2 Lipoproteins

Determination of allelic variants of lipoproteins in patients suffering from aortic stenosis comprises an interesting research topic. Although a higher prevalence of apoE2 [21] and apoE4 [22], has been observed in some studies, these results have not been affirmed by other researchers.

4.4.3 Inflammatory factors

Inflammation is a prerequisite for aortic valve calcification. Specific genetic variants may trigger intense immune response with devastating results. Polymorphisms of the interleukin-10 gene promoter as well as simultaneous presence of the rare chemochine receptor 5 and connective tissue growth factor alleles are associated with severe calcium burden in patients with aortic stenosis [13].

4.4.4 Bone metabolism

Regarding bone metabolism genomics, vitamin D receptor genetic polymorphism has been extensively investigated [23]. High incidence of the B allele has been found in aortic stenosis and is related with reduced calcium absorption, bone resorption and increased expression of parathormone [3, 13].
Runx2, also designated Cbfa1, belongs to the Runt domain family and is the master transcription factor for bone formation inducing transcription of osteoblast-related genes that enhance mineralization such as osteocalcin gene [24]. Trancriptional activity of Runx2 may be suppresed by Notch1 signaling. Recent research demonstrated that a nonsense mutation of the NOTCH1 gene is associated with enhanced calcium deposition in aortic valves probably via reduced inhibition of Runx2 expression [25].
Finally, a polymorphism of the alpha estrogen receptor, in post-menopausal women is related to increase of cholesterol levels and predisposition to aortic valve calcification [26].

4.4.5 Cell cycle proteins

Finally, some cell cycle regulatory proteins are considered to participate in pathophysiologic process. $P21^{WAF1/CIP1}$ (cyclin-dependent proteinkinase inhibitor p21), and 14-3-3 belong to this category and their expression is reduced in areas of calcification [27].

4.5 Bone factors

Osteoblastic phenotype of VICs implies expression of bone proteins exhibiting regulatory or structural role.

Recent evidence suggests that aortic valve calcification is an active process involving chondro-osteogenic pathways. Calcified nodules are composed of hydroxyapatite crystals precipitated on a matrix of collagen, osteopontin (OP) and osteocalcin (OC) [3].

Aortic VICs in areas containing calcific deposits show significantly higher expression of bone regulatory factors such as BMP, Runx2, Osterix in relation to non-calcified areas (Fig. 6) [3,24].

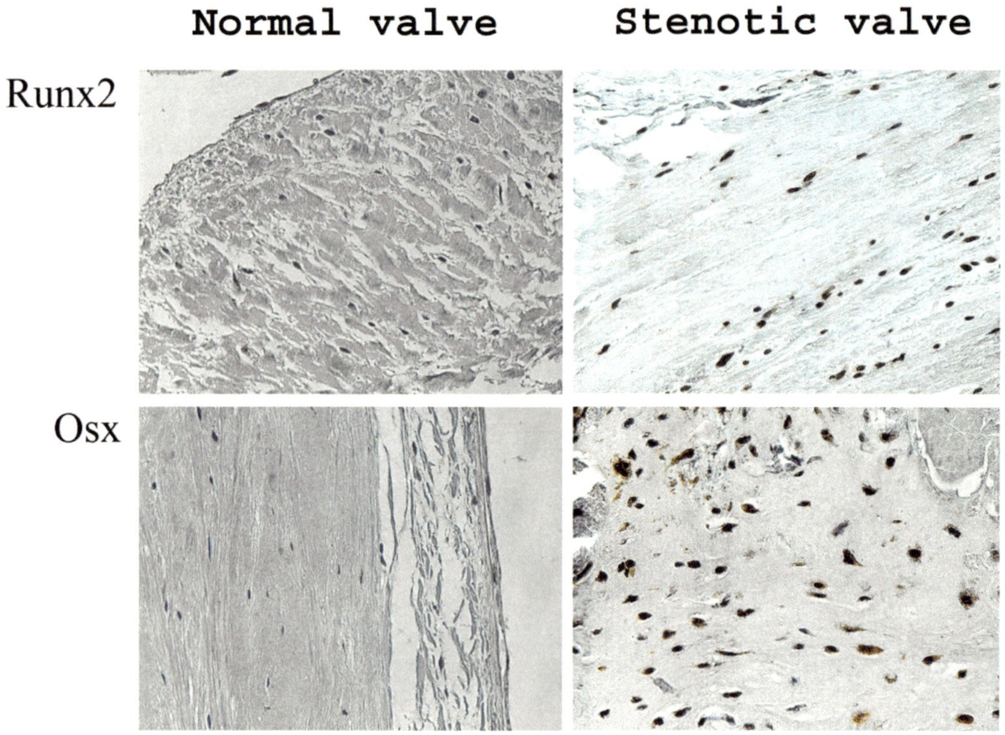

Fig. 6. Runx2 and Osterix immunoreactivity in normal and stenotic aortic valves (x400).

Sox9, a critical regulator of both early and late stages of chondrogenesis, is overexpressed in stenotic aortic valves [24].

Several lines of evidence suggest an important role of the OPG (osteoprotegerin)/RANKL (receptor activator of nuclear factor NF-κB ligand)/RANK (receptor activator of nuclear factor NF-κB) axis in valve pathology [28, 29]. Specifically, in cultured human aortic valve myofibroblasts, RANKL promotes calcium deposition in extracellular matrix and enhances the expression of osteoblast-related genes, promoting osteoblastic phenotype [30].

This phenotype of interstitial cells was also found to be related with high levels of Toll-like receptors (TLR) 2 and 4. Activation of these receptors may lead to increased expression of cytokines and osteogenic factors such as BMP-2 and Runx2 [31].

4.6 Lipids

Initially, Otto et al. noted the association of lipid metabolism with CAS. Accumulation of intracellular and extracellular lipids was constant finding in pathologic specimens [32].

Involvement of the Lrp5 receptor (low-density lipoprotein receptor-related protein 5) in valve calcification has been implicated in several studies [3].

LRP5/Wnt signaling pathway has great importance in bone remodeling. Wnt3a protein is secreted by endothelial cells and has the ability to bind to LDL receptor-related proteins LRP5 or LRP6 complex on the myofibroblast extracellular membrane [33]. This signal results in cytoplasmic accumulation of catenin which subsequently enters nucleus and interacts with proteins of the T-cell factor/lymphoid-enhancer factor-1 family affecting expression of target genes such as cyclin D, Runx2, and Sox9 **(Fig. 7).**

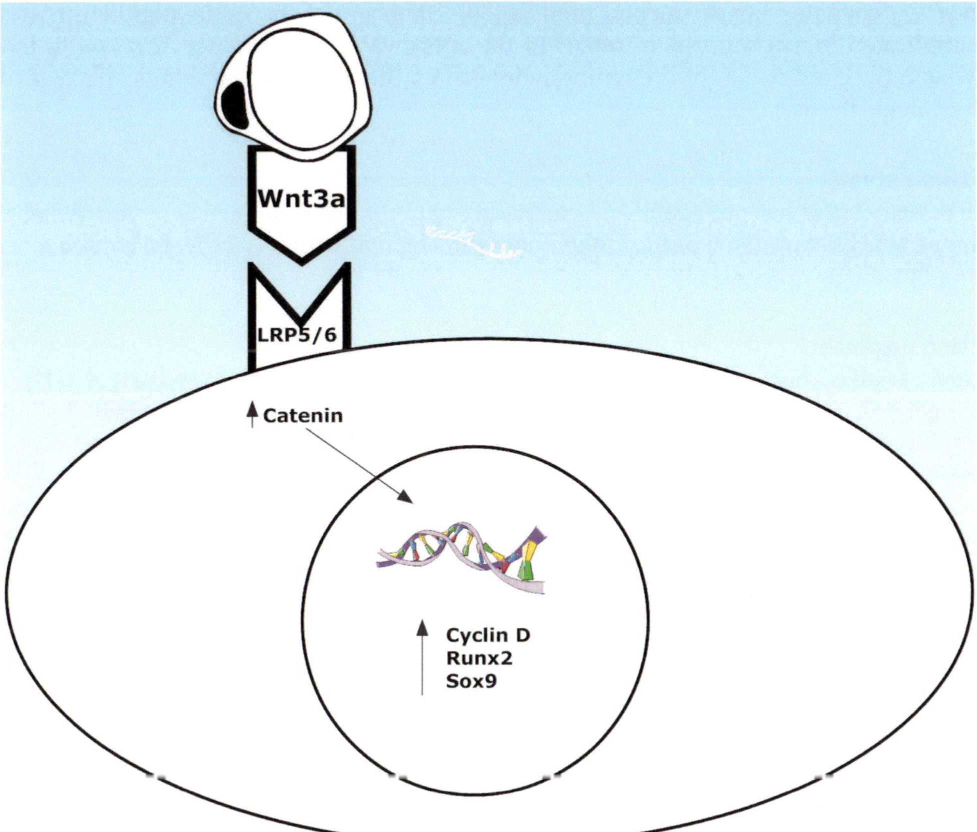

Fig. 7. Effects of LRP5/Wnt signaling pathway on gene expression.

The role of lipid signaling of the LRP5 receptor has been investigated in experimental models of vascular atherosclerosis. Relative deficiency of LRP5 is associated with reduction of intracellular ATP and calcium in response to glucose and thereby decreasing glucose-induced insulin secretion [8]. Interestingly, another study suggested that experimental hypercholesterolemia leads to increased LRP5 receptor expression which promotes cell proliferation and extracellular matrix remodeling. Mineralization, finally, ensues and progressive aortic stenosis is developed [8]. In addition, LRP5 plays significant role in the differentiation process of aortic VICs into osteoblasts, providing another link between lipid metabolism and aortic valve calcification [34].

A high total cholesterol/HDL ratio and small circulating LDL particles (<255A°) seem to be independently associated with rapid development of aortic sclerosis and stenosis.
High levels of angiotensin converting enzyme have been observed in valve lesions presenting increased LDL and apolipoprotein B concentration. It is speculated that plasma lipoproteins promote retention of angiotensin converting enzyme [13, 35].

4.7 Renin-angiotensin system

As we aforementioned, intense angiotensin-converting enzyme localization was observed in fibromyxomatous lesions. Lisinopril managed to attenuate presence of angiotensin-converting enzyme in experimental models [36]. Members of the renin-angiotensin system are implicated in mechanisms of repair of the aortic valve as a normal response to injury. However, hyperactivation of the renin-angiotensin system exerts deleterious effects leading to pathologic fibrosis [1].

4.8 Hemostasis

Role of hemostasis has not been fully elucitaded in CAS. Increased levels of von Willebrand factor as well as expression of fibrinolysis and platelet markers may be just a consequence of pathophysiologic process [13].

4.9 Neoangiosis

Several studies have confirmed neovessel formation in calcified valves [11, 37]. Angiogenesis may be implicated in calcification process by various ways including recruitment of inflammatory cells, transdifferentiation of pericytes of neovessel wall and secretion of cytokines from activated endothelial cells [24].
The whole process is related with increased levels of endothelial nitric oxide synthase, SPARC protein (secreted protein, acidic and rich in cysteine/osteonectin), VEGF and its receptors Flt-1 and Flk-1 [13]. VEGF-A exerts chemotactic activity for human monocytes via its receptor Flt-1, and also promotes their activation and migration [4].
Notably, low grade lesions are characterized by greater neoangiosis relatively to severe lesions suggesting a temporal pattern of the phenomenon in development of aortic stenosis [37].
Considering the fact that neoangiosis is characterized by a short time window as it takes place in days or months, potent therapeutic intervention must be timely and targeted [13].

4.10 Extracellular matrix remodeling

Recent studies have shown overexpression of elastolytic cathepsins S, K, and V and their inhibitor cystatin C in stenotic aortic valves [3].
Matrix metalloproteinases (MMPs) are zinc-dependent endopeptidases that are capable of degrading all kinds of extracellular matrix proteins, but also can process a number of bioactive molecules. Several studies have demonstrated implication of MMP-1, MMP-3, MMP-9 in aortic stenosis [9, 38, 39]. In addition, MMP-1 colocalizes with TNF-a suggesting an association between extracellular matrix remodeling and inflammation [9]. Regarding MMP-2, there is no evidence so far for a potential involvement in progression of disease [40].
It is well known that MMPs activity is depended on their respective tissue inhibitors (TIMPs). There is much confusion about role of TIMPs in pathophysiology of aortic stenosis.

As previous studies [9, 41] have shown conflicting results, further research is needed in order to unravel a possible connection with valve remodeling.

Except MMPs, several other factors with degrading activity such as cathepsins S, K and V overwhelm calcified lesions. Cathepsin S expression is more prominent in severely calcified areas while cathepsin V is related to endothelial cells [42]. Moreover, colocalization of cathepsin G and TGF-1b in mast cells lends further support to hypothesis that inflammation is the underlying cause of calcification [43].

Another extracellular matrix glycoprotein, tenascin-C, presents abundant expression in calcified valves. Tenascin-C is a highly conserved, multifunctional protein implicated in cell proliferation, migration, differentiation, and apoptosis [44]. Emerging evidence suggests that tenascin-C enchances alkaline phosphatase activity and expression of MMPs promoting calcium deposition in degenerative lesions. In contrast, normal valves are deficient or present very low levels of tenascin C [1, 4].

Upregulation of cystatin C, a cysteine protease inhibitor, has been found in calcific human aortic valves. Its presence must not be considered circumstantial as previous study reported increased expression in mature osteoblasts [45].

Extracellular matrix proteins with lytic activity may exert favorable effects in a normal repair process. Nevertheless, overexpression of these factors or defective inhibitory mechanisms are responsible for valve injury [4].

4.11 Inflammation

Inflammation is considered to be the most significant aspect of pathophysiologic process.

Several inflammatory mediators have been observed in diseased valves such as terminal complement complex C5b-9, IL-1b, IL-6, IL-8, TNF-α (tumor necrosis factor-α) and Heat Shock Protein-60 [13].

In addition, high serum levels of soluble endothelial adhesion molecules have been found in patients with severe aortic stenosis who had no history of coronary artery disease. Intercellular adhesion molecule-1, vascular cell adhesion molecule-1 and E-selectin are characteristic representatives indicating an ongoing inflammatory response [4].

There is also intense expression of TGF-b1 [13] which binds to specific proteins of extracellular matrix. Lytic activity of MMPs induces release of TGF-β1 which in turn promotes cellular migration and aggregation as well as apoptosis of VICs [1, 46].

TLR on interstitial cells seem to play critical role in inflammatory response. In vitro studies have demonstrated that peptidoglycan or lipopolysaccharide stimulation of TLR activates NF-kB pathway with subsequent expression of cytokines and bone - related factors [47].

In addition, recent research has shown that aortic VICs in areas containing calcific deposits showed significantly higher Osterix and NFATc1 nuclear immunolocalization compared to non-calcified fibrocellular regions. NFATc1 is a member of a multigene family of transcription factors that belong to the Rel group and control T lymphocyte activation and differentiation [24].

Therefore, inflammation and osteogenesis are indissolubly related.

4.12 Oxidative stress

Oxidative stress has been implicated in aortic stenosis as several research projects have confirmed increase in reactive oxygen species, and a reduction in the expression and activity of antioxidant enzymes catalase and NADPH [48].

4.13 Infectious agents

Great effort has been made by several researchers in order to relate infectious agents with aortic stenosis but data are conflicting.
Bratos-Perez et al. studied aortic valve specimens collected at surgery and indicated the presence of nanobacteria, growing self-replicating calcifying nanoparticles, that potentially represent new pathogens. Their expression has been noticed already in carotid disease and abdominal aorta aneurysms [49].
Nevertheless, role of infectious microorganisms has not been clarified and further evidence is needed.

4.14 Autonomic nervous system

Aortic valve is innervated by adrenergic and cholinergic neural networks. Upregulation of b-adrenergic receptors, especially b2, was observed in areas of calcifcation [50]. In addition, a stable analogue of the purinergic receptor P2Y (ATP-g-S) may cause the transdifferentiation of cultured interstitial aortic valve cells into osteoblasts [51].

5. Treatment effects on pathophysiologic mechanisms

Study of effects of therapeutic strategies on progression of aortic stenosis has provided significant evidence regarding pathophysiology of disease.

5.1 Statins

Role of statins has been studied extensively but findings are inconsistent in patients with moderate to severe degrees of aortic stenosis [13].
Atorvastatin was shown to attenuate leucocyte infiltration and expression of bone regulatory factors in aortic valves of experimental models with hypercholesterolemia [3]. These effects are attributed to modulation of Lrp5 pathway [30] and endothelial nitric oxide synthase [52].
Previous reports suggest that expression of MMPs, in particular MMP-1, MMP-2, MMP-3, and MMP-9, is reduced by VICs and macrophages under the effect of statin treatment [1].
As we aforementioned, TGF-β is an important regulator of cellular proliferation and differentiation and modulator of inflammation and extracellular matrix remodelling. Statins exhibit variable effects on TGF-β expression in aortic valves. Several studies provide evidence that levels of TGF-β in human VICs are reduced with implementation of statin treatment in initial stages of disease [53]. This results in attenuated presence of ALP (alkaline phosphatase) and osteocalcin in calcified lesions [53]. However, these findings were not confirmed in late stages of disease indicating the narrow therapeutic time window of statins [54].
Atorvastatin extenuates the activity of alkaline phosphatase in cultured interstitial aortic cells [48] in contrast to bone tissue where it exerts opposite effect. [55]. Statins, also, reduce the expression of RGS (regulators of G protein-mediated signaling) proteins in calcified valves triggering activation of extracellular-regulated kinases [56] that enhance proliferation of myofibroblasts [13]. Increased expression of BMP-2, a major osteogenic stimulus. has been observed in experimental models treated with HMG-CoA reductase inhibitors [54]. These contradictory findings, called 'statin paradox', suggest that beneficial impact could be time-depended and beyond this time window statins exhibit neutral or even harmful effect. A possible explanation is that different cell populations prevail during several stages of pathophysiologic process resulting in variable response to statin treatment. This could be

related to the results of several trials that failed to demonstrate positive therapeutic effects [13]. In SALTIRE (Scottish Aortic Stenosis and Lipid Lowering Trial, Impact on Regression) and SEAS (simvastatin and ezetimibe in aortic stenosis study) studies, statin therapy had no effect on the rate of progression of aortic stenosis. Further projects such as ASTRONOMER (Aortic Stenosis Progression Observation: Measuring Effects of Rosuvastatin) trial are under way to try to define the role of statins in pathophysiologic process. Meanwhile, there is no indication for statin use specific to aortic stenosis [4].

In conclusion, statins exhibit pleiotropic activities and their role must be further analyzed. Inhibition of the HMG-CoA reductase influences not only cholesterol synthesis but also biosynthesis of isoprenoid compounds that are implicated in inflammation and osteogenesis [13].

5.2 Angiotensin Converting Enzyme Inhibitors (ACEI)

As we discussed earlier, angiotensin converting enzyme exhibits intense presence in diseased valves and there is much evidence regarding its involvement in pathophysiology. Preliminary reports suggest that olmesartan, an angiotensin type 1 receptor antagonist, preserves endothelial integrity and inhibits transdifferentiation of VICs into myofibroblasts or osteoblasts [58].

5.3 Smoking cessation

Smoking, the single most preventable cause of death in Western World, is a leading risk factor not only for atherosclerosis but also for aortic stenosis. Tobacco components, mostly nicotine and acetaldehyde, have the ability to induce TGF-b1 expression in cultured fibroblasts and mast cell activation. These effects are enough to cause increased collagen burden favoring valve calcification [13].

6. References

[1] Mohler 3rd ER: Mechanisms of aortic valve calcification. The American journal of cardiology 94: 1396, 2004.

[2] Ramaraj R and Sorrell VL: Clinical Review: Degenerative aortic stenosis. BMJ 336: 550-555, 2008.

[3] Rajamannan NM: Calcific aortic stenosis: lessons learned from experimental and clinical studies. Arteriosclerosis, thrombosis, and vascular biology 29: 162, 2009.

[4] Yetkin E and Waltenberger J: Molecular and cellular mechanisms of aortic stenosis. International journal of cardiology 135: 4-13, 2009.

[5] Boss Y, Mathieu P and Pibarot P: Genomics:: The Next Step to Elucidate the Etiology of Calcific Aortic Valve Stenosis. Journal of the American College of Cardiology 51: 1327-1336, 2008.

[6] Xu S, Liu AC and Gotlieb AI: Common pathogenic features of atherosclerosis and calcific aortic stenosis: role of transforming growth factor-[beta]. Cardiovascular Pathology 19: 236-247,

[7] Chambers JB: Aortic stenosis. European Journal of Echocardiography 10: i11, 2009.

[8] Rajamannan NM: Mechanisms of aortic valve calcification: the LDL-density-radius theory: a translation from cell signaling to physiology. American Journal of Physiology-Heart and Circulatory Physiology 298: H5,

[9] Kaden JJ, Dempfle CE, Grobholz R, *et al*: Inflammatory regulation of extracellular matrix remodeling in calcific aortic valve stenosis. Cardiovascular Pathology 14: 80-87, 2005.
[10] Hakuno D, Kimura N, Yoshioka M and Fukuda K: Molecular mechanisms underlying the onset of degenerative aortic valve disease. Journal of Molecular Medicine 87: 17-24, 2009.
[11] Chalajour F, Treede H, Ebrahimnejad A, Lauke H, Reichenspurner H and Ergun S: Angiogenic activation of valvular endothelial cells in aortic valve stenosis* 1. Experimental cell research 298: 455-464, 2004.
[12] Chalajour F, Treede H, Gehling UM, *et al*: Identification and characterization of cells with high angiogenic potential and transitional phenotype in calcific aortic valve. Experimental cell research 313: 2326-2335, 2007.
[13] Parolari A, Loardi C, Mussoni L, *et al*: Nonrheumatic calcific aortic stenosis: an overview from basic science to pharmacological prevention. European journal of cardio-thoracic surgery 35: 493-504, 2009.
[14] Ghaisas NK, Foley JB, O'Briain DS, Crean P, Kelleher D and Walsh M: Adhesion molecules in nonrheumatic aortic valve disease: endothelial expression, serum levels and effects of valve replacement* 1. Journal of the American College of Cardiology 36: 2257-2262, 2000.
[15] Diehl P, Nagy F, Sossong V, *et al*: Increased levels of circulating microparticles in patients with severe aortic valve stenosis. THROMBOSIS AND HAEMOSTASIS-STUTTGART- 99: 711, 2008.
[16] Schoen FJ. Cardiac valves and valvular pathology update on function, disease, repair, and replacement. Cardiovascular Pathology 2005;14:189-94.
[17] Taylor PM, Batten P, Brand NJ, Thomas PS, Yacoub MH. The cardiac valve interstitial cell. International Journal of Biochemistry and Cell Biology 2003;35:113-8.
[18] Liu AC, Joag VR, Gotlieb AI. The emerging role of valve interstitial cell phenotypes in regulating heart valve pathobiology. American Journal of Pathology 2007;171:1407.
[19] Oh J, Richardson JA and Olson EN: Requirement of myocardin-related transcription factor-B for remodeling of branchial arch arteries and smooth muscle differentiation. Proceedings of the National Academy of Sciences of the United States of America 102: 15122, 2005.
[20] Combs MD and Yutzey KE: Heart valve development: regulatory networks in development and disease. Circulation research 105: 408, 2009.
[21] Avakian SD, Annicchino Bizzacchi JM, Grinberg M, Ramires JAF and Mansur AP: Apolipoproteins AI, B, and E polymorphisms in severe aortic valve stenosis. Clinical genetics 60: 381-384, 2001.
[22]Novaro GM, Sachar R, Pearce GL, Sprecher DL and Griffin BP: Association between apolipoprotein E alleles and calcific valvular heart disease. Circulation 108: 1804, 2003.
[23] Ortlepp JR, Hoffmann R, Ohme F, Lauscher J, Bleckmann F and Hanrath P: The vitamin D receptor genotype predisposes to the development of calcific aortic valve stenosis. Heart 85: 635, 2001.
[24] Alexopoulos A, Bravou V, Peroukides S, *et al*: Bone regulatory factors NFATc1 and Osterix in human calcific aortic valves. International journal of cardiology 139: 142-149,
[25] Garg V, Muth AN, Ransom JF, *et al*: Mutations in NOTCH1 cause aortic valve disease. Nature 437: 270-274, 2005.
[26] Nordstr m P, Glader CA, Dahlen G, *et al*: Oestrogen receptor α gene polymorphism is related to aortic valve sclerosis in postmenopausal women. Journal of internal medicine 254: 140-146, 2003.

[27] Golubnitschaja O, Yeghiazaryan K, Skowasch D, Schild H and Bauriedel G: p21 WAF1/CIP1 and 14-3-3 σ gene expression in degenerated aortic valves: A link between cell cycle checkpoints and calcification. Amino acids 31: 309-316, 2006.
[28] Steinmetz M, Skowasch D, Wernert N, *et al*: Differential profile of the OPG/RANKL/RANK-system in degenerative aortic native and bioprosthetic valves. JOURNAL OF HEART VALVE DISEASE 17: 187, 2008.
[29] Mallat Z and Tedgui A: Unbalanced RANKL/RANK pathway in aortic valve sclerosis. Journal of molecular and cellular cardiology 36: 17, 2004.
[30] Kaden JJ, Bickelhaupt S, Grobholz R and Haase KK: Receptor activator of nuclear factor [kappa] B ligand and osteoprotegerin regulate aortic valve calcification* 1. Journal of molecular and cellular cardiology 36: 57-66, 2004.
[31] Yang X, Fullerton DA, Su X, Ao L, Cleveland Jr JC and Meng X: Pro-osteogenic phenotype of human aortic valve interstitial cells is associated with higher levels of Toll-like receptors 2 and 4 and enhanced expression of bone morphogenetic protein 2. Journal of the American College of Cardiology 53: 491-500, 2009.
[32] Otto CM, Kuusisto J, Reichenbach DD, Gown AM and O'Brien KD: Characterization of the early lesion of'degenerative'valvular aortic stenosis. Histological and immunohistochemical studies. Circulation 90: 844, 1994.
[33] Rajamannan NM, Subramaniam M, Caira F, Stock SR and Spelsberg TC: Atorvastatin inhibits hypercholesterolemia-induced calcification in the aortic valves via the Lrp5 receptor pathway. Circulation 112: I-229, 2005.
[34] Caira FC, Stock SR, Gleason TG, *et al*: Human degenerative valve disease is associated with up-regulation of low-density lipoprotein receptor-related protein 5 receptor-mediated bone formation. Journal of the American College of Cardiology j. jacc. 2006.2002. 2040v2001, 2006.
[35] O'Brien KD, Shavelle DM, Caulfield MT, *et al*: Association of angiotensin-converting enzyme with low-density lipoprotein in aortic valvular lesions and in human plasma. Circulation 106: 2224, 2002.
[36] Sun YAO, Ratajska A and Weber KT: Inhibition of angiotensin-converting enzyme and attenuation of myocardial fibrosis by lisinopril in rats receiving angiotensin II. The Journal of laboratory and clinical medicine 126: 95-101, 1995.
[37] Soini Y, Salo T and Satta J: Angiogenesis is involved in the pathogenesis of nonrheumatic aortic valve stenosis. Human pathology 34: 756-763, 2003.
[38] Edep ME, Shirani J, Wolf P and Brown DL: Matrix metalloproteinase expression in nonrheumatic aortic stenosis. Cardiovascular Pathology 9: 281-286, 2000.
[39] Fondard O, Detaint D, Iung B, *et al*: Extracellular matrix remodelling in human aortic valve disease: the role of matrix metalloproteinases and their tissue inhibitors. European heart journal 26: 1333, 2005.
[40] Yeghiazaryan K, Skowasch D, Bauriedel G, Schild H and Golubnitschaja O: Could activated tissue remodeling be considered as early marker for progressive valve degeneration? Comparative analysis of checkpoint and ECM remodeling gene expression in native degenerating aortic valves and after bioprosthetic replacement. Amino acids 32: 109-114, 2007.
[41] Satta J, Oiva J, Salo T, *et al*: Evidence for an altered balance between matrix metalloproteinase-9 and its inhibitors in calcific aortic stenosis. The Annals of thoracic surgery 76: 681-688, 2003.
[42] Helske S, Syvaranta S, Lindstedt KA, *et al*: Increased expression of elastolytic cathepsins S, K, and V and their inhibitor cystatin C in stenotic aortic valves. Arteriosclerosis,

thrombosis, and vascular biology 01. ATV. 0000228824.0000201604. 0000228863v0000228821, 2006.
[43] Helske S, Syv ranta S, Kupari M, *et al*: Possible role for mast cell-derived cathepsin G in the adverse remodelling of stenotic aortic valves. European heart journal 27: 1495, 2006.
[44] Wallner K, Li C, Shah PK, *et al*: Tenascin-C is expressed in macrophage-rich human coronary atherosclerotic plaque. Circulation 99: 1284, 1999.
[45] Huh C, Nagle JW, Kozak CA, Abrahamson M and Karlsson S: Structural organization, expression and chromosomal mapping of the mouse cystatin-C-encoding gene (Cst3). Gene 152: 221-226, 1995.
[46] Jian B, Narula N, Li QY and Mohler ER: 3rd and RJ Levy, Progression of aortic valve stenosis: TGF-beta1 is present in calcified aortic valve cusps and promotes aortic valve interstitial cell calcification via apoptosis. Ann Thorac Surg 75: 457-465, 2003.
[47] Meng X, Ao L, Song Y, *et al*: Expression of functional Toll-like receptors 2 and 4 in human aortic valve interstitial cells: potential roles in aortic valve inflammation and stenosis. American Journal of Physiology-Cell Physiology 294: C29, 2008.
[48] Miller JD, Chu Y, Brooks RM, Richenbacher WE, Pe a-Silva R and Heistad DD: Dysregulation of antioxidant mechanisms contributes to increased oxidative stress in calcific aortic valvular stenosis in humans. Journal of the American College of Cardiology 52: 843-850, 2008.
[49] Bratos-P rez MA, S nchez PL, Garc a de Cruz S, *et al*: Association between self-replicating calcifying nanoparticles and aortic stenosis: a possible link to valve calcification. European heart journal 29: 371, 2008.
[50] Osman L, Chester AH, Sarathchandra P, *et al*: A novel role of the sympatho-adrenergic system in regulating valve calcification. Circulation 116: I-282, 2007.
[51] Osman L, Chester AH, Amrani M, *et al*: A novel role of extracellular nucleotides in valve calcification: a potential target for atorvastatin. Circulation 114: I-566, 2006.
[52] Rajamannan NM, Subramaniam M, Stock SR, *et al*: Atorvastatin inhibits calcification and enhances nitric oxide synthase production in the hypercholesterolaemic aortic valve. Heart 91: 806, 2005.
[53] Osman L, Yacoub MH, Latif N, Amrani M and Chester AH: Role of human valve interstitial cells in valve calcification and their response to atorvastatin. Circulation 114: I-547, 2006.
[54] Anger T, Carson W, Weyand M, Daniel WG, Hoeher M and Garlichs CD: Atherosclerotic inflammation triggers osteogenic bone transformation in calcified and stenotic human aortic valves: still a matter of debate. Experimental and molecular pathology 86: 10-17, 2009.
[55] Wu B, Elmariah S, Kaplan FS, Cheng G and Mohler Iii ER: Paradoxical effects of statins on aortic valve myofibroblasts and osteoblasts: implications for end-stage valvular heart disease. Arteriosclerosis, thrombosis, and vascular biology 25: 592, 2005.
[56] Anger T, El-Chafchak J, Habib A, *et al*: Statins stimulate RGS-regulated ERK 1/2 activation in human calcified and stenotic aortic valves. Experimental and molecular pathology 85: 101-111, 2008.
[57] Mundy G, Garrett R, Harris S, *et al*: Stimulation of bone formation in vitro and in rodents by statins. Science 286: 1946, 1999.
[58] Arishiro K, Hoshiga M, Negoro N, *et al*: Angiotensin receptor-1 blocker inhibits atherosclerotic changes and endothelial disruption of the aortic valve in hypercholesterolemic rabbits. Journal of the American College of Cardiology 49: 1482-1489, 2007.

Part 3

Diagnosis and Prognosis

4

Asymptomatic Aortic Stenosis - Prognosis, Risk Stratification and Follow-Up

Paoli Ursula and Dichtl Wolfgang
Medical University Innsbruck, Internal Medicine III / Cardiology, Austria

1. Introduction

Due to an aging population and improved non-invasive cardiac imaging (mainly the wide use of transthoracic echocardiography), the number of patients with asymptomatic aortic stenosis (AS) is continuously increasing. Aortic stenosis is a progressive active disease which can be treated effectively by aortic valve implantation. Therefore, optimal timing of surgery is crucial demanding precise risk stratification to identify high-risk but still asymptomatic patients. Such patients should undergo close clinical follow-up examination or even elective aortic valve replacement.

Whereas severe symptomatic aortic stenosis is a class I indication for valve replacement, the decision to operate on asymptomatic patients remains controversial. Accepted indications for aortic valve replacement for asymptomatic patients with severe aortic stenosis are (a) the need of cardiac surgery for any other reason such as coronary bypass grafting or surgery of the aorta ascendens and (b) if left ventricular systolic dysfunction defined by an ejection fraction below 50% occurs.

The risk of sudden death in asymptomatic severe aortic stenosis without preceding symptoms is a matter of concern, although it is regarded as low (around 1% per year) and below the perioperative mortality of aortic valve replacement. Otherwise, there is a risk of irreversible myocardial damage due to left ventricular hypertrophy and myocardial fibrosis if surgery is performed too late.

The strategy to wait for occurrence of symptoms before indicating aortic valve implantation is further challenged by an increased mortality in patients awaiting surgery after onset of symptoms, by late symptom reporting by many patients and a higher operative risk for more symptomatic patients.

On the other hand, the immediate operative risk, the long-term morbidity and mortality related to the prosthetic aortic valve, and the potential need for re-operation have to be taken into account.

Several risk factors for worse clinical outcome in patients with asymptomatic aortic stenosis have been established in the last years. Hemodynamic parameters such as a peak aortic jet velocity > 5m/s or a mean gradient > 60 mmHg are used to define very severe aortic stenosis, and an increase in peak aortic jet velocity > 0.3 m/s/year define a fast hemodynamic progression rate. Whether such high- risk patients should undergo elective aortic valve implantation even in the asymptomatic state is still a matter of debate and handled differently between European and American Guidelines. Furthermore, interest has

shifted to exercise tolerance, degree of valve calcification, the influence of gender or systemic parameters such as natriuretic peptides. Among these new non-hemodynamic parameters, exercise-induced symptoms are the best validated criterion so far.
Some patients with aortic stenosis have a reduced stroke volume despite preserved left ventricular ejection fraction (referred to as paradoxical low flow aortic stenosis). These patients suffer from more pronounced left ventricular concentric remodelling, smaller left ventricular cavity, increased global left ventricular load, and reduced midwall shortening. They often present with a low transvalvular gradient even though they have a severe stenosis on the basis of valve area, and this situation may lead to an underestimation of stenosis severity and an underutilization of valve replacement.
It remains a clinical challenge to balance risk between watchful waiting and early aortic valve implantation in patients with asymptomatic aortic stenosis. The physician managing these patients has to "look at the valve, listen to the patient" (C. Otto). The decision of aortic valve replacement should be taken by cardiologists who "look globally, think globally" (P. Pibarot, JG. Dumesnil).

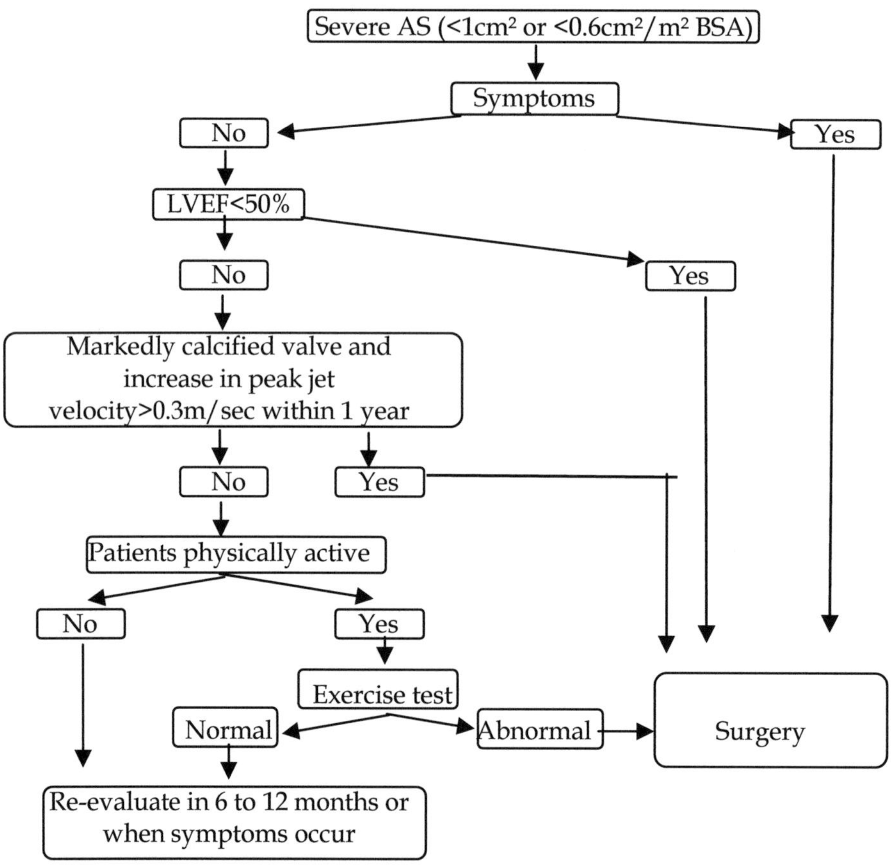

Fig. 1. Management of patients with severe aortic stenosis (AS). BSA denotes body surface area; EF denotes ejection fraction; LV denotes left ventricle (Vahanian & Otto, 2010).

2. Assessment of aortic stenosis

2.1 History

Aortic stenosis proves the outstanding diagnostic power of a well-taken clinical history. Classical symptoms of aortic stenosis are angina pectoris, heart failure, severe cardiac arrhythmia such as ventricular tachycardia and syncope. However, these symptoms are often preceded by a decreased exercise tolerance or dyspnoe on exertion. It is the skill and clinical experience of the physician to discover and interpret these changes correctly in patients who may have a low physical activity also for other reasons (e.g. frailty, pulmonary disease, obesity, de-conditioning).

Patients with congenital valvular stenosis may give a history of a murmur since childhood or infancy. Those with rheumatic stenosis may have a history of rheumatic fever. The influence of sex on the outcome of asymptomatic aortic stenosis is a matter of debate as well. Some studies found that female gender is independently predictive of the midterm development of symptoms (Monin et al., 2009), but guidelines recommendations so far do not differ between genders.

2.2 Physical findings

As usual, anamnesis is followed by physical examination. Typical for aortic stenosis is a systolic ejection murmur, with a maximum in the 2nd ICR right parasternal with radiation in the carotids. In patients with a loud systolic murmur, an echocardiography is indicated. Arterial hypertension is present in many patients and imposes additional load on the left ventricle by increased vascular resistance. This results in lower transvalvular gradients and possible underestimation of stenosis severity, whereas clinical symptoms might occur earlier.

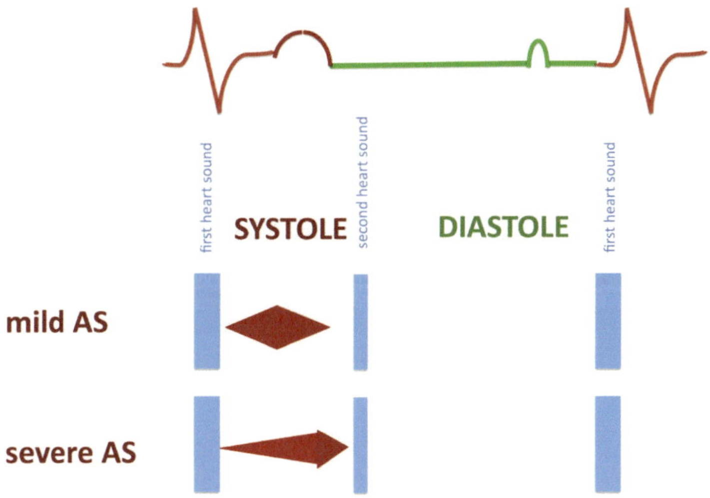

Fig. 2. Systolic murmurs in mild and severe aortic stenosis.

2.3 Echocardiography

Transthoracic echocardiography supplies the most important information for risk stratification of adults with aortic stenosis yielding information about valve anatomy and hemodynamics, the left ventricular response to chronic pressure overload, aortic dilatation and associated valve disease. Only in certain circumstances, a transoesophageal or a 3D-echocardiography is needed, e.g. for improved analysis of valve anatomy (bicuspid valve, planimetry of valve area) or preoperative measurements needed in transcatheter aortic valve implantation (TAVI).

On 2D echocardiography, a stenotic aortic valve is thickened and calcified, with restricted opening of the cusps. Three basic parameters are routinely used to assess the hemodynamic severity of aortic stenosis: jet velocity, mean transaortic pressure gradient and valve area. The aortic jet velocity is measured with continuous wave Doppler from several transducer windows, to obtain the signal most parallel with the direction of stenotic jet flow yielding the highest velocity signal (Figure 2). For this, color-flow imaging may be helpful to guide Doppler beam alignment. Sometimes it is necessary that the patient has to move to a right-supine position using a right parasternal window and a smaller nonimaging continuous-wave Doppler transducer (so-called pencil-probe) which is easier to manipulate between the ribs. In very small or very tall adults, valve area should be indexed for body size, e.g. to avoid that a small person with only a moderate obstruction get the misdiagnosis of a severe aortic stenosis.

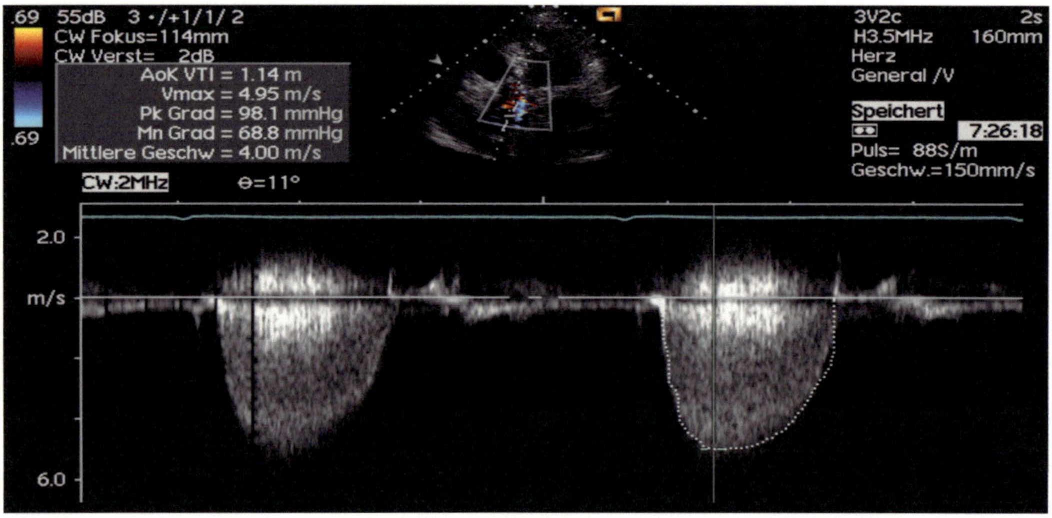

Fig. 3. Using an apical five-chamber view, transvalvular continuous Doppler shows a severe to very severe aortic stenosis, with mean/peak systolic gradients of 69 and 98 mmHg, respectively, and a peak systolic velocity of 4.9 m/s.

There are some caveats in the assessment of aortic stenosis by transthoracic echocardiography. The measurement of the left ventricular outflow tract diameter has to be thoroughly performed from a systolic freeze-frame in the parsternal long-axis view, defined by the distance from where the anterior (right aortic) cusp meets the ventricular septum to the point where the posterior (noncoronary) cusp meets the anterior mitral leaflet. This may be difficult because of heavy calcifications. Furthermore, in patients with atrial fibrillation or flutter, velocities should be averaged from 5 to 10 cardiac cycles.

Whereas systolic left ventricular dysfunction occurs very late in the disease process (mainly in symptomatic patients with very severe aortic stenosis who do not undergo valve replacement for whatever reason), left ventricular diastolic dysfunction is frequently found in an early phase of aortic stenosis. Left ventricular hypertrophy can be found in most cases of severe aortic stenosis.

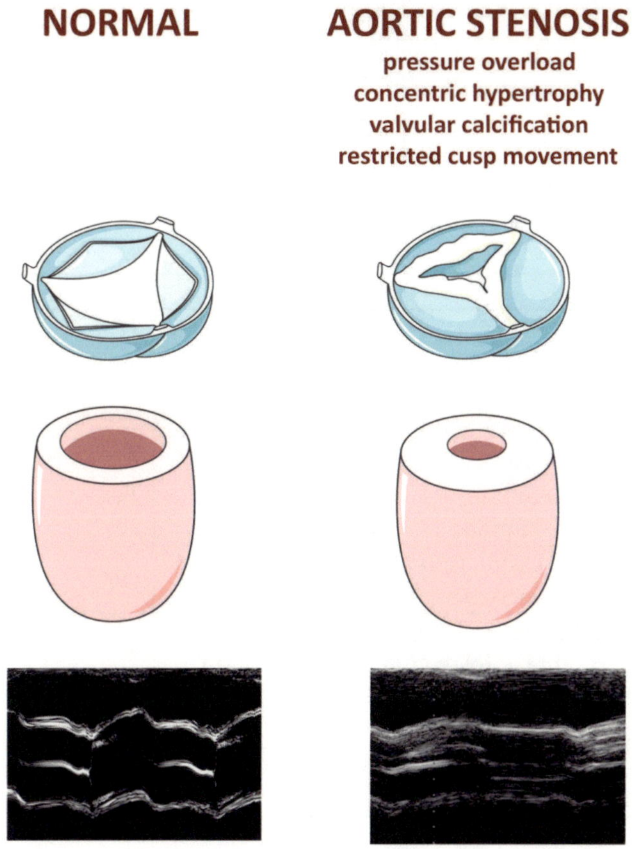

Fig. 4. Left ventricular hypertrophy and restricted aortic cusp movement.

Four echo parameters permit the classification of aortic stenosis severity. Unfortunately, the European Society of Cardiology (ESC) and the American College of Cardiology/ American Heart Association (ACC/AHA) differrently interpret mean gradients, as shown in Table 1 (values in brackets are advised from ACC/AHA). A shortcoming of this classification is that one patient may fall in two different categories, e.g. if he has an aortic jet velocity from 3.1 and an AVA from 1.6 cm^2. Notably, guidelines are based on physiological valve area, as measured by continuity equation, which differs from anatomical valve area.

Additional echo parameters who are not yet used in clinical routine are stroke-work loss and left ventricular strain analysis. Stroke-work loss is the ratio of mean gradient and left ventricular pressure, and a stroke-work loss > 26% results in a major clinical event rate > 30% within the following three months (Bermejo et al., 2003).

Patients with systolic dysfunction and small valve area present with low transvalvular gradients. It is important to differentiate those with a low gradient due to low stroke volume

	Aortic sclerosis	Mild AS	Moderate AS	Severe AS	Very severe AS
Aortic jet velocity (m/s)	< 2.6	2.6 – 3.0	3.0 – 4.0	> 4.0	> 5.0
Mean gradient (mmHg)	-	< 30 (25)	30 - 50 (25-40)	> 50 (40)	> 60
AVA (cm^2)	-	> 1.5	1.0 - 1.5	< 1.0	< 0.6
Indexed AVA (cm^2/m^2)	-	> 0.9	0.6 - 0.9	< 0.6	-

Table 1. Categories of aortic stenosis severity, according to ESC (Vahanian et al., 2007) and ACC/AHA (Bonow et al., 2008) guidelines.

Severe asymptomatic AS	ESC	ACC/AHA
EF < 50%	IC	
Undergoing CABG, aortic surgery or mitral valve surgery	IC	
Exercise test - symptoms - fall in BP to below baseline complex ventricular arrhythmias	 IC IIaC IIbC	 IIbC IIbC /
Predictors of rapid progression (moderate to severe valve calcification, rate of v_{max} increase ≥ 0.3 m/s/year	IIaC	/
Predictors of rapid progression (age, valve calcification, CAD) or if surgery might be delayed at symptom onset	/	IIbC
Severe left ventricular hypertrophy (> 15mm) without arterial hypertension	IIbC	/
Extremly severe AS (AVA < 0.6 m^2, v_{max} > 5 m / s, ΔP_{mean} > 60 mmHg) and operative risk < 1%	/	IIbC
Moderate asymptomatic AS	ESC	ACC/AHA
Hemodynamically unstable	AVR (IB); BAV (IIbC) as bridge to surgery	
Indeterminate severity of AS		
Low-gradient AS with left ventricular dysfunction and contractile reserve	IIaC	/
Low-gradient AS with left ventricular dysfunction but no contractile reserve	IIbC	/

Table 2. Guidelines for aortic valve replacement in asymptomatic patients (Vahanian et al., 2007; Bonow et al., 2008). AVR is recommended in class I indications. AVR is reasonable in class IIa and may be considered in class IIb indications. Note that most indications are based only on a level of evidence C. EF denotes ejection fraction; CABG denotes coronary artery bypass grafting; BP denotes blood pressure; CAD denotes coronary artery disease; BAV denotes balloon aortic valvuloplasty.

(low-gradient, low-flow AS) from those with a cardiomyopathy and concomitant only moderate AS. Dobutamin challenge for low-gradient aortic stenosis and left ventricular dysfunction may result in three pattern of responsiveness: fixed aortic stenosis, relative aortic stenosis and absence of contractile reserve. A fixed aortic stenosis is characterized by an increase in peak velocity > 4 m/s and a mean systolic gradient > 40 mmHg with no change in aortic valve area. These patients may still benefit from valve replacement despite increased perioperative rsik. In contrast, relative aortic stenosis is characterized by a significant increase in calculated aortic valve area (> 0.3 cm^2) without a significant increase in peak velocity or systolic gradients, whereas no variable changed significantly in patients without contractile reserve (lack of increase > 20% of stroke volume).

2.4 Electrocardiogram

Resting ECG in severe aortic stenosis usually shows signs of left ventricular hypertrophy, often accompanied by repolarisation abnormalities (ST-T-wave changes). Left ventricular hypertrophy is an independent predictor for the development of symptoms in asymptomatic severe aortic stenosis. However, the sensitivity for detecting left ventricular hypertrophy by the electrocardiogram is only 40% (Dal-Bianco et al., 2008). Conduction abnormalities are common ranging from first-degree atrio-ventricular block or bundle branch block. Atrial fibrillation is not a typical sign of aortic stenosis and may indicate concomitant mitral valve disease.

2.5 Biomarkers

Natriuretic peptides are secreted from the heart as response to pressure overload. Whereas atrial natriuretic peptide (ANP) is produced in the atria, B-type natriuretic peptide (BNP) is mainly derived from ventricular myocardium. Obviously, increased intraventricular pressure due to significant aortic stenosis is accompanied by elevated plasma levels of BNP and its derivatives such as N-terminal pro BNP. Such an elevation of natriuretic peptides predict adverse clinical outcome, such as occurrence of symptoms in still asymptomatic patients or higher operative mortality or worse post-operative outcome (Bergler-Klein et al., 2004; Pedrazzini et al., 2008). Systemic inflammation, expressed by elevated plasma CRP levels, influence the clinical outcome in advanced stages of aortic stenosis whereas no correlation to the progression from aortic sclerosis to aortic stenosis could be found in the Cardiovascular Health Study (Galante et al., 2001; Novaro et al., 2007).

2.6 Exercise test

An exercise test may be considered for patients with severe AS and equivocal symptoms or for asymptomatic, physically active patients with severe AS and slow progression. A stress test can unmask signs like dyspnoea, angina pectoris, and inadequate rise in blood pressure, complex ventricular arrhythmias or repolarisation abnormalities, and dizziness. Patients suffering from symptoms during exercise have an event-free survival rate of lower than 20% within 2 years, whereas patients with a normal exercise tolerance have a survival rate of over 80% at 5 years (Iung, 2011). A positive exercise test is associated with a 7 times higher clinical event rate (Amato et al., 2001).

The exercise test should be interrupted for limiting dyspnoea and fatigue, any angina or dizziness, > 2mm ST depression, any decrease in systolic blood pressure (> 20 mmHg or a fall compared to baseline), and complex ventricular ectopy. The exercise test should be considered abnormal if exercise tolerance is < 80% according to age- and sex-adjusted levels. The type of exercise test-induced symptom is important for the outcome. Patients with dizziness on exertion have an 83% probability for proximate developing of symptoms, whereas with breathlessness or chest tightness it is only 54%, respectively 50% (Dal-Bianco et al., 2008).

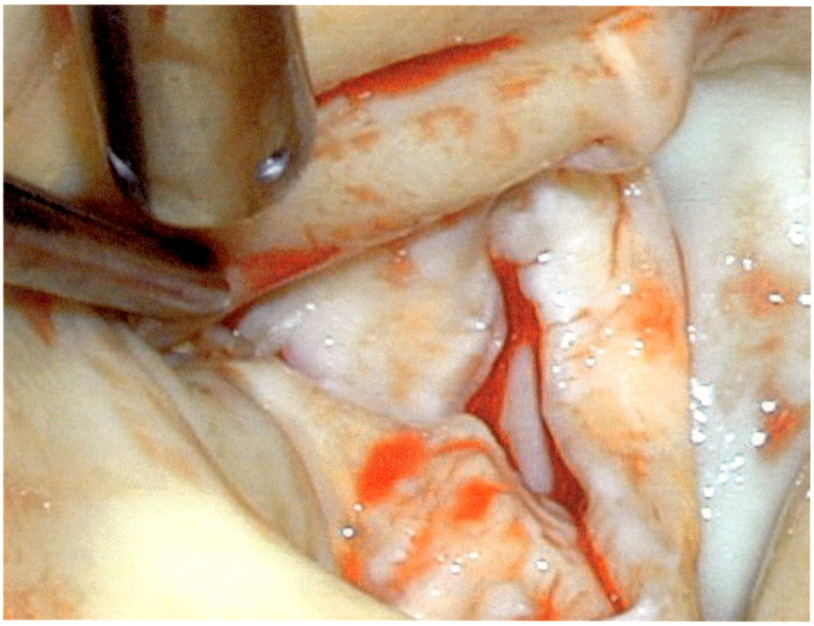

Fig. 5. Intraoperative view of a severely calcified and stenotic aortic valve.

2.7 Cardiac catherization

The role of invasive assessment of aortic stenosis severity has decreased in the last decades, mainly due to the diagnostic power of echocardiography. Passage through a stenotic valve may lead to peripheral embolism. The main indication of cardiac catherization is nowadays to perform coronary angiography at symptom onset. Multislice computed tomography may be used in young patients with a low probabilty of coronary artery disease instead, but this method is limited in older patients because of coronary calcification causing blooming artefacts. Using specific catheters, simultaneous evaluation of the proximal aortic and left ventricular pressures yields the most accurate data. It is important to distinguish the maximum instantenous gradient from the mean and peak-to-peak gradients, when comparing to echocardiographic measurements. Right heart catherization is often performed to assess cardiac output by either the Fick principle or the indicator dilution technique, which allows aortic valve area calculation by the Gorlin formula.

2.8 Chest X-ray

Poststenotic dilatation of the aorta ascendens is often the main chest X-ray finding in patients with aortic stenosis, whereas cardiac silhouette shows no or only minor enlargement. Calcification of the aortic valve is hardly seen on chest X-ray, in contrast to flouroscopy or electron-beam / multislice computed tomography (see below).

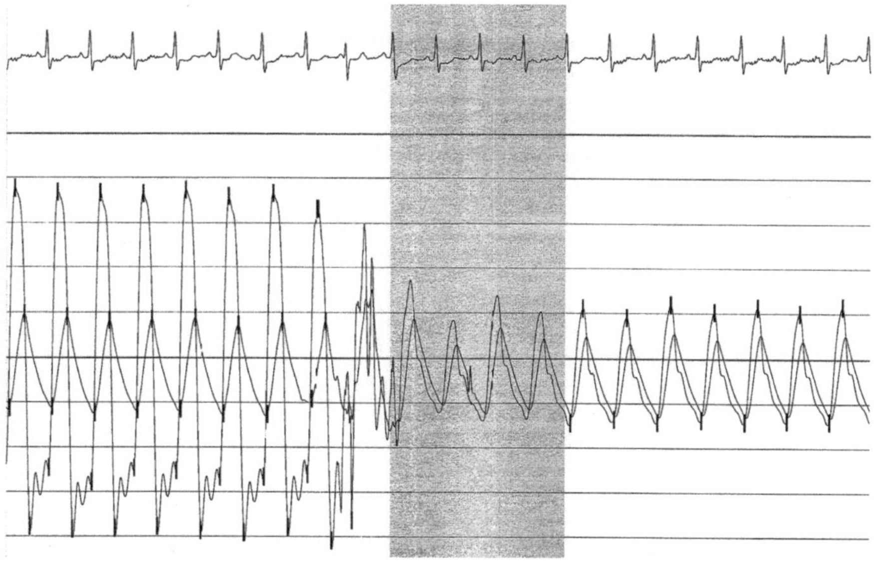

Fig. 6. Invasive assessment of aortic stenosis. Simultaneous measurement of left ventricular and aortic pressures (left side), showing a significant pressure gradient indicating severe aortic stenosis. This gradient disappears after pull-back of the tip of the catheter into the aorta ascendens (right side).

2.9 Cardiac multislice computed tomography and cardiac magnetic resonance

Although limited by the exposure to radiation, its availibity and its use in patients with high heart rate or atrial fibrillation, multislice computed tomography (MSCT) may be helpful in certain clinical situations in patients with aortic stenosis, e.g. diagnosis of coronary artery disease (Figure 3) or better assessment of aortic dilatation / aneurysm. Although lipid-lowering therapy does not halt progression of moderate aortic stenosis, it is certainly indicated in the majority of patients because of concomitant coronary artery disease, as shown in the SEAS study and discussed below. MSCT is superior to quantify aortic valve calcification, although no cut-off point has been established yet influencing clinical decision making. It may also diagnose bicuspid valve morphology, and may even be helpful in assessment of valve area (Feuchtner et al., 2006). Cardiac MRI has been used in patients with asymptomatic aortic stenosis as well, but is not suitable for detection of concomitant coronary disease. Both MSCT and MRI have the limitation that they measure the anatomic and not the functional effective AVA, so the AS severity is often underrated. The velocity- encoded phase contrast imaging is a new magnetic resonance imaging technique, which allows aortic valve area quantification with the continuity equation imitating echocardiographic Doppler quantification. It is helpful in patients with poor echochardiographic windows, obesity, lung disease, or heavily calcified aortic valve (Dal-Bianco et al., 2008).

3. Clinical issues in asymptomatic aortic stenosis

3.1 Prognosis

The natural history of asymptomatic patients with moderate to severe aortic stenosis is not benign. One half of patients with mild-to-moderate aortic stenosis develop severe outflow

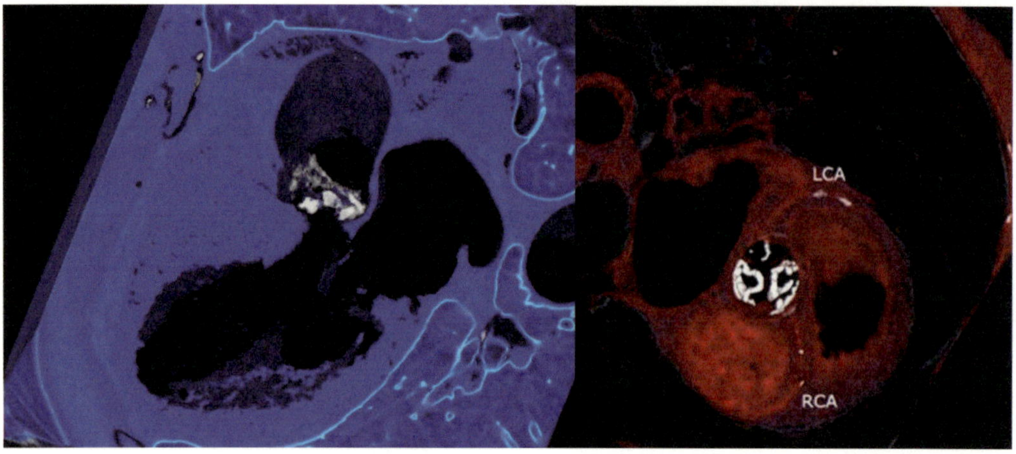

Fig. 7. Cardiac MSCT showing severe aortic valve calcification. On the left panel, poststenotic dilatation of the ascending aorta can be seen, whereas concomitant coronary artery calcification can be detected on the right panel. LCA denotes left coronary artery; RCA denotes right coronary artery.

obstruction within 6 years (Rosenhek et al., 2004). A large prospective study of asymptomatic patients with severe aortic stenosis showed that freedom from cardiovascular death or aortic valve replacement at 1, 2 and 5 years were only 80%, 63% and 20%, respectively. (Pellikka et al., 2005). This is particularly true for patients with very severe aortic stenosis, whose event-free survival is only 64%, 36%, 25% and 12% at 1, 2, 3 and 4 years, respectively (Rosenhek et al., 2009). Furthermore, patients with a peak systolic velocity > 5.5 m/s not referred to elective surgery present with severe symptom onset (defined by NYHA functional class > II), which is associated with a worse perioperative outcome.

A survival analysis from 1968 from Ross and Braunwald showed that patients with aortic stenosis who had developed angina and syncope survived 3 years, patients with dyspnoea 2 years, and patients with heart failure survived only 1 to 2 years. This study included symptomatic patients with heterogeneous AS etiology, thus not only calcific aortic stenosis.

3.2 Noncardiac surgery risk

Aortic stenosis is a risk factor for perioperative mortality and nonfatal myocardial infarction, but it is unclear whether aortic valve surgery should precede noncardiac surgery. Complication rates are depending on the severity of aortic stenosis and the type of noncardiac surgery performed. Perioperative complications may occurr in up to 11% of patients with moderate aortic stenosis and 31% of patients with severe aortic stenosis, as compared to 2% in matched patients without aortic stenosis (Kertai et al., 2004). In experienced centers, low or intermediate risk noncardiac surgery can be performed safely even in patients with severe asymptomatic aortic stenosis with a low myocardial infarction rate of around 3%, if there is prompt vasopressor therapy for hypotensive episodes (Calleja et al., 2010).

3.3 Endocarditis prophylaxis

In 2009, the ESC guidelines concerning antibiotic endocarditis prophylaxis have changed limiting its use to only high-rik patients, such as patients with prosthetic valves, previous infective endocarditis or certain congenital heart disease. Degenerative aortic stenosis is not an indication for antibiotic endocarditis prophylaxis, even if a bicuspid aortic valve is present (Habib et al., 2009).

3.4 Aggressive cardiovascular risk factor intervention

As mentioned above, arterial hypertension puts additional load to the left ventricle in patients with aortic stenosis, and should be carefully treated. However, hypotensive episodes have to be avoided, and regular blood pressure measurements are mandatory. Retrospective studies suggested that lipid-lowering with statins might slow the progression of aortic stenosis, but prospective studies such as SALTIRE (Cowell et al., 2005) or SEAS (Rossebo et al., 2008) could not confirm such a positive effect on aortic valve events in patients with a LDL cholesterol below 140 mg/dl. Nevertheless, the majority of the patients with aortic stenosis need statins because of three reasons:

- **concomitant coronary artery disease**: in SEAS, intensive lipid-lowering therapy with simvastin 40 mg and ezetimibe 10 mg/d daily reduced cardiovascular ischemic events even in patients with baseline LDL cholesterol below 140 mg/dl, mainly driven by a significant reduction in the need of additional bypass grafting when aortic valve replacement became mandatory; notably, LDL cholesterol were reduced by 61.3% to mean 55 mg/dl.
- **hypercholesterolemia**: RAAVE, the only prospective study showing a slowing effect on the hemodynamic progression of aortic stenosis, was performed in hypercholesterolemic patients, defined by a LDL cholesterol above 160 mg/dl (Moura et al., 2007); therefore, such patients should receive statin therapy.
- **early stage of the disease**: a retrospective analysis of 1046 patients (Antonini-Canterin, et al., 2008) could show that statin therapy slowed hemodynamic progression in the early stages of the disease process, e.g. aortic sclerosis or mild aortic stenosis. However, this effect disappeared in patients with more advanced aortic stenosis (defined by a baseline peak aortic velocity between 3 and 4 m/s).

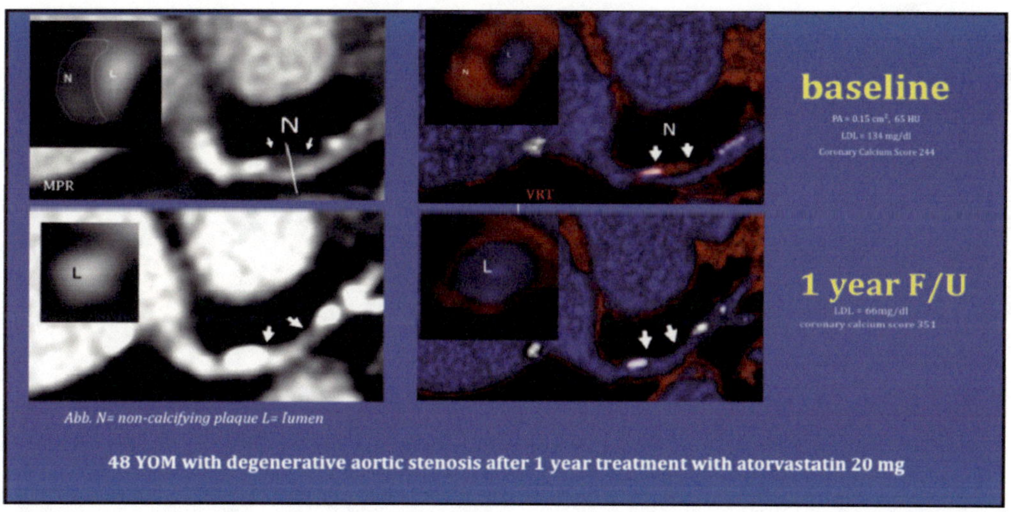

Fig. 8. Cardiac MSCT examinations showing the effects of newly initiated statin treatment on concomitant coronary artery disease. MPR denotes multiplanar reformation; VRT denotes volume-rendering technique; N denotes non-calcified atherosclerotic plaque; YOM denotes year old man.

3.5 Recommended intervals for follow-up examinations

For asymptomatic patients with aortic stenosis, close follow-up is imperative. Clinical evaluation should be performed once a year in patients with mild or moderate aortic stenosis and every 6 months in patients with severe aortic stenosis. Patients need to be questioned thoroughly about symptoms and exercise levels, along with the assessment and treatment of cardiovascular risk factors. Any change in symptoms should prompt the physician to perform a transthoracic echocardiography. Otherwise, intervals between echocardiography examinations are 3 - 5 years in patients with mild aortic stenosis, 1 - 2 years in patients with moderate aortic stenosis and 6 months to 1 year in patient with severe stenosis. In patients with severe asymptomatic aortic stenosis, exercise testing and measurement of natriuretic peptide levels may be helpful.

3.6 Bicuspid aortic valve disease

Bicuspid aortic valve is the most common inherited valve abnormality, affecting 1 - 2% of all individuals. There is a genetic component which may justify familiy testing. Around 40% of patients with bicuspid Aortic valves often suffer from dilatation of the ascending aorta as well, independent of the severity of aortic stenosis and/or insufficiency. A major risk of aortic dilation in these patients is aortic dissection, being 9 times higher for patients with a bicuspid aortic valve than for patients with a tricuspid valve. If the maximum diameter is ≥ 5 cm with a fast progression rate above 0.5 cm^2/year, surgery may be considered even in asymptomatic patients (Class IIaC indication according to ESC guidelines). Therefore, echocardiography should always include measurement of the diameter of the ascending aorta. If dilatation predominates above the sinotubular junction, diagnosis can be missed by transthoracic echocardiography and additional imaging techniques should be considered. Otherwise, management of bicuspid aortic valve disease is similar to that of tricuspid valve disease.

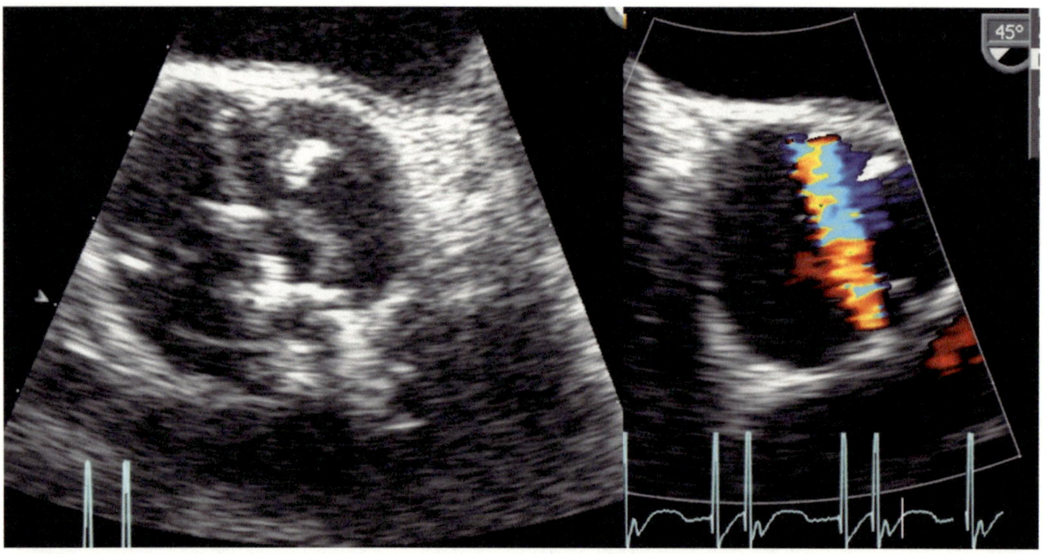

Fig. 9. Using transesophageal echocardiography in a patient with calcific aortic stenosis, a biscupid valve morphology is detected and planimetry of the aortic valve area can be reliably performed.

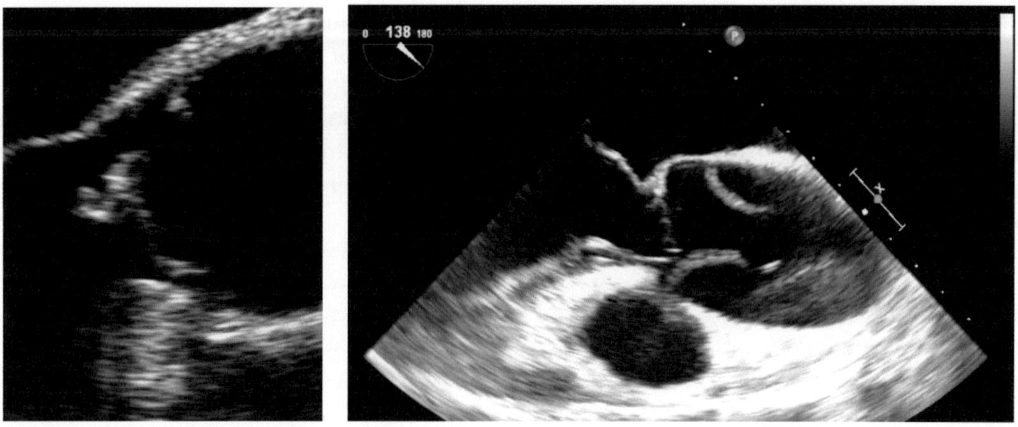

Fig. 10. Complications associated with bicuspid aortic valve disease: endocarditis (left panel) and acute aortic dissection (right panel).

3.7 Balancing risks between earlier surgery and watchful waiting

Besides a positive exercise test, no single risk factor is an absolute criterion to predict poor clinical outcome in patients with asymptomatic severe aortic stenosis so far. Other indicators of high-risk such as rapid hemodynamic progression, heavy valve calcification or increased natriuretic peptide levels should be weightened against the risk of surgery.

Fortunately, operative risk of isolated aortic valve replacement has dramatically declined over the last decades, currently being 2 - 5% in patients < 70 years and 5 - 15% in patients above 70 years. Concomitant bypass surgery increases the perioperative risk by around 5%.

The EuroSCORE or the Society of Thoracic Surgeons predicted risk of mortality (STS-PROM) score are commonly used for the evaluation of the preoperative risk for cardiac surgery. The simple additive EuroSCORE model is easy to use, even at the bedside. In high risk patients, however, the simple additive model often underestimates the risk when certain combinations of risk factors co-exist, and the logististic EuroSCORE should be used. It takes into consideration age, sex, chronic pulmonary disease, extracardiac arteriopathy, neurological dysfunction, previous cardiac surgery, renal insufficiency, active endocarditis, critical preoperative state, as well as cardiac-related factors such as unstable angina, left ventricular function, recent myocardial infarction and pulmonary hypertension.

If a watchful waiting strategy is chosen, the patient should be educated and advised to self-report onset of new symptoms to physician immediately. Patients often reduce subconsciously their physical activity, and so only a stress testing can uncover symptoms.

3.8 The comorbid and elderly patient – considerations on transcatheter aortic valve implantation

A third of patients with severe symptomatic aortic stenosis are not referred for valve replacement. This is mainly a problem for elderly patients, because many physcians ignore the fact that age itself is not a contra-indication to aortic valve implantation. The EuroSCORE or the STS-PROM score are commonly used to estimate the preoperative risk for cardiac surgery. Both scores incorporate various comorbidities such as chronic pulmonary disease and renal insufficiency; if a patient has too grave comorbidities he might be deemed inoperable. The approach to comorbid symptomatic patients is solid risk evaluation in experienced medical centers with a high surgery volume ("heart team").

Interventional cardiologist more and more challenge heart surgeons by the introduction of transcatheter aortic valve implantation (TAVI), and the years to come will show if this new procedure may play a role also in younger patients with moderate preoperative risk.
On the basis of current clinical outcome data, for symptomatic patients with severe aortic stenosis and a life expectancy over 1 year, indications for TAVI are definite contraindications to surgery or when surgery is estimated very high risk and if there are no barriers to TAVI.
The results of TAVI are preliminary and any conclusions carry limitations. It seems that TAVI is practicable and present acceptable clinical and hemodynamic results up to 3 years. However, there are still major limitations for TAVI, e.g. paravalvular leaks causing significant aortic insufficiency, a higher postoperative need for pacemaker implantation or vascular complications. Bicuspid aortic valve morphology is not suitable for TAVI as well. The access for transcatheter aortic valve implantation is retrograde via the femoral or the subclavian artery or antegrade through a transapical approach.

4. Conclusions

Besides coronary artery disease and arterial hypertension, aortic stenosis is the third most common cardiovascular disorder in the Western World, affecting more than four percent of the population above 75 years. It is easy to diagnose by auscultation and subsequent transthoracic echocardiography. Surgical aortic valve implantation (SAVI) offers a very good therapeutic option for symptomatic patients with severe valve obstruction which has a dismal prognosis if left untreated. In contrast, the decision to operate on asymptomatic patients remains a controversity. Unfortunately, there is still no medical therapy available to prevent the development or to delay the progression of aortic stenosis. Probably, medical intervention would be most effective in early stages of the disease, even before obstruction of the left ventricular outflow occurs. This condition called aortic sclerosis is present in 25% of adults over 65 years of age. Currently, around 15% of these patients progress to hemodynamically significant aortic stenosis, and it would be of great importance to stop this active process more effectively in these patients.

5. Acknowledgment

The authors thank Dr. Gudrun Feuchtner, Dr. Hannes Alber and Dr. Maria Wanitschek for support in preparation of Figures 6-8.

6. References

Antonini-Canterin, F.; et al. (2008). Stage-Related Effect of Statin Treatment on the Progression of Aortic Valve Sclerosis and Stenosis. *American Journal of Cardiology,* 102, pp. 738–742.

Amato, MCM.; et al. (2001). Treatment Decision in Asymptomatic Aortic Valve Stenosis: Role of Exercise Testing. *Heart,* 86, pp. 381-386.

Bergler-Klein, J.; et al. (2006). Natriuretic Peptides Predict Symptom-Free Survival and Postoperative Outcome in Severe Aortic Stenosis. *Circulation,* 109, pp. 2302-2308, ISSN 0009-7322.

Bermejo, J.; et al. (2003). Clinical Efficacy of Doppler-Echocardiographic Indices of Aortic Valve Stenosis: A Comparative Test-Based Analysis of Outcome. Journal of the American College of Cardiology, 41, pp. 142-149.

Bonow, RO.; et al. (2008). 008 Focused Update Incorporated Into the ACC/AHA 2006 Guidelines for the Management of Patients With Valvular Heart Disease: A Report of the American College of Cardiology/American Heart Association Task Force on Practice Guidelines. *Journal of the American College of Cardiology,* 52, pp. e1-142.

Calleja, AM.; et al. (2010). Cardiac Risk in Patients Aged > 75 Years With Asymptomatic, Severe Aortic Stenosis Undergoing Noncardiac Surgery. *American Journal of Cardiology,* 105(8), pp. 1159-1163.

Cowell, SJ.; et al. (2005). A Randomized Trial of Intensive Lipid-Lowering Therapy in Calcific Aortic Stenosis. *New England Journal of Medicine,* 352, pp. 2389-2397.

Dal-Bianco, JP.; et al. (2008). Management of Asymptomatic Severe Aortic Stenosis. *Journal of the American College of Cardiology,* 52, pp. 1279-1292, ISSN 0735-1097.

Feuchtner, GM.; et al. (2006). Multislice Computed Tomography for Detection of Patients With Aortic Valve Stenosis and Quantification of Severity. *Journal of the American College of Cardiology,* 47, pp. 1410-1417.

Galante, A.; et al. (2001). C-Reactive Protein is Increased in Patients with Degenerative Aortic Valvular Stenosis. *Journal of the American College of Cardiology,* 38, pp. 1078-1082.

Habib, G.; et al. (2009). Guidelines on the Prevention, Diagnosis, and Treatment of Infective Endocarditis. *European Heart Journal,* 30, pp. 2369-2413.

Iung, B. (2011). Management of Asymptomatic Aortic Stenosis. *Heart,* 97, pp. 253-259.

Kertai, MD. et al. (2004). Aortic Stenosis: An Underestimated Risk Factor For Perioperative Complications In Patients Undergoing Noncardiac Surgery. *American Journal of Medicine,* 116, pp. 8-13.

Monin, JL.; et al. (2009). Risk Score for Predicting Outcome in Patients With Asymptomatic Aortic Stenosis. *Circulation,* 120, pp. 69-75, ISSN 0009-7322.

Moura, LM.; et al. (2007). Rosuvastatin Affecting Aortic Valve Endothelium to Slow the Progression of Aortic Stenosis. *Journal of the American College of Cardiology,* 49, pp. 554 -561.

Novaro, GM.; et al. (2007). Clinical Factors, But Not C-Reactive Protein, Predict Progression of Calcific Aortic-Valve Disease. *Journal of the American College of Cardiology,* 50, pp. 1992-1999, ISSN 0735-1097.

Pedrazzini, GB.; et al. (2008). Comparison of Brain Natriuretic Peptide Plasma Levels Versus Logistic EuroSCORE in Predicting In-hospital and Late Postoperative Mortality in Patients Undergoing Aortic Valve Replacement for Symptomatic Aortic Stenosis. *American Journal of Cardiology,* 102, pp. 749-754.

Pellikka, PA.; et al. (2005). Outcome of 622 Adults With Asymptomatic, Hemodynamically Significant Aortic Stenosis During Prolonged Follow-up. Circulation, 111, pp. 3290-3295.

Rosenhek, R.; et al. (2004). Mild and Moderate Aortic Stenosis. Natural History and Risk Stratification By Echocardiography. *European Heart Journal,* 25, pp. 199-205.

Rosenhek, R.; et al. (2009). Natural History of Very Severe Aortic Stenosis. *Circulation;* 121, pp. 151-156, ISSN 0009-7322.

Ross, J Jr. & Braunwald, E. (1968). Aortic Stenosis. *Circulation;* 38, pp. 61-67.

Rossebo, AB.; et al. (2008). Intensive Lipid Lowering with Simvastatin and Ezetimibe in Aortic Stenosis. *New England Journal of Medicine,* 359, pp. 1343-1356.

Vahanian, A.; et al. (2007). Guidelines on the Management of Valvular Heart Disease. The Task Force on the Management of Valvular Heart Disease of the European Society of Cardiology. *European Heart Journal,* 28, pp. 230-268.

Vahanian, A. & Otto, CM. (2010). Risk Stratification of Patients With Aortic Stenosis. *European Heart Journal,* 31, pp. 416-423.

5

Stress Testing in Patients with Asymptomatic Severe Aortic Stenosis

Asim M. Rafique, Kirsten Tolstrup and Robert J. Siegel
Cedars-Sinai Heart Institute,
University of California
United States of America

1. Introduction

The natural history of valvular aortic stenosis (AS) is characterized by a protracted symptom free period during which morbidity and mortality are very low. During this period the average decrease in the aortic valve area is about 0.1 cm^2 per year (1-4), although it is impossible to predict the rate of progression in an individual patient. For this reason, regular clinical follow-up is standard of care in all patients with asymptomatic mild to moderate AS (1). The onset of symptoms such as: angina, syncope, or heart failure significantly changes prognosis, with an average survival of 60% at 1 year and has increased risk of sudden cardiac death (5-7).

2. Identifying high risk asymptomatic patients with severe AS

Aortic valve replacement (AVR) is the current standard treatment for patients with severe AS who have symptoms or left ventricular (LV) systolic dysfunction (1, 2). However, the best treatment strategy in asymptomatic patients with severe AS and preserved LV systolic function is debated (8). Conservative approach with a watchful waiting is generally favored although the utility of early elective AVR has been debated in subset of high risk patients. Several predictors have been proposed which predict poor outcomes in patients with asymptomatic severe AS. These include stress testing, severity of AS, rapid homodynamic progression of AS, elevated left atrial pressure as assessed by E/E′ using tissue Doppler imaging or atrial natriuretic peptide (NPA). Of these stress testing is the most validated way of identifying asymptomatic patients who may benefit from AVR (9-10).

3. Importance of stress testing

Improved life expectancy has resulted in there being more elderly patients with AS, in whom the true symptoms may be underestimated (11). Given the slow progression of disease, patients may reduce their level of physical activity to avoid or minimize symptoms and be unaware of subtle changes in effort tolerance or attribute it to deconditioning or a physical impact due to aging. The accurate determination of symptoms is crucial; as symptoms increase the risk of sudden death worsens as well as protend an overall worst prognosis (12-13).

Valvular heart disease has a varying dynamic components which depend on loading conditions, ventricular contractility, ventricular contractile reserve, volume-dependent compliance of heart chambers, and ventricular arterial coupling. The current primary role of stress testing in asymptomatic severe aortic stenosis is to provide an objective assessment of functional capacity which is of the utmost importance in patients who often adapt and reduce their physical activity, thus masking the symptoms. In addition, exercise testing can identify changes in valvular as well as ventricular function and the changes in the valve gradient with the changes in forward flow and to differentiate true vs. pseudo aortic stenosis in the setting of low cardiac output.

4. Indications of stress testing

Valve replacement is indicated in the presence of symptoms and severe aortic stenosis. In such patients, stress testing is contraindicated. In contrast, exercise testing is recommended in asymptomatic patients with severe aortic stenosis. Exercise testing is strongly advocated in the European guidelines and is a grade IIb recommendation in the American College of Cardiology/American Heart Association (ACC/AHA) 2006 guidelines (1, 2). There is no prospective clinical trial on the use of stress testing in asymptomatic patients with severe AS as an indicator for aortic valve replacement. However, several retrospective small clinical studies have evaluated the predictive value of stress testing in asymptomatic severe AS (14-26), as shown in figure 1 which has been adapted from the American Journal of Cardiology (9). In this meta-analysis there were no sudden deaths in the patients with normal stress test results after 1 year of follow-up, while 5% with abnormal stress test results had sudden cardiac death. Overall, 52 of 253 patients (21%) with normal stress test results had adverse cardiac events, compared with 156 of 238 (66%) with abnormal stress test results. Stress testing can be used for risk stratification and for deciding on the timing of AVR in asymptomatic patients with severe AS.

Study or Subgroup	Normal Stress Test	Abnormal Stress Test	Weight	Odds Ratio M-H, Random, 95% CI
Alborino 2002	2/12	14/18	7.1%	0.06 [0.01, 0.38]
Amato 2001	3/22	35/44	11.4%	0.04 [0.01, 0.17]
Das 2005	10/79	26/46	22.3%	0.11 [0.05, 0.27]
Lancellotti 2005	4/43	14/26	13.3%	0.09 [0.02, 0.32]
Marechaux 2007	10/26	20/24	12.6%	0.13 [0.03, 0.47]
Peidro 2007	10/35	37/67	22.5%	0.32 [0.13, 0.78]
Takeda 2001	13/36	10/13	10.9%	0.17 [0.04, 0.73]
Total	**52/253**	**156/238**	**100.0%**	**0.12 [0.07, 0.21]**

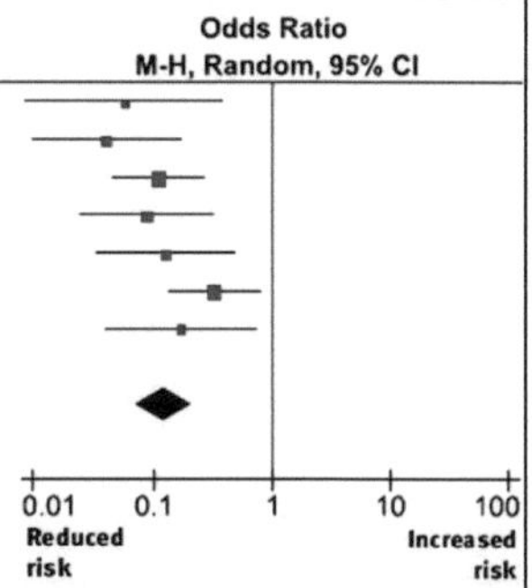

Heterogeneity: Tau² = 0.13; Chi² = 8.08, df = 6 (P = 0.23); I² = 26%
Test for overall effect: Z = 7.63 (P < 0.00001)

A

Fig. 1. Utility of stress testing in predicting cardiac events in patients with Severe AS

5. Prevalence of stress testing

The results of the Euro Heart Survey on Valvular Heart Disease revealed that stress testing is underused in Europe. Only about 5.7% of asymptomatic patients with severe AS undergo exercise testing (27). The reason for the low usage of stress testing include: concern about safety, lack of awareness of its utility and lack of randomized, prospective trials. Stress testing is considered low risk when performed in asymptomatic patients under medically supervised conditions (9).

6. Types of stress test

A symptom-limited exercise test is more physiologic than a dobutamine test and may be performed safely. Treadmill or upright bicycle ergometry are the most frequent tests and the choice is based on individual experience or equipment available in a given laboratory. Symptom-limited graded bicycle exercise in a semi-supine position may be preferable since it allows continuous two dimensional and Doppler echocardiographic examinations. Dobutamine stress echocardiography may be used to assess aortic valve compliance by plotting effective orifice area against flow at each stage of the dobutamine test. However, in asymptomatic patients with severe aortic stenosis it is less likely to be helpful in identifying patients with occult symptoms. In asymptomatic patients with severe AS exercise testing should be repeated every 6 months for severe aortic stenosis and every year for moderate aortic stenosis (14). Testing should be performed in laboratory equipped with a resuscitation cart in the presence of a physician so that potential complications can be treated effectively.

7. Parameters to be evaluated on stress testing

Total exercise time, maximum workload, peak heart rate and blood pressure and the reason for stopping the test are recorded. The criteria of an abnormal exercise test provided in the European recommendations are listed in table 1. It is essential to record the development of symptoms carefully, such as objective dyspnea, angina, dizziness or near-syncope. When Doppler echocardiography is obtained during exercise, aortic velocity–time integral can be regularly recorded from the same window to assess changes in mean pressure gradient.

The assessment of exercise capacity often identifies symptoms that patient has not reported and has important prognostic significance as outlined in multiple clinical studies but simple stress testing fails to identify patients at higher risk for rapid disease progression (9). A representative example of ST changes during stress testing in a patient with AS is shown in figure 2.

8. Pathophysiology during exercise

Multiple studies have shown that the LV response to exercise is abnormal in apparently asymptomatic AS (24-29). Patients with apparently asymptomatic AS with symptoms detected during exercise testing have lower peak myocardial oxygen consumption and lower peak stroke index than those patients who remained asymptomatic (24). Studies have shown that normal increases in stroke volume on exercise in patients with mild and

Symptoms during exercise: dyspnea, angina, syncope or near syncope
Fall in blood pressure or <20 mm Hg rise in systolic blood pressure during exercise
<80% of normal level of exercise tolerance
>2 mm ST segment depression during exercise (horizontal or down sloping, in comparison to baseline, not attributable to other causes)
Ventricular arrhythmias

Table 1. Criteria of an abnormal exercise test in patients with asymptomatic aortic stenosis

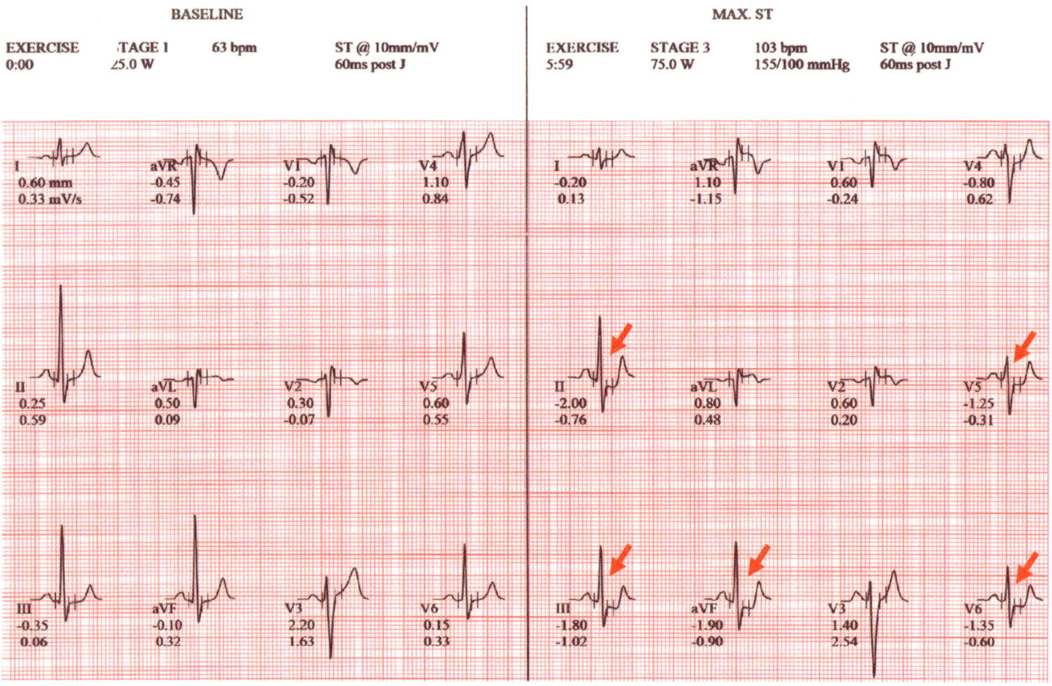

Fig. 2. A representative example of ST changes in infero-lateral leads during stress testing in a patient with AS

moderate AS but stroke volume was significantly decreased in symptomatic patients with severe AS both at rest and on exercise. Otto et al observed a decrease in stroke volume on exercise in asymptomatic patients with AS using Doppler echocardiography (15). Severe calcification has been reported to sometimes represent or be associated with a faster progression of the AS and a higher risk for the rapid progression to symptoms and events (8). Lancellotti et al demonstrated that an abnormal exercise response in patients with asymptomatic AS was mediated by impaired contractile reserve and a relatively large increase in gradient (21). Mare´chaux et al. showed the utility of risk stratification based on the increase in the mean pressure gradient of >18mmHg as the most predictive of outcomes (24). Peak exercise LV ejection fraction is another parameter for risk stratification in patients with asymptomatic AS, if LVEF does not increase by ≥5% it indicates impaired contractile reserve, and it is suggestive of limited LV functional reserve (23). Aortic physiology due to altered compliance may play a role in the pathophysiology and progression of the disease, and this may become evident on stress testing. Some authors have noted a blunted fall in systemic vascular resistance associated with exercise induced symptoms (24-26). In short, AS, coronary disease and reduced aortic compliance exist as a continuum, and stress testing can play the critical role of revealing symptoms and subsequent referral for intervention.

9. Clinical utility of stress testing

The current ESC guidelines recommend AVR in patients who develop cardiac symptoms (class I) or who develop asymptomatic hypotension (class IIa) or asymptomatic ventricular arrhythmias (class IIb) during the exercise test (2). In contrast, the ACC/AHA guidelines recommend AVR if symptoms or hypotension appear during the exercise test (class IIb) (1).The divergent recommendations can be explained by the lack of definitive evidence from prospective clinical trials and subsequent different interpretation by the two groups. While, exercise stress testing is recommended in the management of asymptomatic patients with severe AS, exercise stress echocardiography is not routinely recommended in the current guidelines.

No randomized trial has been conducted in patients with asymptomatic severe aortic stenosis (30). The risk of sudden death is low and is usually considered to be lower than the risk of operation. However, the mortality is rather high early after the onset of symptoms or if the patient is on a surgical waiting list. In some patients, symptoms are not identified, especially in elderly subjects who are rather inactive (31). On the other hand, dyspnea and chest pain may be non-specific. Exercise testing can identify a limited exercise capacity and unmask symptoms in about one-third of the apparently asymptomatic patients (32-33). The development of symptoms during exercise seems to be more predictive than the other criteria, but this needs to be confirmed. A significant increase in mean transaortic pressure gradient predicts a higher risk of cardiac events and has been shown to provide incremental prognostic information over clinical, resting Doppler echocardiographic and exercise testing (21,24). Further studies using novel echocardiographic techniques may provide additional understanding of the hemodyamics in patients with severe asymptomatic AS and refine the utility of stress testing in risk stratification of AS patients for AVR either surgical or by newer percutaneous techniques (34).

In summary, stress testing appears to be of value in unmasking the symptoms in otherwise asymptomatic patients who may have denial or who unconsciously limit their activity secondarily to progressive AS. In addition, in elderly patients, symptoms may not be identified because of inactivity, thus in these groups of asymptomatic patients stress testing readily provides an objective assessment of functional status.

10. References

[1] American College of Cardiology/American Heart Association Task Force on Practice Guidelines; Society of Cardiovascular Anesthesiologists; Society for Cardiovascular Angiography and Interventions; Society of Thoracic Surgeons, Bonow RO,

Carabello BA, Kanu C, de Leon AC Jr, Faxon DP, Freed MD, Gaasch WH, Lytle BW, Nishimura RA, O'Gara PT, O'Rourke RA, Otto CM, Shah PM, Shanewise JS, Smith SC Jr, Jacobs AK, Adams CD, Anderson JL, Antman EM, Faxon DP, Fuster V, Halperin JL, Hiratzka LF, Hunt SA, Lytle BW, Nishimura R, Page RL, Riegel B. ACC/AHA 2006 guidelines for the management of patients with valvular heart disease: a report of the American College of Cardiology/American Heart Association Task Force on Practice Guidelines. Circulation 2006;114:e84–e231.

[2] Vahanian A, Baumgartner H, Bax J, Butchart E, Dion R, Filippatos G, Flachskampf F, Hall R, Iung B, Kasprzak J, Nataf P, Tornos P, Torracca L, Wenink A, Priori SG, Blanc JJ, Budaj A, Camm J, Dean V, Deckers J, Dickstein K, Lekakis J, McGregor K, Metra M, Morais J, Osterspey A, Tamargo J, Zamorano JL, Zamorano JL, Angelini A, Antunes M, Fernandez MA, Gohlke-Baerwolf C, Habib G, McMurray J, Otto C, Pierard L, Pomar JL, Prendergast B, Rosenhek R, Uva MS, Tamargo J. Guidelines on the management of valvular heart disease: the Task Force on the Management of Valvular Heart Disease of the European Society of Cardiology. Eur Heart J 2007;28:230–268.

[3] Otto CM, Pearlman AS, Gardner CL. Hemodynamic progression of aortic stenosis in adults assessed by Doppler echocardiography. J Am Coll Cardiol 1989;13:545–550.

[4] Wagner S, Selzer A. Patterns of progression of aortic stenosis: a longitudinal hemodynamic study. Circulation 1982;65:709–712.

[5] Ross J Jr., Braunwald E. Aortic stenosis. Circulation 1968;38:61–7.

[6] Schwarz F, Baumann P, Manthey J, Hoffmann M, Schuler G, Mehmel HC, Schmitz W, Kübler W. The effect of aortic valve replacement on survival. Circulation 1982;66:1105–1110.

[7] Iivanainen AM, Lindroos M, Tilvis R, Heikkila J, Kupari M. Natural history of aortic valve stenosis of varying severity in the elderly. Am J Cardiol 1996;78:97–101.

[8] Zamorano JL, Goncalves A. Exercise echocardiography in aortic stenosis: one more piece in the puzzle. Eur Heart J. 2010 Jun;31(11):1295-7.

[9] Rafique AM, Biner S, Ray I, Forrester JS, Tolstrup K, Siegel RJ. Meta-analysis of prognostic value of stress testing in patients with asymptomatic severe aortic stenosis. Am J Cardiol 2009;104:972–977.

[10] Biner S, Rafique AM, Goykhman P, Morrissey RP, Naghi J, Siegel RJ. Prognostic value of E/E' ratio in patients with unoperated severe aortic stenosis. JACC Cardiovasc Imaging. 2010 Sep;3(9):899-907. PubMed PMID: 20846623.

[11] Nkomo VT, Gardin JM, Skelton TN, Gottdiener JS, Scott CG, Enriquez-Sarano M. Burden of valvular heart diseases: a population-based study. Lancet 2006;368: 1005–1011.

[12] Bouma BJ, van Den Brink RB, van Der Meulen JH, Verheul HA, Cheriex EC, Hamer HP, Dekker E, Lie KI, Tijssen JG. To operate or not on elderly patients with aortic stenosis: the decision and its consequences. Heart 1999;82:143–148.

[13] Bach DS, Siao D, Girard SE, Duvernoy C, McCallister BD Jr, Gualano SK. Evaluation of patients with severe symptomatic aortic stenosis who do not undergo aortic valve replacement: the potential role of subjectively overestimated operative risk. Circ Cardiovasc Qual Outcomes. 2009;2(6):533-539.

[14] Chambers J, Das P. Treadmill exercise in apparently asymptomatic aortic stenosis. Heart. 2001 Oct;86(4):361-2.

[15] Otto CM, Burwash IG, Legget ME, Munt BI, Fujioka M, Healy NL, Kraft CD, Miyake-Hull CY, Schwaegler RG. Prospective study of asymptomatic valvular aortic stenosis. Clinical, echocardiographic, and exercise predictors of outcome. Circulation. 1997 May 6;95(9):2262-70.

[16] Das P, Rimington H, Chambers J. Exercise testing to stratify risk in aortic stenosis. Eur Heart J 2005;26:1309–1313.

[17] Alborino D, Hoffmann JL, Fournet PC, Bloch A. Value of exercise testing to evaluate the indication for surgery in asymptomatic patients with valvular aortic stenosis. J Heart Valve Dis 2002;11:204–209.

[18] Amato MC, Moffa PJ, Werner KE, Ramires JA. Treatment decision in asymptomatic aortic valve stenosis: role of exercise testing. Heart 2001;86:381–386.

[19] Atwood JE, Kawanishi S, Myers J, Froelicher VF. Exercise testing in patients with aortic stenosis. Chest 1988;93:1083–1087.

[20] Takeda S, Rimington H, Chambers J. Prediction of symptom-onset in aortic stenosis: a comparison of pressure drop/flow slope and haemodynamic measures at rest. Int J Cardiol 2001;81:131–137.

[21] Lancellotti P, Lebois F, Simon M, Tombeux C, Chauvel C, Pierard LA. Prognostic importance of quantitative exercise Doppler echocardiography in asymptomatic valvular aortic stenosis. Circulation 2005;112:I377–1382.

[22] Peidro R, Brion G, Angelino A. Exercise testing in asymptomatic aortic stenosis. Cardiology 2007;108:258–264.

[23] Marechaux S, Ennezat PV, LeJemtel TH, Polge AS, de Groote P, Asseman P, Nevière R, Le Tourneau T, Deklunder G. Left ventricular response to exercise in aortic stenosis: an exercise echocardiographic study. Echocardiography 2007;24:955–959.

[24] Maréchaux S, Hachicha Z, Bellouin A, Dumesnil JG, Meimoun P, Pasquet A, Bergeron S, Arsenault M, Le Tourneau T, Ennezat PV, Pibarot P. Usefulness of exercise-stress echocardiography for risk stratification of true asymptomatic patients with aortic valve stenosis. Eur Heart J. 2010 Jun;31(11):1390-7.

[25] Weisenberg D, Shapira Y, Vaturi M, Monakier D, Iakobishvili Z, Battler A, Sagie A. Does exercise echocardiography have an added value over exercise testing alone in asymptomatic patients with severe aortic stenosis? J Heart Valve Dis. 2008 Jul;17(4):376-80.

[26] Kusljugic Z, Barakovic F, Dilic M, Dizdarevic-Hudic L, Smajic E, Caluk J, Avdic S, Mulic S, Isabegovic M, Avdagic M, Kovacevic-Divkovic K, Bijedic A. The role of exercise test in stratifying the risk of asymptomatic patients with moderate/severe aortic stenosis. Med Arh. 2010;64(5):269-273.

[27] Iung B, Baron G, Butchart EG, Delahaye F, Gohlke-Bärwolf C, Levang OW, Tornos P, Vanoverschelde JL, Vermeer F, Boersma E, Ravaud P, Vahanian A. A prospective survey of patients with valvular heart disease in Europe: The Euro Heart Survey on Valvular Heart Disease. Eur Heart J 2003;24:1231–1243.

[24] Rajani R, Rimington H, Chambers JB. Treadmill exercise in apparently asymptomatic patients with moderate or severe aortic stenosis: relationship between cardiac index and revealed symptoms. Heart. 2010 May;96(9):689-95.

[25] Laskey WK, Kussmaul WG 3rd, Noordergraaf A. Systemic arterial response to exercise in patients with aortic valve stenosis. Circulation 2009;119: 996e1004.

[26] Vekshtein VI, Alexander RW, Yeung AC, et al. Coronary atherosclerosis is associated with left ventricular dysfunction and dilatation in aortic stenosis. Circulation 1990;82:2068e74.

[27] Lancellotti P, Donal E, Magne J, Moonen M, O'Connor K, Daubert JC, Pierard LA. Risk stratification in asymptomatic moderate to severe aortic stenosis: the importance of the valvular, arterial and ventricular interplay. Heart. 2010Sep;96(17):1364-71.

[28] Dalsgaard M, Kjaergaard J, Pecini R, Iversen KK, Kober L, Moller JE, Grande P, Clemmensen P, Hassager C. Predictors of exercise capacity and symptoms in severe aortic stenosis. Eur J Echocardiogr. 2010 Jul;11(6):482-7.

[29] Leurent G, Donal E, de Place C, Chabanne C, Gervais R, Fougerou C, le Helloco A, Daubert JC, Mabo P, Laurent M. Argument for a Doppler echocardiography during exercise in assessing asymptomatic patients with severe aortic stenosis. Eur J Echocardiogr. 2009 Jan;10(1):69-73.

[30] McCann GP, Steadman CD, Ray SG, Newby DE; on behalf of the British Heart Valve Society. Managing the asymptomatic patient with severe aortic stenosis: randomised controlled trials of early surgery are overdue. Heart. 2011 Mar 12.

[31] Shah RV, Desai NR, O'Gara PT. Asymptomatic severe aortic stenosis: silence of the lambs? Circulation. 2010 Oct 26;122(17):1734-9.

[32] Picano E, Pibarot P, Lancellotti P, Monin JL, Bonow RO. The emerging role of exercise testing and stress echocardiography in valvular heart disease. J Am Coll Cardiol. 2009 Dec 8;54(24):2251-60.

[33] Rosenhek R, Zilberszac R, Schemper M, Czerny M, Mundigler G, Graf S, Bergler-Klein J, Grimm M, Gabriel H, Maurer G. Natural history of very severe aortic stenosis. Circulation. 2010 Jan 5;121(1):151-6.

[34] Lancellotti P, Donal E, Magne J, O'Connor K, Moonen ML, Cosyns B, Pierard LA. Impact of global left ventricular afterload on left ventricular function in asymptomatic severe aortic stenosis: a two-dimensional speckle-tracking study. Eur J Echocardiogr. 2010 Jul; 11(6):537-43.

6

Analog Simulation of Aortic Stenosis

M. Sever[1], S. Ribarič[2], F. Runovc[3] and M. Kordaš[2]
[1] *Department of Internal Medicine, University Clinical Center Ljubljana, Ljubljana,*
[2]*Institute of Pathophysiology, Faculty of Medicine, University of Ljubljana, Ljubljana,*
[3]*Faculty of Natural Sciences and Engineering, University of Ljubljana, Ljubljana,*
Slovenia

1. Introduction

In cardiovascular physiology mathematical and analog simulations are well known (Beneken, 1965; Defares et al.; 1963, Grodins; 1959; Kordaš et al., 1968; Milhorn, 1966; Osborn,1967;). However, in analog modelling physical electrical models have been replaced by computer analysis of electronic analog circuitry. Then they have been applied to various physiological systems (Bošnjak & Kordaš, 2002; Dolenšek et al., 2005), to study also cardiovascular physiology (Rupnik et al., 2002), including mechanisms of compensation (Podnar et al., 2002) and principles of homeostasis, i. e. negative feedback mechanisms (Podnar et al., 2004). Recently, the equivalent circuit simulating the cardiovascular system was further upgraded to simulate, as close as possible, conditions in man in vivo. First, the intrathoracic pressure was made slightly negative and undulating at the rate of respiration. Second, the homeostasis included not only a control of venous tone and contractility of left and right ventricle, but also the control of heart rate. Third, the mean arterial pressure was - in some conditions - reset from the normal to a higher operating level (simulating increased sympathetic tone). By using these approaches recently various clinical conditions were simulated: acute left ventricle failure (myocardial infarction), aortic stenosis and exercise in man with aortic stenosis (Sever et al., 2007), and consequences of aortic and of mitral regurgitation (Dolenšek et al., 2009).
In present simulations it is attempted to extend both recent simulations quoted above. The consequences, induced by exercise in patients with aortic stenosis are to be studied in more detail. To meet this end, in aortic stenosis i) the aortic and mitral flows are studied and ii) mechanism of exhaustion, induced by exercise, are simulated.

2. Methods

Analysis of the equivalent circuit is performed by using Electronics Workbench Personal version 5.12 (Adams, 2001).
As in previous simulations four targets are modulated by negative feedback: venous tone, contractility of right ventricle, contractility of left ventricle, and heart rate. Essentially, the present equivalent circuit is the same as reported (Sever et al., 2007). The resetting of mean arterial pressure includes procedures whereby its resting value, "clamped" at about 98 mm Hg is shifted and then "clamped" again at a higher level. Heart rate control is the same as described in Sever and coworkers (Sever et al., 2007); the duration of the systole is constant,

200 ms in all simulation conditions. Mitral and aortic valve are simulated by diode D1. Input to the left ventricle is slightly modified as published (Dolenšek et al., 2009). Contractility modulation is the same as described in Sever and coworkers (Sever et al., 2007); via negative feedback it can be increased from 1 to about 8 "units of contractility". The time constant for myocardial contractility modulation control is increased from 1 s to 5 s.
Aortic stenosis is simulated as described (Sever et al., 2007). Exercise is simulated by decreasing arteriolar and capillary resistance by 50 % and by resetting mean arterial pressure. Then, via negative feedback, heart rate, myocardial contractility and venous capacitance are adjusted accordingly. Exhaustion of LV sympathetic drive is simulated by decreasing myocardial contractility modulation factor from about 8 to 1. Mild LV failure is simulated by decreasing the nominal contractility by about 50 %.
Results are expressed graphically as described (Sever et al., 2007; Dolenšek et al., 2009), as the time course of equivalent variables. Thus electrical variables voltage, current, resistance, capacitance and charge correspond to physiological variables pressure, blood flow, resistance, capacitance and volume (for details refer to Sever et al., 2007; Dolenšek et al., 2009). The acronyms used are listed below:

AoP	aortic pressure
CO	cardiac output
CVV	"contractible" volume of veins
EDVLV	end-diastolic volume of left ventricle
EFLV	left ventricle ejection fraction
ESVLV	end-systolic volume of left ventricle
ESVRV	end-systolic volume of right ventricle
ICT	isovolumetric contraction time
IRT	isovolumetric relaxation time
ITP	intrathoracic pressure
LV, LVV	left ventricle, volume of left ventricle
LAtP	left atrial pressure
LVP	left ventricular pressure
MAoP	mean arterial pressure
SVLV	stroke volume of the left ventricle
Sy	LV contractility modulation; inothropic (homeostatic) sympathetic effect on LV

Note that negative and undulating ITP affects slightly almost all variables. To allow comparison before and after a disturbance occurs, the time course of variables are recorded at the same instant of the heart cycle, defined here as the height of inspiration.

3. Results

All results are presented graphically showing the time course of variables which are of interest to be studied.
The transition of normal conditions into conditions affected by exercise are shown in Fig. 1A. The transition of normal conditions into conditions of aortic stenosis, exercise and exhaustion are shown in Fig. 2A.
The time course of these variables is also shown for systole and part of diastole. Effects of exercise are shown in Figs. 1B, C. Effects of exercise in aortic stenosis and after exhaustion are shown in Figs. 2B, C, D, E.

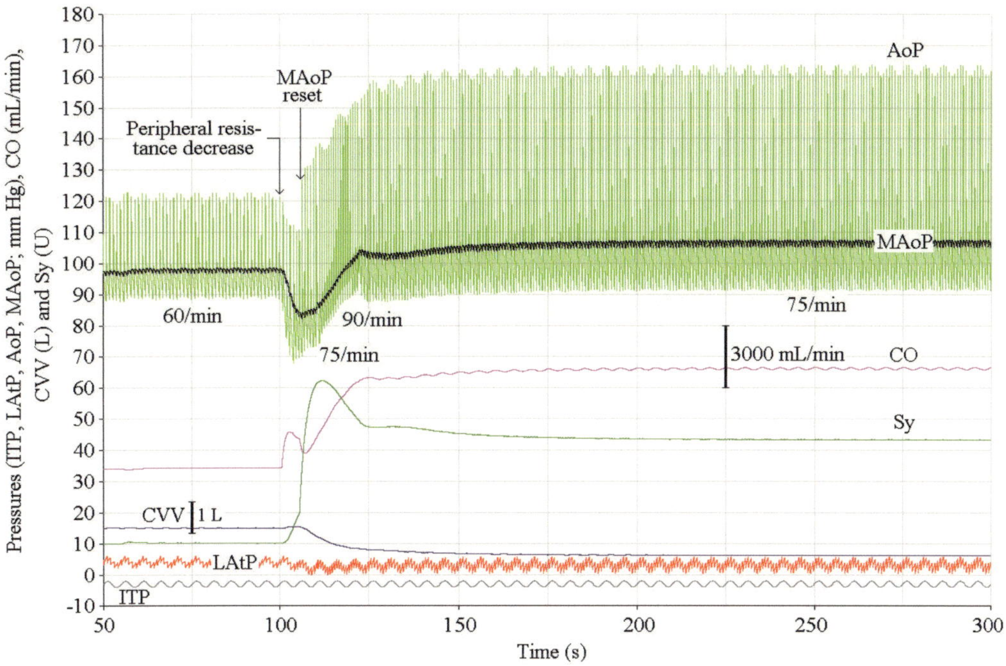

Fig. 1A. The time course of AoP, MAoP, heart rate, CO, Sy, CVV, LAtP and ITP in normal (resting) conditions and after peripheral resistance decrease (exercise; by 50 %, at 100.5 s. MAoP is reset at 105.5 s). Transiently the heart rate is increased from 60/min to 75/min and 90/min, until in steady state conditions it stabilises at 75/min. Note that despite venoconstriction (decreased CVV) LAtP is decreased. This is because Sy is increased, resulting in a strong LV contraction increase. Consequently, systolic AoP and pulse pressure is increased. There is little change in diastolic AoP. Because peripheral resistance is decreased MAoP is about 108 mm Hg and CO almost doubled.

Changes in cardiovascular variables (AoP, MAoP, CO, CVV, LAtP and ITP) in normal (resting) conditions, after peripheral resistance decrease (exercise) and after resetting of MAoP are presented in Fig. 1A. Initially (50 s - 100 s), all variables are in steady state. After peripheral resistance decrease (100 s - 300 s) the initial brief AoP and MAoP decrease are offset by MAoP reset (increased sympathetic tone). Due to venoconstriction (CVV decrease) and huge increase in Sy the force and rate of LV contraction are increased. Heart rate is increased. Consequently, CO and the systolic LVP and AoP are strongly increased.

Fig. 1B displays the time course of AoP, MAoP, LVP, LAtP, ICT, IRT, aortic and mitral flow, and various LV variables during systole and part of diastole in resting conditions (58.7 s - 59.3 s). Note that the relatively large aortic flow in early systole.

The time course of the same variables, as in Fig. 1B, during systole and part of diastole after peripheral resistance decrease (exercise; 193.3 s - 193.9 s) is shown in Fig. 1C. Comparing Figs. 1B and 1C the following changes show up: due to vigorous LV contraction ICT is drastically shortened. Aortic flow is huge and occurs early in systole. Therefore SVLV is increased, but EDVLV decreased. Consequently the early diastolic LVP is negative!

The values of AoP, MAoP, CO, CVV, LAtP and ITP in normal (resting) conditions, after induction of aortic stenosis, after peripheral resistance decrease (exercise) and resetting

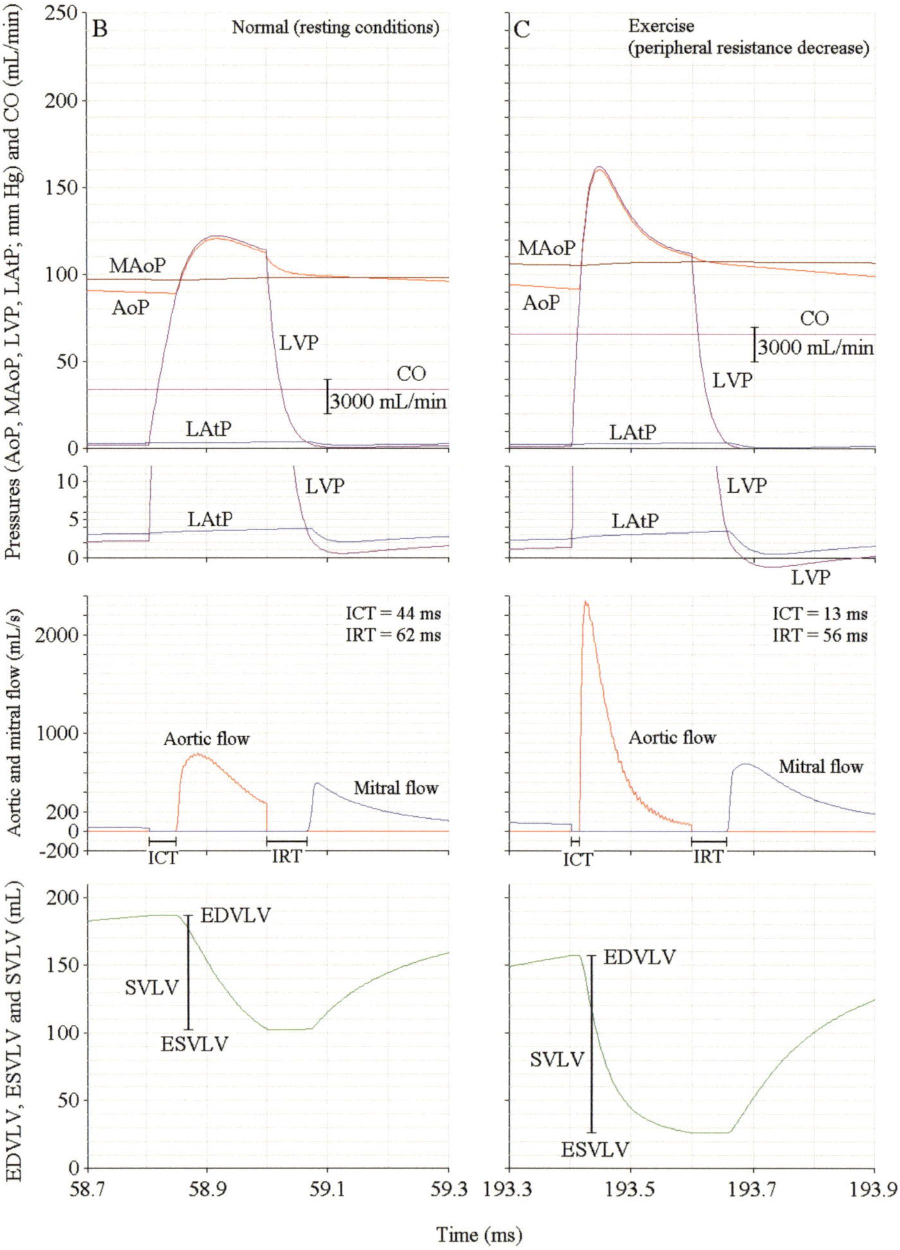

Fig. 1B, C. AoP, MAoP, LVP, LAtP, CO, (upper two blocks), aortic and mitral flow (middle block), and left ventricular volumes (bottom block) recorded during systole and part of diastole. B: Normal (resting) conditions (58.7 s - 59.3 s). Note the peak aortic flow in mid-systole and peak mitral flow in early diastole. C: Exercise (peripheral resistance decrease and MAoP reset; 193.3 s - 193.9 s). Due to a vigorous LV contraction ICT is decreased, EDVLV and ESVLV decreased and SVLV increased. Peak aortic flow occurs early in systole. Consequently, early diastolic LVP is slightly negative.

MAoP and, finally, after exhaustion of LV sympathetic drive and mild LV failure are shown in Fig. 2A. Initially (50 s - 70.5 s), all variables are in steady state. After aortic stenosis (at 70.5 s) the recorded variables are affected only transiently. After peripheral resistance decrease (100 s - 300 s) the initial brief AoP and MAoP decrease are offset by MAoP reset (increased sympathetic tone). Due to venoconstriction (CVV decrease) and huge increase in Sy the force and rate of LV contraction are increased. Heart rate is increased. Consequently, CO and the systolic LVP and AoP are strongly increased. At 200.5 s and 205.5 s, respectively, as Sy is decreased due to exhaustion and mild LV failure occurs, AoP, MAoP and CO decrease and LAtP is strongly increased.

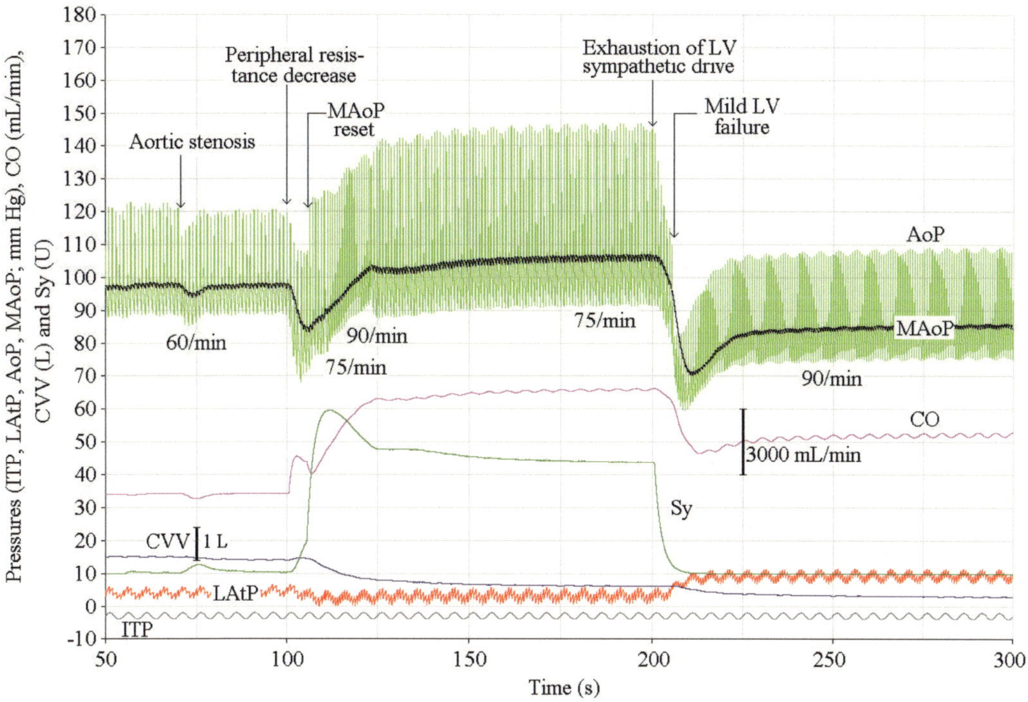

Fig. 2A. The time course of AoP, MAoP, heart rate, CO, Sy, CVV, LAtP and ITP in normal (resting) conditions, after aortic stenosis (0.08 U, at 70.5 s), after peripheral resistance decrease (exercise) and MAoP reset (by 50 % at 100.5 s and 105.5 s, respectively). Exhaustion of LV sympathetic drive and mild LV failure occur at 200.5 s and 205.5 s, respectively. Note that aortic stenosis has a small and transient effect, mainly in AoP only. The abrupt decrease in peripheral resistance results in a transient AoP and MAoP decrease and increase in heart rate from 60/min to 75/min. CO moderately increased, little change in CVV and LAtP. However, the resetting in MAoP results in a large Sy and CO increase. Heart rate is further increased (90/min). In steady state conditions of exercise the AoP and pulse amplitude are increased, MAoP about 108 mm Hg, CO almost doubled, LAtP slightly decreased, heart rate 75/min. Exhaustion of LV sympathetic drive (Sy decrease) and mild LV failure result in a AoP and MAoP decrease and a large LAtP increase. Heart rate is increased, CO is below exercise level, but above resting state level.

Fig. 2C shows the time course of cardiovascular variables (i.e. AoP, MAoP, LVP, LAtP, EDVLV, ESVLV and SVLV) during systole and part of diastole after aortic stenosis (93.7 s - 94.3 s). Note a relatively large aorto-ventricular pressure gradient. LAtP and EDVLV are slightly increased and ICT decreased. Aortic flow is evenly distributed through mid- and late systole. Fig. 2B is identical to Fig. 1B and is displayed together with Fig. 2C to illustrate the changes during aortic stenosis.
The changes in AoP, MAoP, LVP, LAtP, EDVLV, ESVLV and SVLV values induced by exercise in aortic stenosis are shown in Fig. 2D. The aorto-ventricular gradient is further increased. Due to vigorous LV contraction ICT is strongly decreased, therefore the peak of aortic flow occurs early in systole. Consequently, LAtP is slightly decreased and in early diastole LVP becomes negative. The effect of exhaustion of sympathetic drive and mild LV failure is simulated in Fig. 2E. Note the persistence of the aorto-ventricular gradient. ICT is slightly lengthened and, consequently, aortic flow proceeds late in systole. LAtP and EDVLV are increased.

4. Discussion

4.1 General comments

It should be pointed out that in present circuit i) a flow-dependent decrease in pulmonary vascular resistance is not simulated and ii) the control of peripheral (arteriolar) resistance is not included into the negative feedback. In principle it would be possible to include both features. However, this would considerably contribute to the complexity of the circuitry, without contributing very much to the understanding of underlying physiological mechanisms.
But despite the simplifications described above the negative feedback (incorporating the control of venous volume, of contractility of RV and LV, and of heart rate) seems to be quite similar to that controlling the human cardiovascular system (Berne & Levy, 1997; 1998; Germann & Stanfield, 2004; Guyton, 1966; Guyton et al., 1973; Guyton & Hall, 1996; Kusumoto, 2000).

4.2 Specific comments

It is well known that in man the resting MAoP can be reset from the normal to a higher level and then maintained by homeostatic mechanisms until required (e.g. in increased sympathetic tone, as a conditioned reflex before exercise, or during exercise; (Berne & Levy; 1997; Topham & Warner, 1967)). The resetting mechanism should include procedures whereby the resting MAoP, "clamped" at about 98 mm Hg is shifted and then "clamped" again at a higher level.
If MAoP is reset the main change is a temporary increase in heart rate and a moderate, steady state increase in CO and very slight decrease in CVV (Fig. 1A). Compared with resting conditions (MAoP about 98 mm Hg) it is clear that the increase of MAoP (to about 120 mm Hg) is due to a combination of slight venoconstriction and increased force of contraction of left ventricle (decreased early diastolic pressures, decreased EDVLV, strongly increased SVLV and its ejection fraction; Fig. 1B).
Animal experiments showed that in exercise the initiating factor is a decrease in peripheral resistance in working muscles, therefore MAoP is decreased. Consequently, through homeostatic mechanisms cardiac output is increased and MAoP reset to a higher level (Topham & Warner, 1967).

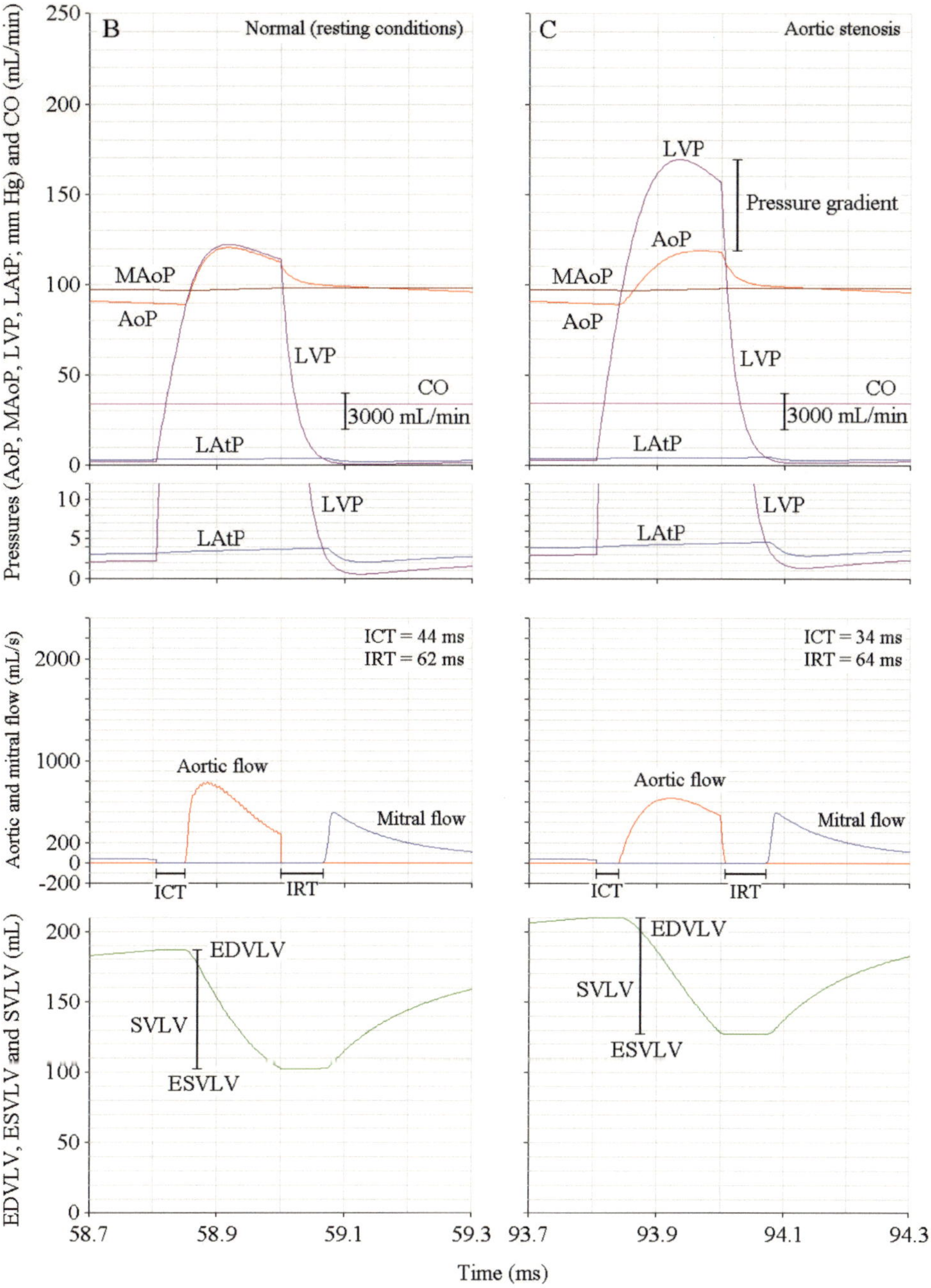

Fig. 2B, C: AoP, MAoP, LVP, LAtP, CO (upper two blocks), aortic and mitral flow (middle block), and left ventricular volumes (bottom block) recorded during systole and part of diastole. B: Normal (resting) conditions (58.7 s - 59.3 s). Note the peak aortic flow in mid-systole and peak mitral flow in early diastole. C: Aortic stenosis (93.7 s - 94.3 s). Note a pressure gradient (about 50 mm Hg) between AoP and LVP. A slight LAtP and EDVLV increase and ICT decrease. Peak aortic flow is shifted to late systole.

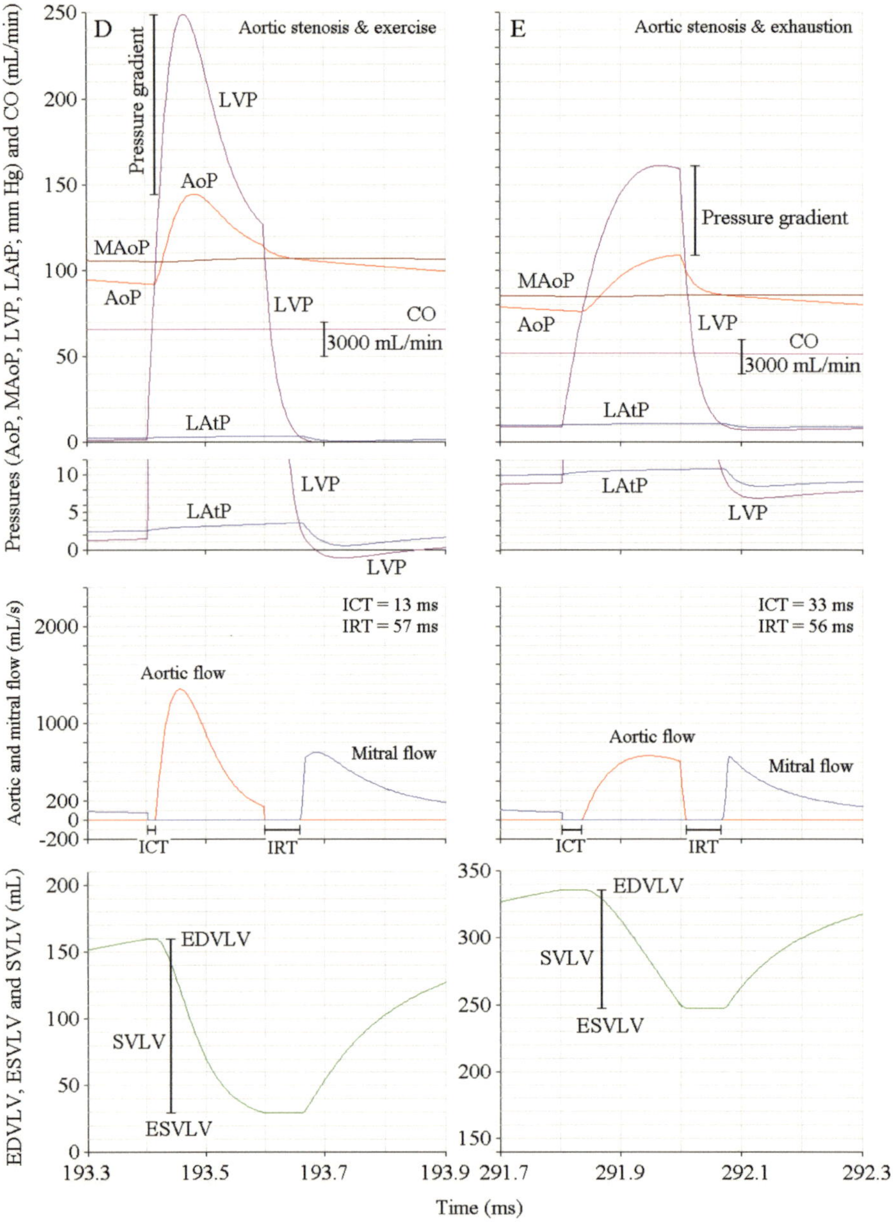

Fig. 2D, E: AoP, MAoP, LVP, LAtP, CO (upper two blocks), aortic and mitral flow (middle block), and left ventricular volumes (bottom block) recorded during systole and part of diastole. D: Aortic stenosis and exercise (193.3 s - 193.9 s). Note a huge pressure gradient (about 100 mm Hg) between AoP and LVP. Due to a vigorous LV contraction ICT is further decreased; peak aortic flow in about mid-systole. Early diastolic LVP slightly negative. E: Aortic stenosis, exhaustion and mild LV failure (291.7 s - 292.3 s). The pressure gradient (about 50 mm Hg) persists. Note a strong LAtP and EDVLV increase. Peak aortic flow is in late systole.

In this investigation exercise is simulated by decreasing arteriolar and capillary resistance by 50 % and by resetting MAoP (Fig. 1A, B, C). Transient phenomena in these variables are over in about 30 s. Steady state conditions are established where AoP, MAoP, CO and heart rate are about 160/92 mm Hg, 108 mm Hg, 9930 ml/min and 75/min, respectively. Strongly decreased CVV and slightly decreased LAtP. The time course of AoP, MAoP, LVP, LAtP, CO and SVLV during the early part of the heart cycle are shown in Fig. 1B, C. Compared to resting conditions the force and rate of contraction of left ventricle is highly increased, thus increasing SVLV and its ejection fraction. Qualitatively, simulation results described are quite similar to those obtained in experimental animal (Topham & Warner, 1967). Quantitatively, compared to simulation, the main dissimilarity is the fact that in experimental animal and man in exercise the range of heart rate is large, about 60/min to 180/min (Topham & Warner, 1967; Berne & Levy, 1997). In this simulation the range of heart rate is much less (60/min - 75/min - 90/min); in steady state conditions heart rate is 75/min. If the range of heart rate is increased (60/min - 90/min - 120/min) in steady state conditions heart rate is 90/min. However, results are similar in both heart rate settings (cf. also Table 1). In steady state conditions AoP, MAoP, CO and heart rate are about 150/95 mm Hg, 109 mm Hg, 10100 ml/min and 90/min, respectively. This is because in this model the heart rate/cardiac output curve is very flat, as shown earlier (Podnar et al., 2002); an increase in heart rate from 90/min to 120/min results in a comparatively small increase in CO.

At rest + aortic stenosis				
HR	LVP	MAoP	AoP	CO
in steady state conditions				
min^{-1}	(mm Hg)			ml/min
60	170/3	98	118/90	5145

Exercise + aortic stenosis					
HR		LVP	MAoP	AoP	CO
Maximum during transient	in steady state conditions				
min^{-1}	min^{-1}	(mm Hg)			ml/min
90	75	248/1.5	106	145/92	9900
120	90	220/1.0	108	137/95	10125

Table 1. The effect of aortic stenosis (at rest and in exercise) on heart rate (HR), pressure in the left ventricle (LVP: ventricular maximum/end-distolic), mean aortic pressure (MAoP), aortic pressure (systolic/diastolic; AoP) and cardiac output (CO).

Aortic stenosis is a chronic disturbance compensated by long-term cardiovascular control mechanisms. Clinically, it can be subdivided into valvular, subvalvular, and supravalvular variant. However, for a successful simulation of these variants additional data - on magnitude and on the distribution – of resistance and elastance (capacitance) would be required. As they are not available, present simulations apply to the valvular variant of aortic stenosis only.

If the patient featuring aortic stenosis is exercised the short-term control mechanisms are invoked. Thus, it would be of interest to make use of the present equivalent electronic circuit, to modify it according to this pathology. Data obtained by simulation could be compared with data obtained in clinical examination in man. A similarity in results could show a wider applicability of analogue simulation and possibly contribute to the understanding of homeostasis in this particular situation. In man, the effect of aortic stenosis on cardiovascular variables was studied at rest, in exercise and in conditions of pharmacologically induced decreased peripheral resistance (Anderson et al., 1969; Arshad et al., 2004; Bache et al., 1971; Diver et al., 1988; Huber et al. 1981; Peterson et al., 1978; Vanoverschelde et al., 1992).

Simulation of this clinical condition is shown in Fig. 2A. On increasing aortic resistance only a transient, small decrease in AoP shows up. Shortly afterwards exercise (decrease in peripheral resistance) results in a decrease in AoP and MAoP and increase in heart rate to 75/min. However, as soon as MAoP is reset heart rate is further increased to 90/min. Consequently, AoP and pulse amplitude increase. In steady state conditions heart rate is 75/min, AoP and MAoP are about 145/92 mm Hg and 106 mm Hg, respectively. CO is almost doubled, CVV strongly and LAtP slightly decreased. However, as soon as the sympathetic drive is decreased and mild LV failure induced, CO is decreased and LAtP strongly increased.

The time course of AoP, MAoP, LVP, LAtP, CO and SVLV during the early part of a heart cycle is shown for normal conditions in Fig. 2B and for aortic stenosis in Fig. 2C. It results in an increased force and velocity of contraction of left ventricle. This is shown by a decrease in ICT. The ventriculo-aortic pressure gradient is about 50 mm Hg. Because LAtP is slightly increased, EDVLV is slightly increased and CO is almost normal. Note that aortic stenosis results in a slower time course of aortic flow.

If in this condition peripheral resistance is decreased and MAoP reset (Fig. 2D) the ventriculo-aortic pressure gradient is increased to almost 100 mm Hg. LAtP is almost normal, EDLVL decreased and its ejection fraction strongly increased. Aortic flow is increased, but featuring a much slower time course.

Data obtained in patients (Anderson et al., 1969; Bache et al., 1971; Diver et al., 1988; Huber et al. 1981; Peterson et al., 1978; Vanoverschelde et al., 1992) showed that in some patients exercise resulted in a large, while in other patients in a very small increase in heart rate. It would be thus of interest to asses - at the same aortic resistance - the effect of heart rate on the ventriculo-aortic pressure gradient, aortic pressure and pulse pressure. Therefore, beside the frequency range 60/min, 75/min and 90/min another simulation is performed in which range of frequencies 60/min, 90/min and 120/min is used. Data obtained in steady state conditions and during transient phenomenon are summarised in Table 1.

Ventriculo-aortic pressure gradient, aortic pressure, pulse pressure and cardiac output are affected by heart rate, but differences are relatively small.

Investigations on aortic stenosis in patients showed that the average left ventricular end-diastolic pressure (LVEDP) was 12 mm Hg at rest and 20 mm Hg in exercise (Bache et al., 1971). But individual patient data showed that LVEDP at rest may have been quite low (3 mm Hg; Anderson et al., 1969). This is very close to that LVEDP recorded in simulations above. However, almost as a rule, in exercising patients LVEDP regularly increased (7 mm Hg; Anderson et al., 1969) in some patients quite high, 36 mm Hg (Bache et al., 1971) or even 41 mm Hg (Anderson et al., 1969). In simulations however, in aortic stenosis and exercise

LVEDP does not change or is slightly decreased. In explaining this simulation phenomenon it should be remembered that LVEDP is a variable depending on various (homeostatically controlled) parameters. If in exercise predominantly the contractility of LV is increased, LVEDP tends to decrease. On the contrary, if in exercise venoconstriction predominates, LVEDP will tend to increase. In patients with aortic stenosis in exercise the latter compensatory mechanism is more likely to occur.
It is clear that simulation data agree well - qualitatively, sometimes even quantitatively - with data obtained in patients (Anderson et al., 1969; Bache et al., 1971; Diver et al., 1988; Huber et al. 1981; Peterson et al., 1978; Vanoverschelde et al., 1992) or in patients with hypertrophic cardiomyopathy and outflow tract gradient (Geske et al., 2007, 2009; Sorajja et al. 2008).
Exhaustion of LV sympathethetic drive and mild LV failure is simulated in Fig. 2A and 2D. As expected, the aorto-ventricular gradient persists and pulmonary congestion is quite pronounced. EDVLV is increased and aortic flow with a very slow time course. It seems that these changes contribute to the understanding of homeostasis and its failure in exercise, the syncope, a frequent complication.

5. Conclusions

A computer analysis of an equivalent electronic circuit is developed to simulate the human cardiovascular system and its homeostatic control. Thus the response of the system can be studied if the latter is acted upon by various disturbances. In present simulation these are
- exercise in normal conditions and
- exercise in a subject featuring aortic stenosis, including exhaustion of compensatory mechanisms.

Exercise is simulated by a decrease in peripheral resistance and by an increase in sympathetic tone (resetting the mean aortic pressure to a higher level).
In exercise in normal conditions, through negative feedback, cardiac output, systolic aortic pressure, force and frequency of left ventricle contraction, are increased. The time course of aortic flow reflects changes of left ventricle contraction dynamics. Mean aortic pressure is mildly increased. There is almost no change in diastolic aortic pressure.
In exercise in aortic stenosis, through negative feedback, similar changes occur as described above. However, in these conditions the dominant feature is a large aorto ventricular pressure gradient, almost doubling the systolic left ventricular pressure. It can be assumed that the latter results in an exhaustion of sympathetic (inothropic) mechanism(s). The final result is a decrease in aortic pressure, a sluggish aortic flow and pulmonary congestion.
It seems that consequences of i) exercise and ii) exercise in aortic stenosis can be qualitatively successfully simulated (resembling actual clinical conditions), including an exhaustion of compensatory mechanisms. Quantitatively, however, there are minor differences, because many quantitative data on human cardiovascular system are still lacking.

6. References

Adams, J. (2001). *Mastering Electronics Workbench*. McGraw-Hill, ISBN 978-0071344838, New York.

Anderson, F.L.; Tsagaris, T.J.; Tikoff, G.; Thorne, J.L.; Schmidt, A.M. & Kuida, H. (1969). Hemodynamic effects of exercise in patients with aortic stenosis. *The American Journal of Medicine,* Vol.46, pp. 872-885, ISSN 0002-9343

Arshad, W.; Duncan, A.M.; Francis, D.P.; O'Sullivan, C.A.; Gibson, D.G. & Henein, M.Y. (2004). Systole-diastole mismatch in hypertrophic cardiomyopathy is caused ba stress induced left ventricular outflow tract obstruction. *American Heart Journal,* Vol.148, pp. 903-909, ISSN 0002-8703

Bache, R.J.; Wang, Y. & Jorgensen, C.R. (1971) Hemodynamic effects of exercise in isolated valvular aortic stenosis. *Circulation,* Vol.44, pp. 1003-1013, ISSN 0009-7322

Beneken, J.E.W. (1965) *A mathematical approach to cardiovascular function. The uncontrolled human system.* Institute of Medical Physics, Da Costakade 45, Utrecht.

Berne, R.M. & Levy, M.N. (1998). *Physiology,* 4th ed. ISBN 0-8016-6465-9, St. Louis: Mosby.

Berne, R.M. & Levy, M.N. (1997). *Cardiovascular physiology,* 7th ed., ISBN 0-8151-0901-6, Mosby, St. Louis.

Bošnjak, R. & Kordaš, M. (2002). Circulatory effects of internal jugular vein compression: a computer simulation study. *Medical & Biological Engineering & Computing,* Vol.40, No.4, pp. 423-431, ISSN 0140-0118

Diver, D.J.; Royal, H.D.; Aroesty, J.M.; McKay, R.G.; Ferguson, J.J., Warren, S.E. & Lorell, B.H. (1988). Diastolic function in patients with aortic stenosis: Influence of left ventricular load reduction. *Journal of the American College of Cardiology,* Vol.12, pp. 642-648, ISSN 0735-1097

Defares, J.G.; Osborn, J.J. & Hara, H.H. (1963). Theoretical synthesis of the cardiovascular system. Study I: The controlled system. *Acta Physiologica et Pharmacologica Neerlandica,* Vol.12, pp. 189-265, ISSN 0001-6748

Dolenšek, J.; Runovc, F. & Kordaš, M. (2005). Simulation of pulmonary ventilation and its control by negative feedback. *Computers in Biology and Medicine,* Vol.35, No.3, pp. 217-228, ISSN 0010-4825

Dolenšek, J.; Podnar, T.; Runovc, F. & Kordaš, M. (2009). Analog simulation of aortic and of mitral regurgitation. *Computers in Biology and Medicine,* Vol.39, pp. 474-481, ISSN 0010-4825

Germann, W. & Stanfield, C. (2004). *Principles of human physiology,* 2nd ed. Pearson Education Ltd., Harlow, 2004.

Geske, J.B.; Sorajja, P.; Nishimura, R.A. & Ommen, R.S. (2007). Evaluation of left ventricular filling pressures by Doppler Echocardiography in patients with hypertrophic cardiomyopathy: Correlation with direct left atrial pressure measurement az cardiac catheterization. *Circulation,* Vol.116, pp. 2702-2708, ISSN 0009-7322

Geske, J.B.; Sorajja, P.; Ommen, R.S. & Nishimura, R.A. (2009). Left ventricular outflow tract gradient variability in hypertrophic cardiomyopathy. Clinical Cardiology, Vol.32, pp. 397-402, ISSN 0160-9289

Grodins, F.S. (1959) Integrative cardiovascular physiology: A mathematical synthesis of cardiac and blood vessels haemodynamics. *The Quarterly Review of Biology,* Vol.34, No.2, (June), pp.93-116, ISSN 0033-5770

Guyton, A.C. (1966). *Textbook of medical physiology*. W.B. Saunders Company, Philadelphia.

Guyton, A.C.; Jones, C.E. & Coleman, T.G. (1973) *Circulatory physiology: Cardiac output and its Regulation*. ISBN 978-0721643601, W.B. Saunders, Philadelphia

Guyton, A.C. & Hall, J.E. (1996). Textbook of medical physiology. 9th ed. ISBN 978-0721659442, W.B Saunders Company

Huber, D.; Grimm, J.; Koch, R. & Krayenbuehl, H.P. (1981) Determinants of ejection performance in aortic stenosis. *Circulation*, Vol.64, pp. 126-134, ISSN 0009-7322

Kordaš, M.; Trontelj, J. & Leonardis, S. (1968). An electrical model of blood circulation. *Medical & Biological Engineerin*, Vol.6, No.4, pp. 449-451, ISSN 0025-696X

Kusumoto, F. (2000). Cardiovascular Disorders: Heart Disease. In: *Pathophysiology of disease. An introduction to clinical medicine*, McPhee, S.J.; Lingappa, V.R.; Ganong, W. & Lange, J.D. (Eds.), 222-257, Lange Medical Books/McGraw-Hill, ISBN 0-07-112004-1, New York

Milhorn, H.T. (1966). *The application of control theory to physiological systems*. Saunders, Philadelphia, London

Osborn, J.J.; Hoehne, W. & Badia, W. (1967). Ventricular function in the basic regulation of the circulation: Studies with a mechanical analog. In: *Physical bases of circulatory transport. Regulation and exchange*, Reeve, E.B. & Guyton, A.C, (Eds.), 47-60, W.B. Saunders, Philadelphia

Peterson, K.L.; Tsuji, J.; Johnson, A.; DiDonna, J. & LeWinter, M. (1978). Diastolic left ventricular pressure-volume and sterss-strain relation in patients with valvular aortic stenosis and left ventricular hypertrophy. *Circulation*, Vol.58, pp. 77-89, ISSN 0009-7322

Podnar, T.; Runovc, F. & Kordaš, M. (2002). Simulation of cardiovascular physiology: the diastolic function(s) of the heart. *Computers in Biology and Medicine*, Vol.32, pp. 363-377, ISSN 0010-4825

Podnar, T.; Runovc, F.; Milisav, I. & Kordaš, M. (2004) Simulation of some short-term control mechanisms in cardiovascular physiology. *Computers in Biology and Medicine* Vol.34, pp. 35-49, ISSN 0010-4825

Rupnik, M.; Runovc, F.; Sket, D. & Kordaš, M. (2002). Cardiovascular physiology: Simulation of steady state and transient phenomena by using the equivalent electronic circuit. *Computer Methods and Programs in Biomedicine*, Vol. 67, pp. 1-12, ISSN 0169-2607

Sever, M.; Podnar, T.; Runovc, F. & Kordaš, M. (2007). Analog simulation of two clinical condition: (1) Acute left ventricle failure; (2) exercise in patient with aortic stenosis. *Computers in Biology and Medicine*, Vol.37, pp. 1051-1062, ISSN 0010-4825

Sorajja, P.; Nishimura, R.A.; Ommen, S.R.; Charanjit, S.R., Gersh, B.J. & Holmes, D.R. (2008). Effect of septal ablation on myocardial relaxation and left atrial pressure in hypetrophic Cardiomyopathy. JACC: Cardiovascular Interventions, Vol.1, pp. 552-560, ISSN 1936-8798

Topham, S. & Warner, H.R. (1967). The control of cardiac output during exercise, In: *Physical bases of circulatory transport. Regulation and exchange*. Reeve, E.B & Guyton, A.C. (Eds.), 77-90, W. B. Saunders, Philadelphia

Vanoverschelde, J.L.; Essamri, B.; Michel, X.; Hanet, C.; Cosyns, J.R.; Detry, J-M.R. & Wijns, W. (1992). Hemodynamic and volume correlates of left ventricular diastolic relaxation and filling in patients with aortic stenosis. *Journal of the American College of Cardiology*, Vol. 20, pp. 813–821, ISSN 0735-1097

Part 4

Surgical and Interventional Treatments

7

Minimally Invasive Aortic Valve Surgery - New Solutions to Old Problems

Juan Bustamante, Sergio Cánovas and Ángel L Fernández
Hospital Universitario La Princesa, Madrid
Hospital General Universitario de Valencia &
Hospital Clinico Universitario de Santiago de Compostela
Spain

1. Introduction

Aortic stenosis is the most frequent valvulopathy in the western world and basically affects people over 60 years old. It is currently the most common cause of valve replacement in Europe and North America (Schmitto et al., 2011) and its incidence increases with age. (Lung et al., 2003) 25% of people over 65 suffer sclerosis of the aortic valve which can be detected in image tests such as echocardiography and 3% of those over 75 develop aortic stenosis (Lindroos et al., 1993; Stewart et al., 1997).

Approximately 16% of patients with aortic valve sclerosis develop stenosis within the space of 7 years. (Cosmi et al., 2002) This rate of progression is variable and has been related with factors common to those for arterial sclerosis. The average reduction in the valve area has been stated as being around 0.1 cm^2 per year. (Otto et al., 1997) and the annual increase in gradient as about 10 mmHg.

Rheumatic etiology is not common in the more developed countries and its origin is usually degenerative. In approximately half of the cases there usually exists a bicuspid aortic valve basis. Bicuspid aortic valve valvulopathy affects 2% of the population (Kurtz & Otto, 2010) and constitutes the most frequent congenital anomaly. Aortic valve stenosis is more prevalent in men than women (Chambers et al., 2009).

This disease normally remains asymptomatic for a long time and represents a low sudden death risk of less than 1%. When stenosis becomes symptomatic, however, the prognosis is much worse. The symptoms usually appear at the end of the disease with three of them being typical and each one of them determining a state which is both evolutionary and prognostic: dyspnea (due to heart faillure), angina and syncope. In aortic stenosis there co-exist three physiological phenomena: cardiac ischemia, elevated pressure in the left ventricle and diminished cardiac output.

Diminished tolerance to exercise is generally the first symptom of aortic stenosis and could be the result of the three previously mentioned phenomena. A careful medical history investigation is necessary in order to obtain this information as the earliest clinical signs may be insidious and may not be accompanied by dyspnea as such, and may be consciously or unconsciously disguised by the patient in the progressive restriction of their day-to-day activity as the disease develops.

The classic symptoms of aortic stenosis, angina, syncope and dyspnea due to cardiac insufficiency, are associated with high mortality (survival rate of 4-5 years, 2-3 years and 1-2 years respectively). These symptoms do not need to appear with a specific time sequence (Lester et al ., 1998).

The commencement of the symptoms predicts an increase in mortality in the evolution of the disease and constitutes as such an indication for surgical treatment. Symptoms are not always related with the seriousness of the stenosis; that is to say with the valve area and the transvalvular gradients. Otto et al (Otto et al., 1997) in a 123 asymptomatic patient study established, by means of a uni-variant analysis, baseline aortic velocity, the ratio of increase in velocity and the functional class as being the predictive factors for the commencement of symptoms. Pellikka et al (Pellikka et al., 2005) and Rosenhek et al (Rosenhek et al., 2000) point out the jet velocity and the severity of valve calcification as indications of a bad prognosis.

	Severe Aortic Stenosis	Moderate Aortic Stenosis	Mild Aortic Stenosis	Aortic sclerosis
Aortic jet velocity (m/s)	>4	3-4	2.6-3	<2.6
Mean gradient (mmHg)	>50 (40)	30–50 (25–40)	<30 (25)	-
Indexed AVA (cm^2/m^2)	<0.6	0.6-0.9	>0.9	-
AVA (cm^2)	<1	1-1.5	>1.5	-
Velocity ratio	<0.25	0.25–0.50	>0.50	-

Table 1. Classification of the severity of aortic stenosis.

Based on the ASE/EAE Recommendations for Quantitation of Stenosis Severity, (Baumgartner et al., 2009) ESC Valve Guidelines, (Vahanian et al., 2007) and American College of Cardiology/American Heart Association (ACC/ AHA) Valve Guidelines. (Bonow et al., 2008) ACC/AHA guidelines use lower mean gradient cutoffs as indicated in parentheses. The ESC definitions apply only in the presence of normal flow conditions. The velocity ratio is included in the ASE/EAE guidelines only.

2. Minimally invasive surgical approaches

These can be divided into two basic groups: those that have been classified as mini-sternotomies, and those that are carried out by means of a mini-thoracotomy.

Minimally invasive surgery, as has already been pointed out, is more of a concept than a specific a surgical approach and its aim is to minimise the degree of surgical intrusiveness. Thus, such approaches are numerous, with some having been described previously in the historical background review. Their outcomes generally overlap and the decision to adopt one or other technique largely depends on the clinical characteristics of the patient in question or the experience and expertise of the centre where the technique is carried out. The table below summarises the various possible techniques.

Partial sternotomy	
	Para-sternal incision (Cohn et al., 1997; Navia & Cosgrove 1996)
	Trans-sternal incision (Cohn et al., 1997)
	Upper sternotomy (Byrne et al., 2000)
	T mini-sternotomy (Stamou et al., 2003)
	V-shaped incision (Corbi et al., 2003)
	Inverted L incision (Stamou et al., 2003)
	Reversed L incision (Detter et al., 2002)
	J incision (Cohn et al., 1997; Doll et al., 2002)
	Reversed C incision
	Inverted T incision (Farhat et al., 2003)
Thoracotomy	
	Right anterior thoracotomy 2° or 3° inter-costal space (Burfeind et al., 2002)
	Right anterior thoracotomy 4° or 5° inter-costal space (Sharony et al., 2003)
Video-assisted vision	
	Port access (Galloway et al., 1999)
Video-direct vision	
	AESOP 3000 (Computer Motion, Goleta, CA) (Falk et al., 1998)
	Da Vinci System (Intuitive Surgical, Sunnyvale, CA) (Carpentier et al., 1998)
	Zeus (Computer Motion, Goleta, CA) (Cohn et al., 1997)

Table 2. Minimally Invasive Approaches.

At present, a partial upper sternotomy is the most frequently used incision for a minimally invasive approach to the aortic valve. (Ehrlich et al., 2000). In the case of a thoracotomy approach, this is usually carried out via a parasternal incision over the second and third inter-costal space, which is of 6 to 10 centimetres long, and then proceeds with the re-sectioning of the costal cartilages, finally arriving at the pericardial aperture (Cohn et al., 1997).
Other approaches include a partial upper sternotomy with central cannulation, transverse sternotomy, limited sternotomy with a J-incision, right-sided partial sternotomy, reversed L sternotomy, and a limited right thoracotomy for aortic valve replacement (AVR). (Cosgrove et al., 1998; Izzat et al., 1998; Konertz et al., 1996; Svensson et al., 1996; Svensson et al., 1997; Tam et al., 1998; Walther et al., 1999). The most frequently used techniques can be seen in the following figures.

3. Background to minimally invasive surgery

Surgical treatment of valvulopathies was one of the most important medical advances of the twentieth century. This advance began in 1923 with the closed mitral commissurotomy of Cutler and has continued until the present day with the implanting of more complex hemodynamic prostheses with approaches different from the conventional ones. Aortic valve replacement has permitted thousands of lives to be saved since it was first successfully carried out by Harken and Starr in 1960 (Harken et al., 1961; Starr & Edwards, 1961).
Cardiac surgery for the treatment of valvulopathies has also advanced considerably through the improvement of various aspects such as circulatory support, myocardial protection measures and, of course, the development of new surgical approaches that have come to be called minimally invasive, which tend to be less surgically intrusive and which will be dealt with later in this text.

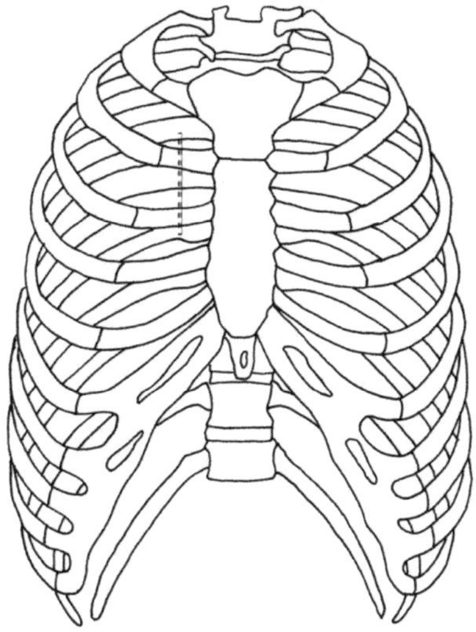

Fig. 1. Right anterior thoracotomy 2°

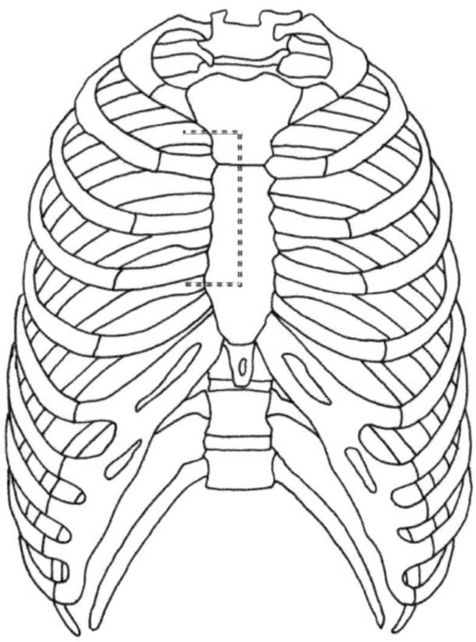

Fig. 2. Reversed C incision 3° inter-costal space

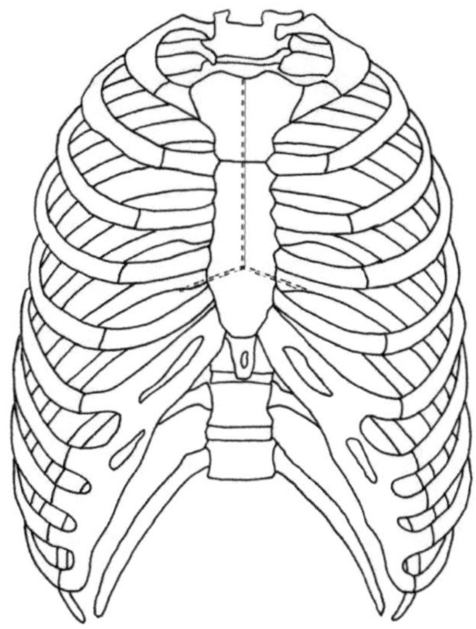

Fig. 3. T mini-sternotomy

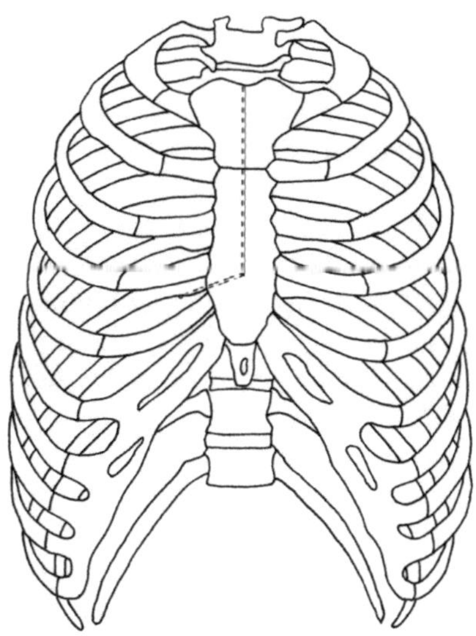

Fig. 4. Reversed L incision

Initially it was in other fields of surgery such as obstetrics, thoracic surgery, urology or general surgery where minimally invasive approaches were developed but they have finally been incorporated into the area of cardiac surgery with their late incorporation largely being due to the very characteristics of this speciality (Cohn et al., 1997).

The traditional approach to the treatment of aortic valvulopathy was based on sternotomy with arterial cannulation in the ascendant aorta and venous cannulation in the right atrium. As time passed and surgical techniques developed and improved the objective of reducing surgical aggression by means of using minimally invasive approaches arose. Normal sternotomy has the advantage of a direct view of all the cardiac structures and likewise access to them when compared with other approaches.

It has recently been postulated that the use of partial sternotomy in its various forms or mini-thoracotomy, by virtue of being a less intrusive method, could minimise the risk of infection in the wound, loss of blood and postoperative pain without putting surgical results at risk. (Cuenca et al., 1998).

Minimally invasive surgery in the realm of cardiac pathologies began with the use of slight thoracotomies without extra-corporal circulation in order to carry out myocardial re-vascularisation, without circulatory support, fundamentally on the front face of the heart (Benetti et al., 1991; Buffolo et al., 1996; Arom et al., 1996, Subramanian et al., 1995; Califiore et al., 1997).

At the same time the system of Port-Access from Heartport, Inc., Redwood City, CA, (Stevens et al., 1996) was being developed for the carrying out of myocardial re-vascularisation with cardiac arrest and endovascular clamping. Eventually the development of minimally invasive techniques was incorporated into the treatment of valvulopathies.

The development of minimally invasive approaches for the treatment of mitral and aortic pathologies has occurred simultaneously, but here the focus is on aortic approaches.

In contrast with minimally invasive myocardial re-vascularisation surgery, which requires special resources and exhaustive training, aortic valvulopathy treatment, originally described by Dr. Cosgrove of the Cleveland Clinic, does not require either special equipment or extensive training.

Thus it was that minimally invasive surgery began to be incorporated into the field of cardiac surgery in the 1990s. Some of the first reports of this approach were made by Cosgrove, Minale and Hirose. In the following years the application of the technique and the means for carrying it out had improved considerably, as will later be seen, guaranteeing good results that were comparable with those obtained through a traditional surgical approach.

In 1996 Cosgrove and Sabik described a technique with which it was possible to effect aortic valve replacement by means of a mini-thoracotomy through a right parasternal incision 10 cm long. In the technique that they described they performed the peripheral cannulation by means of the femoral artery and vein. The incision ran from the lower edge of the second rib cartilage to the upper edge of the fifth rib cartilage. Then the main pectoral muscle was dissected and the third and fourth rib cartilages were resected. The internal mammary artery was bound just below the second and above the fifth rib cartilage. The inter-costal muscles and the pleura were opened at the edge of the sternum and the pericardium was incised allowing the ascendant aorta to be exposed (Cosgrove & Sabik, 1996).

About the same time, Hirose described left side thoractomy for the treatment of aortic valvulopathy (Hirose et al., 1994).

Since then there has been a growing interest in minimally invasive approaches due to the results observed. In 1997 Minale et al reported on a series of 27 patients where a right parasternal technique with an 8 cm long incision was used. This group accessed the thoracic cavity through the third inter-costal space. The internal mammary artery was tied and sectioned. These authors carried out cannulation on the ascendant aorta and the atrial appendage in order to avoid dissecting the femoral vessels and the morbidity that goes with this (Minale et al., 1997).

In 1998 Izzat described another process for the treatment of aortic valvulopathy by means of upper T mini-sternotomy. In the first series that he published he included 9 patients. This technique was carried out by making a 6 cm vertical incision from two finger widths below the sternal fork to the area adjacent to the fourth rib. They performed an upper mini-sternotomy and it was extended laterally and caudally to the level of the third inter-costal space. One of the potential benefits of this procedure was to avoid tying the mammary vessels as well as not having to dissect femoral vessels. It had the advantage that, in case of any complications related with the technique, it could be extended and converted into a complete sternotomy in a short space of time (Izzat et al., 1998).

Other similar approaches with the same aim were also described at that time, such as that of Konertz et al, which proposed a technique by means of a sternotomy in J in order to reduce intrusion (Konertz et al., 1996).

Rodriguez et al described a series of 25 patients upon whom the technique of an inverted 'L' mini-sternotomy through an upper sternal incision for cardiac operations was used. An 8 cm vertical incision was made and then extended laterally to the right to the level of the third or fourth inter-costal space (Rodríguez et al., 1996).

While surgeons have been developing new focal points for surgical techniques, the medical industry has also been capable of putting specifically designed stents, instruments, devices and equipment at their disposal for this therapeutic technique, allowing it to be simplified and improving its results as well as broadcasting them and making them more accessible.

4. Characteristics of minimally invasive surgery

4.1 Definition

The Society of Thoracic Surgeons National Database defines minimally invasive surgery as "any procedure that has not been performed with a full sternotomy and cardiopulmonary bypass support. All other procedures, on or off pump with a small incision or off pump with a full sternotomy are considered minimally invasive." (STS National Database, 2003).

This definition can lead to contradictions depending on the type of approach and the different forms of cannulation used to carry out the surgery. For example, should a mitral valve replacement via a mini-thoracotomy with peripheral femoral and jugular cannulation be considered a minimally invasive procedure? Faced with this problem Chitwood suggests that the concept of minimally invasive surgery is not limited to a specific approach, but is a philosophy in surgical treatment which aims to reduce the degree of surgical aggression (Chitwood & Gulielmos, 2003).

In the case of coronary pathology the focus of minimally invasive surgery is on surgical approaches and the extraction of transplants using endoscopic systems, but it also includes circulatory support. The intention is to avoid extra-corporal circulation which is one of the most serious surgical aggressions due to the inflammatory response it provokes. However, in the case of valve surgery, extra-corporal circulation is necessary in order to be able to carry out the surgical procedure, so a less invasive approach is not possible. Attempts to reduce aggression have therefore been centred on the surgical approaches.

There are many options in terms of ways to carry out the procedure using a minimally invasive approach. We must consider, for example, the location of the cannulations (central or peripheral), the type of aortal clamping (external or endovascular) and the form of administering the cardioplegia (antegrade, retrograde or direct via the coronary ostium). All these variants make it difficult to compare results between the different published studies, due to the heterogeneity, not only of the procedures, but also of the sample groups analysed.

4.2 Anaesthesia - Cannulation

Preoperative preparation in patients about to undergo a minimally invasive procedure is similar to that for conventional surgery, with some small differences such as: 1) selective pulmonary intubation in some of the approaches, this tends to be restricted to approaches via mini-thoracotomy for treating mytral tricuspid and congenital pathologies, and some processes involving tumours. 2) The necessity to monitor the pressure curve in both radial arteries if an endoclamp® is used. 3) In the case of approach via mini-thoracotomy the patient should be placed in the supine position with a slight elevation of the right hemithorax by placing the roll at the level of the right shoulder in order to facilitate exposure.

The routine use of transesophageal echocardiography is necessary not only to assess the results of the intervention and the purging of air from the cardiac cavities but also to monitor the correct positioning of the cannulas. It is also necessary to install external defibrillator paddles as, given the size of the incision, it may not be possible to insert even paediatric paddles. It is also necessary to consider the possible limits to their effectiveness due to the poor contact with the epicardial surface (Woo et al., 2007).

4.3 Cannulation

Cannulation will depend on the type of procedure undertaken, the approach used and the experience of the team. In the beginning peripheral cannulation was used, as described by Cosgrove. That approach required the dissection of the femoral vessels. Many groups opt for direct cannulation in mininvasive procedures both with partial sternotomy and with mini-thoracotomy to avoid morbidity and reduce surgical aggression. On the other hand, as surgical teams have gained experience it has been possible to apply central cannulation without significant reduction to visibility in the operating field, and without significant increase in technical difficulty.

Direct

The cannulation of the ascendant aorta, close to the aortic arch, is to facilitate exposure selecting a zone free of plaques.

Peripheral

Through an incision in the femoral region the femoral vessels are dissected, isolating the vessels and proceeding to direct cannulation. Another option is percutaneous cannulation (Seldinger technique). It must be borne in mind that in the case of carrying out the procedure by Heart Port and endovascular clamping using endoclamp, larger gauge cannulas, for example 23 F, may be necessary. In these cases it is important to carefully assess the vascular tree using a transesophageal echocardiogram, to rule out the existence of arteriosclerosis or aortic aneurysm. Some teams recommend a prior arteriograph or angio-CT scan. It is important to consider the patient's body surface area, which will be in accordance with the diameter of the vascular tree.

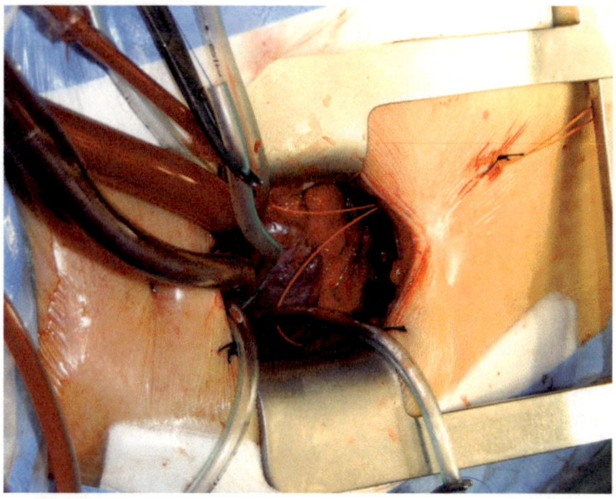

Fig. 5. Image showing central cannulation through a mini-sternotomy in the ascendant aorta and superior vena cava.

4.4 Field of vision

The operating field is reduced, and with it the accessibility of the different structures. This means that the surgeon must be more dexterous. Different studies have shown that minimally invasive approaches are a safe therapeutic option and that the results of the procedure need not be affected. In the case of approach via mini-thoracotomy, the procedure is guided by a video camera, with the video thoracoscope being placed via another access port, generally at the level of the second inter-costal space. The use of articulated arms enables the image to be stabilised correctly (Lopez- Gude et al., 2010). In the case of patients operated on using the mini-sternotomy it is possible to improve the operating field through the insertion of stitches in the valvular commisures that exercise traction in order to elevate the valvular plane, this technique enables an approximation of almost 5 cm with respect to the plane of the incision (Aris et al., 1997).

4.5 Transesophageal echocardiogram

Tranesophageal ecocardiography plays a determining role in minimally invasive surgery for a number of reasons, including (Chitwood, 2001):

1. Diagnosis of aortic intramural pathology. The presence of atheromatous plaques at the level of the arch has been related to the occurrence of ictus in the postoperative period in cardiac patients with cannulation in the ascendant aorta (Katz et al., 1992; Stern et al., 1999). As with other interventionist therapeutic procedures such as, for example, the insertion of an intra aortic balloon counter pulsation pump, we should conduct a risk-benefit analysis according to the base pathology: atheroma, aneurysm, collagenopathy or calcification.
2. Monitoring of the placing of the retrograde cardioplegia cannula. Many teams place this cannula percutaneously, guided by echography through the internal jugular vein (Kort et al., 2001) For the correct assessment of the positioning the longitudinal, transverse or bicaval axis is used (Kronzon et al., 1995). If, on the echocardiogram, the coronary sinus gives the impression of being dilated it is necessary to exclude the persistence of the superior vena cava using an injection of agitated saline via the upper left peripheral venal access. The scope is used for definitive confirmation of the positioning.

3. Whether or not the cannula is placed percutaneously it is vital to asses it using echocardiography because we will not have other information, for example that obtained by palpation. Monitoring pressure has not been demonstrated to be sufficient to ensure correct positioning.
4. Positioning of the femoral venous cannula and its progression towards the right atrium.
5. Assessment of air in cavities before the patient is weaned off cardiopulmonary by-pass to avoid gas embolism and the dysrhythmias resulting from the entry of air in the right heart.
6. Analysis of the segmental contractility and assessment of cardiac function.
7. In patients where the mini-sternotomy approach is used, on occasion it is observed that when weaning from cardiopulmonary by-pass the right ventricle is under-filled, combined with an increase in central venal pressure. This phenomenon is due to a compression of the front face of the right ventricle by an undivided lower sternum on the anteriorly retracted heart. This can be assessed using echocardiography.
8. The result of the valve surgery in the case of both valve repair and replacement.
9. Location of the level of sternal division, the assessment of the location of the aortic ring provides orientation as to whether we should extend the sternotomy into the third or fourth inter-costal space with a view to improving access (Sardari et al., 1997).

4.6 Aortic cross clamp

4.6.1 External clamping

Aortic clamping in order to be able to carry out the surgical procedure can be done using external pincers (the conventional or classic method) both in the mini-sternotomy or mini-thoractotomy, or using endoluminal clamping with the aid of an inflatable balloon, the endoclamp®. In the case of treatment for aortic pathology this latter method is not used but we will take this opportunity to review some of the concepts.

In aortic valvulopathy treatment using minimally invasive surgery, aortic clamping in the case of the mini-sternotomy would be done directly with a conventional clamp. In the case of patients treated via the mini-thoracotomy with Port Access, the Cosgrove flexible aortic cross-clamp or the Glauber tend to be used, via an incision at the level of the third inter-costal space.

4.6.2 Endoclamp®

The endoclamp is introduced via the femoral arterial cannula. It presents a series of advantages and disadvantages as against external clamping. The endoclamp® is positioned at the level of the sinotubular junction and enables the administration of antegrade cardioplegia. The endoclamp® is also equipped with a vent that enables root venting of the air retained in the cardiac cavities. To facilitate placing the endoclamp® and to avoid its possible migration during positioning 0.25 mg/kg of adenosine are administered. The position and correct inflation of the clamp are monitored using echocardiography or radiology.

In the case of patients where endovascular clamping is used, which is fundamentally those patients with mitral tricuspid valvulopathies, it is important to be aware that the correct positioning of the clamp is necessary in order to avoid its migration and the possible occlusion of the brachiocephalic trunks which may cause neurological damage as it compromises circulation. That is why it is so important to monitor both radial arteries as well as having a trans-cranial Doppler to assess correct cerebral perfusion.

The principal complication that can be present with the use of the endoclamp® is aortic dissection which, although it has reduced in frequency as teams have gained experience (1.3% initially as against 0.2% currently), nonetheless has a very high morbimortality (Galloway et al., 1999).

5. Profile of candidates for minimally invasive surgery: indications and contraindications

In principle any patient is a candidate for minimally invasive approaches because of the possible benefits. The different published studies discuss patient profiles in which the application of the technique may be more beneficial.

5.1.1 Elderly

The elderly are a group which has been singled out for the special benefits that minimally invasive surgery can have, given the rapid recovery of patients and the improved clinical evolution. Sharony et al, in a retrospective case-control study of elderly patients (average age 75.3 years) observed a reduction in hospitalisation. Overall, elderly patients are considered to be a high risk group for surgery as expressed in the different risk scales such as the EUROSCORE (Nashef et al., 2002). It is in this type of patient that minimally invasive surgery is thought to be potentially most beneficial. (Sharony et al., 2003).

5.1.2 Re-intervention in coronary patients

It is a widely accepted opinion that reoperations are associated with an increase in morbidity and mortality not only derived from patient-specific clinical factors (i.e. old age and increased comorbidities) but also from the complexity of the surgical technique due to the absence of pericardial closure after initial heart surgery and the development of adhesions. Reoperation status remains an independent predictor of operative death after adjusting for confounding factors. The aorta, right ventricle, and bypass grafts may adhere to the underside of the sternum and can be easily injured during reoperation. In-hospital mortality for patients undergoing cardiac reoperation is higher than that of patients undergoing primary surgical interventions (Yap et al., 2009; Yau et al.., 2000) Previous surgical revascularization is a predictive factor for early mortality (Van Eck et al., 2002).

Many authors have proposed reduced approaches with a view to minimising this risk (Byrne et al., 2000; Byrne et al., 1999; Svensson et al., 2001; Tabata et al., 2008). Gaeta et al., in a study of 16 patients with LIMA to LAD analyse the mini-sternotomy as an alternative to the complete sternotomy with a view to reducing the incidence of complications associated with the dissection. Byrne JG et al analyse the results of 39 patients who, following prior revascularization required reintervention due to the development of aortic valvulopathy. In the series of patients analysed they observed a significant reduction in blood loss and in the need for hemoderivatives. It is possible that minimally invasive approaches avoid the potential damage caused by dissecting the structures of the mediastinum as the focus is on the ascendant aorta and partially on the right atrium (Byrne et al., 2000). Myocardial protection was carried out via antegrade or retrograde cardioplegia observing that it was not necessary to dissect and exclude the coronary transplants for correct myocardial protection, as body temperature was reduced (20 degrees in the case of patients with LIMA to LAD and 25 degrees in all cases) and cold cardioplegia was administered, the heart received optimal protection (Byrne et al., 1999).

5.1.3 Contraindications

There are no clearly defined contraindications however it is not recommended to use minimally invasive surgery in cases where the technical difficulty or risk would be increased without justification (von Segesser et al., 1999; Lopez- Gude et al., 2010; Ehrlich et al., 2000):

1. Patients with significant esophageal stricture of any etiology, which means echocardiography monitoring cannot be used.
2. Patients with pectum excavatum
3. Patients with morbid obesity
4. Patients in which it is intended to use the endoclamp® and who present aortic regurgitation of a grade greater than I and diameter of the sinotubular junction greater than 35 mm
5. Patients in whom assistance via peripheral cannulation is proposed and who have a history of peripheral arteriosclerosis.
6. In patients where there is documented existence of aortic pathologies such as aneurysms, atheromatous plaques, intramural hematomas or certain collagenopathies the use of the endoclamp may be inadvisable
7. Cardiac ischemia
8. Short or long ascendant aorta
9. Calcifications in the ascendant aorta or porcelain aorta
10. Small aortic ring to which it is planned to apply techniques for expanding the ring

6. Advantages of minimally invasive approaches in the treatment of aortic stenosis

The principal advantages of minimally invasive surgery are associated with the results it obtains, that is to say, to the clinical benefits derived from the technique as well as other benefits fundamentally related to the field of management: the reduction of time spent in intensive care units and overall hospitalisation or possible cosmetic effects.
The first published study in which minimally invasive surgical procedures were carried out saw a reduction in the average hospitalisation time, the need for hemoderivatives and a faster functional recovery. Nevertheless they also observed an increase in surgery time (extra-corporal circulation and aortic clamping) (Frazier et al., 1998).
There are significant discrepancies between the results of some of the studies listed. Some can be explained by the characteristics of the sample studied, as they deal with samples that are not clinically comparable, or the techniques applied are not superimposable. Others can be explained as due to failings in the design of the study.
The interest that minimally invasive surgery has awoken is based on the idea that these less intrusive approaches mean less surgical aggression and therefore less postoperative pain, less hospitalisation time, faster functional recovery and greater cosmetic benefits as the size of scars is reduced (Rao et al., 1993; Wang et al., 2003; Klokocovnik, 1998; Szwerc et al., 1999; Aris et al., 1999; Bonacchi et al., 2002; Caffarelli & Robbins., 2004).
Results have changed since the early days of the application of minimally invasive techniques leading, as we will see, to the construction of a safe and effective surgical option for the treatment of aortic valvulopathy. Below we analyse some of the aspects in which minimally invasive surgery offers certain advantages in comparison with conventional treatment.

6.1 Blood loss

One of the potential advantages attributed to minimally invasive surgery is the reduction of post-operative bleeding, and therefore the need for hemoderivatives. Many studies support this, including Cosgrove et al, Tam et al, Bonachi et al and Macchler et al. One of the limitations of these studies was that the analysis of the effects of minimally invasive approaches on blood loss were carried out without adjusting for pre-operative risk factors or without conducting a multivariant analysis in order to clarify this issue. (Cosgrove et al., 1998; Tam & Almeida, 1998; Bonacchi et al., 2002; Machler et al., 1999). There is a generalised consensus about the possible reduction of bleeding rates, however there is also discordant data on the subject. Stamou et al. conducted a study analysing a sample of 511 patients in which 455 (89%) were treated using sternotomy and 56 (11%) underwent mini-AVR. The aim of the study was to compare perioperative clinical outcomes, transfusion requirements, and early mortality in patients who had mini-AVR versus conventional AVR by using a risk stratification model to adjust for potential differences between the two groups. Nevertheless after adjusting for risk factors the conclusion was reached that there were no differences in the rate of bleeding observed between the two groups (odds ratio [OR] of transfusion postoperatively =0.94, 95% confidence interval [CI] =0.42 to 2.12], p =0.88; OR of transfusion intraoperatively =0.79, 95% CI =0.45 to 1.40, p =0.42).

This data contrasts with that of Dogan et al, who found, in a randomised study, that there was a reduction in the amount of surgical drainage in the group of patients treated using minimally invasive approaches.

It seems that the evidence of the different studies, even with the methodological limitations to the design and the variability of the groups studied, suggests a reduction in surgical drainage and therefore in the need for hemoderivatives in the immediate postoperative period.

6.2 Pain

The reduction of pain felt by the patient and the demand for analgesics in the immediate postoperative period assessed according to different subjective scales is another aspect that has been analysed at great length, and in principle there is consensus as to the benefits of minimally invasive techniques. There is a certain amount of variation in the ways in which this assessment has been made, however, despite these variations, the results agree. Studies by Candaele et al or Bonacchi et al are among those that record this benefit in comparison with conventional approaches (Candaele et al., 2003; Bonacchi et al., 2002; Liu et al.., 1999).

The upper partial sternotomy offers the comfort factor of sternotomy over thoracotomy and prevents complications of other distentions at the costovertebral joint or brachial plexus traction at the thoracic inlet. This causes a reduction in the pain felt by the patient. (Von Segesser et al., 1999).

6.3 Pulmonary function

As the integrity of the thorax is maintained and pain, which is one of the factors that most affects movement in the thorax, is reduced, it is logical to expect that the parameters of pulmonary function will be less affected by minimally invasive approaches. Various authors have analysed this aspect and the results suggest that there is a smaller fall in respiratory parameters using spirometry following intervention with minimally invasive approaches (Moustafa et al., 2007).

Nevertheless, as with the other results obtained pertaining to minimally invasive techniques there are certain discrepancies in this regard (Calderon et al., 2009). Aris et al, in a randomised study of 40 patients did not find any benefits in the respiratory parameters, patients showed a reduction of 26% and 33% in FVC and of 22% and 35% in FEV1 in minimally invasive groups as against sternotomy ones. (Aris et al., 1999) In this analysis it is possible differences were not observed between the groups due to the size of the sample studied.

6.4 Duration of hospital stay and functional recovery

One of the objectives of minimally invasive approaches is to reduce surgical aggression and thus favour functional recovery. The benefit of these approaches in terms of the impact on the duration of hospitalization is quite uniform, and the majority of authors observe benefits in the reduction of the average hospital stay both in time spent in intensive care and total time in hospital. In this vein we find the results of Bonacchi et al, Brinkman et al, Grossi et al, Moustafa M A et al or Liu J et al (Bonacchi et al., 2002; Brinkman et al., 2010; Grossi et al., 2001; Moustafa et al., 2007; Liu et al., 1999).

Patients operated on using minimally invasive surgery present, in general terms, less time on mechanical ventilation than patients operated on in the conventional way. It is important to remember that the most significant risk factor in the development of respiratory infection complications is the duration of intubation. It is possible that through minimally invasive surgery there may be a reduction in the incidence of certain infectious complications such as the pneumonia associated with mechanical ventilation. As with other aspects analysed, more studies are required with larger sample sizes in order to confirm what seems, a priori, to be the case.

Once again, Aris' study does not show differences in the duration of the hospitalisation (6.3 ± 2.3 days as against 6.3 ± 2.4; p=0.8) (Aris et al., 1999) and again, this could be due to the size of the sample analysed. Other studies, such as Ehrlich, report a reduction in time spent in the ICU but do not observe differences related to the surgical approach in the total time spent in hospital (Ehrlich et al., 2000).

Comparative studies have demonstrated that there are no differences in early mortality between minimally invasive approaches and a complete sternotomy (Liu et al., 1999; Machler et al., 1999).

6.5 Reduction of infections, cosmetic effects

Grossi et al observe an incidence of infection of 0.9% for minimally invasive approaches as against 5.7% in cases of patients with the approach by sternotomy, p=0.05. It has been observed that this difference increases in elderly patients (1.8 and 7.7% respectively) (Grossi et al., 2001). Other authors observe that in comparison with the classical approach there is a lesser incidence of infectious complications (Lee et al., 2000; Tabata et al.b, 2008).

Associated with this, a cosmetic benefit is observed, which traditionally has been one of the great advantages of these approaches in the case of young patients. In the following images we can see how the incision to be able to treat valvulopathy is considerably reduced in both the approaches using the mini-sternotomy and those using the mini-thoracotomy.

In the first images we can see the cosmetic benefits of the mini-thoracotomy technique and in the following image the reduced scar size for mini-sternotomy.

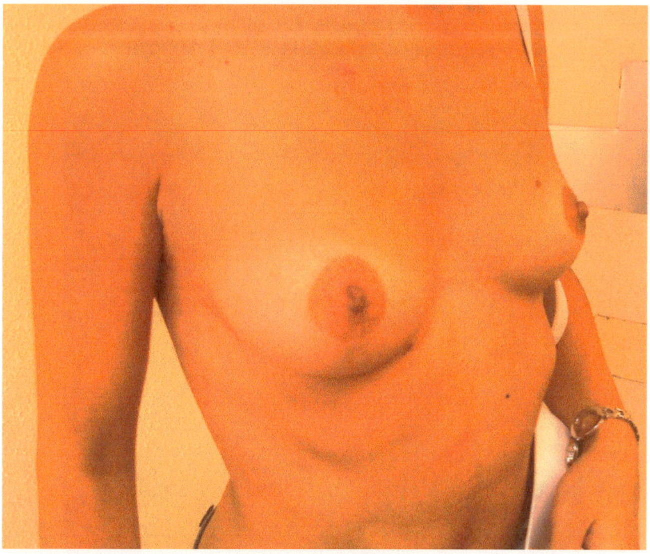

Fig 6. Image showing the mini-thoracotomy approach.

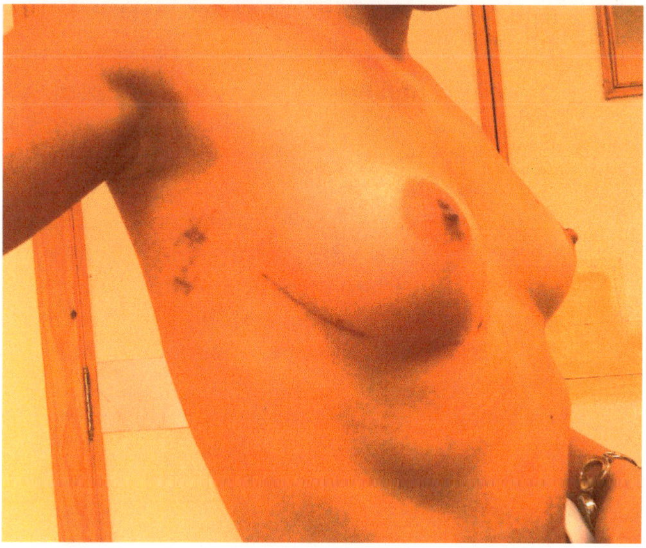

Fig. 7. Images showing the mini-thoracotomy approach in the treatment of mitral valvulopathy.

6.6 Costs

These techniques are a paradigm for the future in terms of cost-effectiveness. If superimposable clinical results can be guaranteed with both approaches, the use of minimally invasive surgery with less aggression, less postoperative complications, faster functional recovery and better cosmetic effects overlaps with the objective of more effective medical management.

Furthermore, these patients recover faster and can therefore incorporate themselves into working life faster and with fewer rehabilitation requirements. It is estimated that the costs

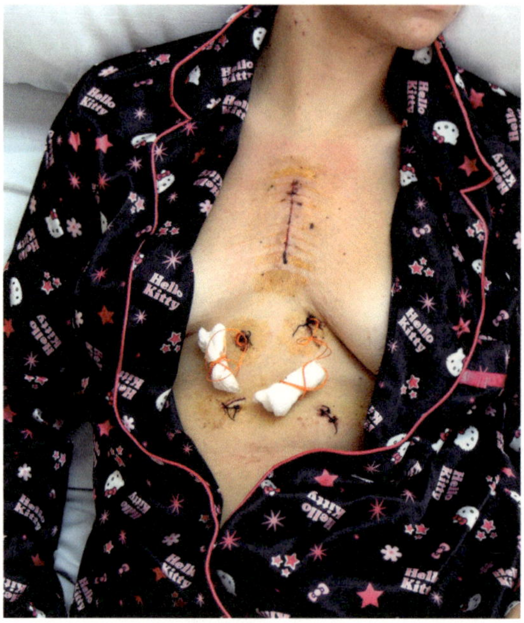

Fig. 8. Image showing the mini-sternotomy appropach

of post-hospital care surpass tens of millions of dollars in the United States and these costs are rising. If operations can be carried out more efficiently in terms of management of hospital resources and the need for post-hospital care (rehabilitation) can be reduced, this could be important for health management. (Cohn et al., 1997)

Many studies have analysed the impact that treatments using minimally invasive approaches can have on health costs. It is clear that if these approaches reduce hospitalization and the incidence of certain complications requiring expensive treatments, the average cost of the procedures will be reduced. Cohn LH indicates that it is possible to observe a reduction of up to 20% of the cost per diagnostic team if minimally invasive approaches are applied. Nevertheless, studying the cost effectiveness of these options is extremely complex as it is affected by a large number of factors many of which are difficult to quantify in economic terms in normal clinical practice, such as the hours the operating theatre is in use or the time taken by the surgeon to carry out the surgical procedure. Studies more in this vein would be necessary, rather than studies of clinical benefits, which at the end of the day are far more important for the patient and the doctor. Nevertheless, in terms of better use of resources the question of costs should not be forgotten. Table 3 shows the results observed in various different studies over the potential benefits of minimally invasive surgery.

MI, minimally invasive; C, convencional; CPB cardiopulmonary bypass time; ICU intensive care unit

7. Disadvantages of minimally invasive approaches in the treatment of aortic stenosis

A number of factors have been highlighted as potential disadvantages of minimally invasive surgery as compared with the conventional approach, particularly noteworthy are:

Study	Year	Study desing	Patients, n	Drainage bleed	Pain	Transfusion	CPB	Cross clamp time	ICU stay	Lengh of stay	Intubation	Respiratory reserve	Reoperation for bleeding
Aris et al.	1999	Randomized	20(MI)/20(C)	NS	NS	-	NS	0.005	NS	NS	NS	NS	-
Bonacchi et al.	2002	Randomized	40(MI)/40(C)	0.004	0.001	<0.0001	NS	NS	0.04	0.029	0.006	<0.05	NS
Brinkman et al.	2010	Case-control	90(MI)/360(C)	-	-	NS	NS		0.01	0.033	-	-	NS
Machler et al.	1999	Randomized	60(MI)/60(C)	<0.001	<0.05	-	NS	NS	-	-	<0.001	-	NS
Moustafa et al.	2007	Randomized	30(MI)/30(C)	0.001	0.001	0.001	0.031	0.044	0.001	0.001	0.001	0.001	-
Liu et al.	1999	Case-control	86(MI)/78(C)	<0.05	-	-	NS	NS	-	<0.01	<0.05	-	-
Sharony et al.	2003	Case-control	189(MI)/189(C)	-	-	-	NS	NS	-	<0.001	-	-	NS
Doll et al.	2002	Case-control	176(MI)/258(C)	0.04	-	<0.05	NS	0.03	<0.05	<0.05	<0.05	-	NS

Table 3. Summary of studies and results observed

7.1 Operating theatre time

Here again, we find inconsistent results, the explanation for which ultimately lies with the type of patient operated on and the centre's level of experience. Tabata et al observe in their study that within the period analysed, 1996 to 2006, three distinct time frames emerge (1996 to 1999, 2000 to 2003 and 2004 to 2006) in terms of the time taken to do a cardiopulmonary by-pass, as the learning curve for this procedure was reduced. (Tabata et al., 2008) It is known that the learning curve plays a determinant role in the results of minimally invasive surgery and, of course, in the time spent in theatre. Volume of cases is fundamental in acquiring the dexterity and confidence to carry out these interventions.

When considering the time taken to carry out surgery we should distinguish between the time taken to do the cardiopulmonary by-pass, the time required for aortic clamping and finally the overall surgery time. In terms of the first two, results diverge, due to the explanations given above. Nevertheless in terms of the overall in-theatre time there is more agreement that this is extended due to the characteristics of the surgical approach and the time required for hemostasis among other reasons.

Studies that support an increase in the time for cardiopulmonary bypass and aortic clamping are Farhat et al, Detter et al, de Vaumas et al, and Stamou et al. (Farhat et al, 2003; Detter et al., 2002; de Vaumas et al., 2003; Stamou et al., 2003); contradictory results can be found in Corbi et al., Sharony et al or the randomised study by Bonachi et al. (Corbi et al., 2003; Sharony et al., 2003; Bonachi et al., 2002).

7.2 De-airing

De-airing can be slower and more difficult with the resulting risk of gas embolism, fundamentally at a cerebral level, and the dysrhythmias that are a consequence of gas embolism in the right of the heart. This is due to the fact that there is no direct access to the heart to be able to carry out manual manoeuvres that help to eliminate residual air from the cardiac cavities. A number of measures have been proposed to minimise this risk and facilitate the purging of air (Woo et al., 2007; Gaeta et al., 2010):

1. Administer retrograde cardioplegia
2. Volume loading the heart earlier
3. Early restart of pulmonary ventilation while the aortotomy is being closed

4. Terminating venting earlier
5. Rotating the operating table upward and on the Leith side
6. The use of CO_2 is useful in the treatment of aortic valvulopathy, with it being effective as almost the only measure applied to a flow of 2l/ min

If one is meticulous in the application of these techniques, the problems associated with purging the air are significantly reduced and there is no reason to expect serious disturbances from it.

7.3 Technical difficulties

Another aspect that has been assessed is the increase in technical complexity which could put the effectiveness of the surgical procedure at risk. However, in this respect, many authors have indicated that aortic valve surgery can be carried out with an increase in technical complexity that surgeons can accommodate to without undue efforts in the learning curve, and that results for both approaches are similar (Liu et al., 1999; Machler et al., 1999). Sharony et al indicate that the results for both approaches are similar in the actuarial survival curve at three years.

Below we bring together the results of some of the studies that have been carried out in the treatment of aortic valvulopathy with the results observed in each of the aspects that have been considered here.

8. Conclusions

Minimally invasive surgery, both in the treatment of cardiac ischemia and in valvulopathies, has been the subject of considerable developments and improvements in recent years thanks to the perfecting of surgical techniques and the support that the industry has provided for carrying out those techniques.

Minimally invasive surgery is a safe and effective therapeutic option in the treatment of aortic valvulopathy that can be compared with conventional treatment, and which, in some centres, represents a not unimportant percentage (majority). It currently has similar results, with a reduction in bleeding rates, pain perceived by the patient, infection of surgical wounds, duration of hospitalisation, functional recovery and significant cosmetic effects.

The necessary skills to be able to conduct the procedure are not very demanding and are easily reproduced. Limitations due to the surgical field exposed, procedural challenges and potential pitfalls are easily overcome with the right knowledge and strategies.

9. References

Arís, A., Padró, J.M., & Cámara, M.L. (1997) Minimally invasive aortic valve replacement. *Rev Esp Cardiol.* 1997 Nov; 50(11):778-81.

Aris, A., Camara, M.L., & Montiel, J. (1999) Ministernotomy versus median sternotomy for aortic valve replacement: a prospective randomized study. *Ann Thorac Surg* 1999; 67:1583–7.

Arom, K.V., Emery, R.W., & Nicoloff, D.M. (1996) Mini-sternotomy for coronary artery bypass grafting. *Ann Thorac Surg* 1996; 61: 1.271- 1.272.

Baumgartner, H., Hung, J., & Bermejo, J. (2009) American Society of Echocardiography, European Society of Echocardiography. Echocardiographic assessment of valve stenosis: EAE/ASE recommendations for clinical practice. *Eur J Echocardiogr* 2009; 10: 1–23.

Benetti, F.J., Naselli, G., & Wood, M. (1991) Direct myocardial revascularization without extracorporeal circulation. Experience in 700 patients. *Chest* 1991; 100: 312-316.

Bonacchi, M., Prifti, E., & Giunti, G. (2002) Does ministernotomy improve postoperative outcome in aortic valve operations? A prospective randomized study. *Ann Thorac Surg* 2002; 73:460–5.

Bonow, RO, Carabello, BA, & Chatterjee, K. (2008) American College of Cardiology/American Heart Association Task Force on Practise Guidelines. 2008 focused update incorporated into the ACC/AHA 2006 guidelines for the management of patients with valvular heart disease: a report of the American College of Cardiology/American Heart Association Task Force on Practise Guidelines (Writing Committee to revise the 1998 guidelines for the management of patients with valvular heart disease). Endorsed by the Society of Cardiovascular Anesthesiologists, Society for Cardiovascular Angiography and Interventions, and Society of Thoracic Surgeons. *J Am Coll Cardiol* 2008; 52:e1–e142.

Brinkman, W.T., Hoffman, W., & Dewey, T.M. (2010) Aortic valve replacement surgery: comparison of outcomes in matched sternotomy and PORT ACCESS groups. *Ann Thorac Surg*. 2010 Jul; 90(1):131-5.

Buffolo, E., Silva de Andrade, J.C., & Rodrigues, J.N. (1996) Coronary atery bypass grafting without cardiopulmonary bypass. *Ann Thorac Surg* 1996; 61: 63-66.

Burfeind, W.R., Glower, D.D., & Davis, R.D. (2002) Mitral surgery after prior cardiac operation: port-access versus sternotomy or thoracotomy. *Ann Thorac Surg*. 2002 Oct; 74(4):S1323-5.

Byrne, J.G., Aranki, S.F., & Couper, G.S. (1999) Reoperative aortic valve replacement: partial upper hemisternotomy versus conventional full sternotomy. *J Thorac Cardiovasc Surg* 1999; 118: 991–7.

Byrne, J.G., Karavas, A.N., & Adams, D.H. (2000) Partial upper re sternotomy for aortic valve replacement or re-replacement after previous cardiac surgery. *Eur J Cardiothorac Surg* 2000; 18: 282–6.

Caffarelli, A.D. & Robbins, R.C. (2004) Will minimally invasive valve replacement ever really be important? *Curr Opin Cardiol* 2004; 19:123–7.

Calderon, J., Richebe, P., & Guibaud, J.P. (2009) Prospective randomized study of early pulmonary evaluation of patients scheduled for aortic valve surgery performed by ministernotomy or total median sternotomy. *J Cardiothorac Vasc Anesth*. 2009 Dec; 23(6):795-801.Califiore, A.M., Teodori, G., & Di Giammarco, G. (1997) Minimally invasive coronary artery bypass grafting on a beating heart. *Ann Thorac Surg* 1997 63:S72-S75.

Candaele, S., Herijgers, P., & Demeyere, R. (2003) Chest pain after partial upper versus complete sternotomy for aortic valve surgery. *Acta Cardiol* 2003, 58:17–21.

Carpentier, A., Loulmet, D., & Aupècle, B. (1998) Computer assisted open heart surgery. First case operated on with success *C R Acad Sci III*. 1998 May; 321(5):437-42.

Chambers, J.B. (2009) Aortic stenosis. *Eur J Echocardiogr*. 2009 Jan; 10(1):i11-9.

Chitwood, W.R. Jr. (2001) Minimally invasive aortic valve surgery: What is "port access"? *Am Heart J.* 2001 Sep; 142(3):391-2.

Chitwood, W.R. Jr. & Gulielmos V. (2003) What is minimally invasive cardiac surgery? CTSnet Web site. 2003. Available at: http://www.ctsnet.org/doc/7525.

Cohn, L.H., Adams, D.H., & Couper, G.S. (1997) Minimally invasive cardiac valve surgery improves patient satisfaction while reducing costs of cardiac valve replacement and repair. *Ann Surg.* 1997 Oct; 226(4):421-6; discussion 427-8.

Connolly, H.M., Oh J.K., & Orszulak, T.A. (1997) Aortic valve replacement for aortic stenosis with severe left ventricular dysfunction: prognostic indicators. *Circulation* 1997; 95:2395- 400.

Corbi, P., Rahmati, M., & Donal, E. (2003) Prospective comparison of minimally invasive and standard techniques for aortic valve replacement: initial experience in the first hundred patients. *J Card Surg* 2003, 18:133–139

Cosgrove, D.M. 3rd. & Sabik, J.F. (1996) Minimally invasive approach for aortic valve operations. *Ann Thorac Surg.* 1996 Aug; 62(2):596-7.

Cosgrove, D.M., Sabik, J.F., & Navia, J.L. (1998) Minimally invasive valve operations. *Ann Thorac Surg* 1998; 65:1535–8.

Cosmi, J.E., Tunick, P.A., & Rosenzweig, B.P. (2002) The risk of development of aortic stenosis in patients with 'benign' aortic valve thickening. *Arch Intern Med* 2002; 162:2345-7.

Cuenca, J., Rodríguez-Delgadillo, M.A., & Valle, J.V. (1998) Is the femoral cannulation for minimally invasive aortic valve replacement necessary? *Eur J Cardiothorac Surg.* 1998 Oct; 14 Suppl 1:S111-4.

Detter, C., Deuse, T., & Boehm, D.H. (2002) Midterm results and quality of life after minimally invasive vs. conventional aortic valve replacement. *Thorac Cardiovasc Surg* 2002, 50:337–341.

Doll, N., Borger, M.A., & Hain, J. (2002). Minimal access aortic valve replacement: effects on morbidity and resource utilization. *Ann Thorac Surg.* 2002 Oct; 74(4):S1318-22.

Ehrlich, W., Skwara, W., & Klövekorn, W. (2000) Do patients want minimally invasive aortic valve replacement? *Eur J Cardiothorac Surg.* 2000 Jun; 17(6):714-7.

Falk, V., Walther, T., & Autschbach, R. (1998) Robot-assisted minimally invasive solo mitral valve operation. *J Thorac Cardiovasc Surg.* 1998 Feb; 115(2):470-1.

Farhat, F., Lu, Z., & Lefevre, M. (2003) Prospective comparison between total sternotomy and ministernotomy for aortic valve replacement. *J Card Surg* 2003, 18:396–401

Frazier, B.L., Derrick, M.J., & Purewal, S.S. (1998) Minimally invasive aortic valve replacement. *Eur J Cardiothorac Surg.* 1998 Oct; 14 Suppl 1:S122-5.

Gaeta, R., Lentini, S., & Raffa, G. (2010) Aortic valve replacement by ministernotomy in redo patients with previous left internal mammary artery patent grafts. *Ann Thorac Cardiovasc Surg.* 2010 Jun; 16(3):181-6.

Galloway, A.C., Shemin, R.J., & Glower, D.D. (1999) First report of the Port Access International Registry. *Ann Thorac Surg.* 1999 Jan; 67(1):51-6; discussion 57-8.

Grossi, E.A., Galloway, A.C., & Ribakove, G.H. Impact of minimally invasive valvular heart surgery: a case-control study. *Ann Thorac Surg.* 2001 Mar; 71(3):807-10.

Harken, D.E., Soroff, H.S., & Taylor, W.H. Aortic valve replacement, in Merendino KA (ed): Prosthetic Valves for Cardiac Surgery. Springfield, IL, Thomas, 1961, pp 508-526

Hirose, H., Umeda, S., & Mori, Y. (1994) Another approach for aortic valve replacement through left thoracotomy. *Ann Thorac Surg*. 1994 Sep; 58(3):884-6.

Izzat, M.B., Yim, A.P., & El-Zufari, M.H. (1998) Upper T ministernotomy for aortic valve operations. *Chest* 1998; 114:291–4.

Katz, E.S., Tunick, P.A., & Rusinek, H. (1992) Protruding aortic arch atheromas predict stroke in elderly patients undergoing cardiopulmonary bypass: experience with intraoperative transesophageal echocardiography. *J Am Coll Cardiol* 1992; 20:70-7.

Klokocovnik, T. (1998) Aortic and mitral replacement through a minimally invasive approach. *Tex Heart Inst J* 1998; 25:166–9.

Konertz, W., Waldenberger, F., & Schmutzler, M. (1996) Minimal access valve surgery through superior partial sternotomy: a preliminary study. *J Heart Valve Dis*. 1996 Nov; 5(6):638-40.

Kort, S., Applebaum, R.M., & Grossi, E.A. (2001) Minimally invasive aortic valve replacement: echocardiographic and clinical results. *Am Heart J*. 2001 Sep; 142(3):476-81.

Kouchoukos, N.T., Davila-Roman, V.G., & Spray, T.L. (1994) Replacement of the aortic root with a pulmonary autograft in children and young adults with aortic-valve disease. *N Engl J Med* 1994; 330:1– 6.

Kronzon, I., Tunick, P.A., & Jortner, R. (1995) Echocardiographic evaluation of the coronary sinus. *J Am Soc Echocardiogr* 1995; 8:518-26.

Kurtz, C.E. & Otto, C.M. (2010) Aortic stenosis: clinical aspects of diagnosis and management, with 10illustrative case reports from a 25-year experience. *Medicine* (Baltimore). 2010 Nov; 89(6):349-79.

Kvidal, P., Bergstrom, R., & Horte, L.G. (2000) Observed and relative survival after aortic valve replacement. *J Am Coll Cardiol* 2000; 35: 747–56.

Lee, J.W., Lee, S.K., & Choo, S.J. (2000) Routine minimally invasive aortic valve procedures. *Cardiovasc Surg*. 2000 Oct; 8(6):484-90.

Lester, S.J., Heilbron, B., & Gin, K. (1998) The natural history and rate of progression of aortic stenosis. *Chest*. 1998 Apr; 113(4):1109-14.

Lindroos, M., Kupari, M., & Heikkala, J. (1993) Prevalence of aortic valve abnormalities in the elderly: an echocardiographic study of a random population sample. *J Am Coll Cardiol* 1993; 21:1220-5.

Liu, J., Sidiropoulos, A., & Konertz, W. (1999) Minimally invasive aortic valve replacement (AVR) compared to standard AVR. *Eur J Cardiothorac Surg*. 1999 Nov; 16 Suppl 2:S80-3.

Lopez- Gude, M.J., Garcia, D., & Forteza, A. (2010) Heart PortTM access technique for valvular surgery. *Cir. Cardiov*. 2010; 17(4):345-50.

Lund, O. (1990) Preoperative risk evaluation and stratification of long-term survival after valve replacement for aortic stenosis: reasons for earlier operative intervention. *Circulation* 1990; 82:124 –39.

Lung, B., Baron, G., & Butchart, E.G. (2003) A prospective survey of patients with valvular heart disease in Europe: the Euro Heart Survey on valvular heart disease. *Eur Heart J* 2003; 24:1231–1243.

Machler, H.E., Bergmann, P., & Anelli-Monti, M. (1999) Minimally invasive versus conventional aortic valve operations: a prospective study in 120 patients. *Ann Thorac Surg* 1999, 67:1001–1005

Minale, C., Reifschneider, H.J., & Schmitz, E. (1997) Single access for minimally invasive aortic valve replacement. *Ann Thorac Surg*. 1997 Jul; 64(1):120-3.

Moustafa, M.A., Abdelsamad, A.A., & Zakaria, G. (2007) Minimal vs median sternotomy for aortic valve replacement. *Asian Cardiovasc Thorac Ann*. 2007 Dec; 15(6):472-5.

Murphy, E.S., Lawson, R.M., & Starr, A. (1981) Severe aortic stenosis in patients 60 years of age or older: left ventricular function and 10-year survival after valve replacement. *Circulation* 1981; 64:II184–8.

Nashef, S.A., Roques, F., & Hammill, B.G. (2002) EurpSCORE Project Group: Validation of European System for Cardiac Operative Risk Evaluation (EuroSCORE) in North American cardiac surgery. *Eur J Cardiothorac Surg* 2002, 22:101–105

National Adult Cardiac Surgical Database Report 1999–2000. The United Kingdom Cardiac Surgical Register. Accessed 10 May 2006. http://www. scts.org/file/NACSDreport2000ukcsr.pdf

Navia, J.L. & Cosgrove, D.M. Minimally invasive mitral valve operations. *Ann Thorac Surg*. 1996 Nov; 62(5):1542-4.

Otto, C.M., Burwash, I.G., & Legget, M.E. (1997) Prospective study of asymptomatic valvular aortic stenosis. Clinical, echocardiographic, and exercise predictors of outcome. *Circulation* 1997; 95:2262-70.

Pellikka, P.A., Sarano, M.E., & Nishimura, R.A. (2005) Outcome of 622 adults with asymptomatic, hemodynamically significant aortic stenosis during prolonged follow-up. *Circulation*. 2005 111:3290–3295.

Rao, P.N. & Kumar, A.S. (1993) Aortic valve replacement through right thoracotomy. *Tex Heart Inst J* 1993; 20:307–8.

Rodríguez, J.E., López, M.J., & Carrascal, Y. (1996) Aortic valve replacement via ministernotomy. *Rev Esp Cardiol. 1996* Dec; 49(12):928-30.

Rosenhek, R., Binder, T., & Porenta, G. (2000) Predictors of outcome in severe, asymptomatic aortic stenosis. *N Engl J Med*. 2000; 343:611–617.

Sardari, F.F., Schlunt, M.L., & Applegate, R.I. (1997) The use of transesophageal echocardiography to guide sternal division for cardiac operations via mini-sternotomy. *J Cardiac Surg* 1997; 12:67±70.

Schmitto, J.D., Mohr, F.W., & Cohn, L.H. (2011) Minimally invasive aortic valve replacement: how does this perform in high-risk patients? *Curr Opin Cardiol*. 2011 Mar; 26(2):118-22.

Sharony, R., Grossi, E.A., & Saunders, P.C. (2003) Minimally invasive aortic valve surgery in the elderly: a case-control study. *Circulation* 2003, 108:43II–47II

Smith, N., McAnulty, J.H., & Rahimtoola, S.H. (1978) Severe aortic stenosis with impaired left ventricular function and clinical heart failure: results of valve replacement. *Circulation* 1978; 58:255- 64.

Stamou, S.C., Kapetanakis, E.I., & Lowery, R. Allogeneic blood transfusion requirements after minimally invasive versus conventional aortic valve replacement: a risk-adjusted analysis. *Ann Thorac Surg* 2003, 76:1101–1106

Starr, A. & Edwards, M.L. (1961) Mitral replacement: Clinical experience with a ball valve prosthesis. *Ann Surg* 1961 154:726-740.

Stern, A., Tunick, P.A., & Culliford, A.T. Protruding aortic arch atheromas: risk of stroke during heart surgery with and without aortic arch endarterectomy. *Am Heart J* 1999; 138:746-52.

Stevens, J.H., Burdon, T.A., & Siege1, L.C. Port-access coronary artery bypass with cardioplegic arrest: Acute and chronic studies. *Ann Thorac Surg* 62:435-441,1996

Stewart, B.F., Siscovick, D., & Lind, B.K. Clinical factors associated with calcific aortic valve disease: Cardiovascular Health Study. *J Am Coll Cardiol* 1997; 29:630-4.

STS National Database: Spring 2003 Executive Summary. Durham, NC: Duke Clinical Research Institute; 2003.

STS national database: STS U.S. cardiac surgery database: 1997 Aortic valve replacement patients: preoperative risk variables. Chicago, Society of Thoracic Surgeons; 2000. Accessed 10 May 2006. http:// www.ctsnet.org/doc/3031

Subramanian, V.A., Sani, G., & Benetti, F.J. (1995) Minimally invasive coronary bypass surgery: a multi-center report of preliminary clinical experience. *Circulation* 1995; 92 (Supl 1): 645.

Svensson, L.G. (1997) Minimal-access "J" or "j" sternotomy for valvular, aortic, and coronary operations or reoperations. *Ann Thorac Surg* 1997; 64:1501–3.

Svensson, L.G. & D'Agostino, R.S. (1998) Minimal-access aortic and valvular operations, including the "J/j" incision. *Ann Thorac Surg* 1998; 66:431–5.

Svensson, L.G., Nadolny, E.M., & Kimmel, W.A. (2001) Minimal access aortic surgery including re-operations. *Eur J Cardiothorac Surg* 2001; 19: 30–3.

Szwerc, M.F., Benckart, D.H., & Wiechmann, R.J. (1999) Partial versus full sternotomy for aortic valve replacement. *Ann Thorac Surg* 1999; 68:2209–13.

Tabata, M., Khalpey, Z., & Shekar, P.S. (2008a) Reoperative minimal access aortic valve surgery: minimal mediastinal dissection and minimal injury risk. *J Thorac Cardiovasc Surg*. 2008 Dec; 136(6):1564-8. Epub 2008 Oct 23.

Tabata, M., Umakanthan, R., & Cohn, L.H. (2008b) Early and late outcomes of 1000 minimally invasive aortic valve operations. *Eur J Cardiothorac Surg*. 2008 Apr; 33(4):537-41. Epub 2008 Feb 5.

Tam, R.K. & Almeida, A.A. (1998) Minimally invasive aortic valve replacement via partial sternotomy. *Ann Thorac Surg* 1998; 65:275–6.

Vahanian, A., Baumgartner, H., & Bax, J. (2007) Task Force on the Management of Valvular Hearth Disease of the European Society of Cardiology; . ESC Committee for Practice Guidelines. *Eur Heart J* 2007; 28:230–268.

Van Eck, F.M., Noyez, L., & Verheugt, F.W. (2002) Preoperative prediction of early mortality in redocoronary artery surgery. *Eur J Cardiothorac Surg*. 2002; 21:1031-6.

de Vaumas, C., Philip, I., & Daccache, G. (2003) Comparison of minithoracotomy and conventional sternotomy approaches for valve surgery. *J Cardiothorac Vasc Anesth* 2003, 17:325–328.

von Segesser, L.K., Westaby, S., & Pomar, J. Less invasive aortic valve surgery: rationale and technique. *Eur J Cardiothorac Surg*. 1999 Jun; 15(6):781-5.

Walther, T., Falk, V., & Metz, S. (1996) Pain and quality of life after minimally invasive versus conventional cardiac surgery. *Ann Thorac Surg* 1999; 67:1643–7.

Wang, W.L., Cai, K.C., & Zeng, W.S. (2003) Experience in using three different minimally invasive approaches in cardiac operations. *Med Sci Monit* 2003; 9:109–13.

Woo, Y.J., Seeburger, J., & Mohr, F.W. (2007) Minimally invasive valve surgery. *Semin Thorac Cardiovasc Surg*. 2007 Winter; 19(4):289-98.

Yap, C.H., Sposato, L., & Akowuah, E. (2009) Contemporary results show repeat coronary artery bypass grafting remains a risk factor for operative mortality. *Ann Thorac Surg*. 2009; 87:1386-91.

Yau, T.M., Borger, M.A., & Weisel, R.D. (2000) The changing pattern of reoperative coronary surgery: trends in 1230 consecutive reoperations. *J Thorac Cardiovasc Surg*. 2000; 120:156-63.

8

Technical Modifications for Patients with Aortic Stenosis and Calcified Ascending Aorta During Aortic Valve Replacement

Masanori Hirota, Joji Hoshino, Yasuhisa Fukada, Shintaro Katahira, Taichi Kondo, Kenichi Muramatsu and Tadashi Isomura
Department of Cardiovascular Surgery, Hayama Heart Center, Kanagawa, Japan

1. Introduction

Aortic stenosis (AS) is the most prevalent valvular heart disease in developed countries[1]. Aortic valves deteriorate due to degenerative processes, and calcification is the most frequent cause of AS. Clinical factors related to aortic valve calcification are similar to those for atherosclerosis, and the prevalence of calcified aortic valves increases with age[2]. As a consequence, AS is associated with a high risk of cardiovascular morbidity and mortality in the elderly[3]. To achieve longer life expectancy, aortic valve replacement (AVR) is recommended as a definitive treatment for calcified aortic valves[4,5]. Although the operative mortality of isolated AVR is low, the surgical risk is increased in elderly patients due to concomitant procedures and/or comorbidities associated with advanced age[6]. Thus, it is very important to plan a careful strategy for co-existing atherosclerotic lesions, especially in the ascending aorta.

Atherosclerotic change in the ascending aorta is one of the potential causes of postoperative stroke, which results in higher morbidity and mortality[7,8]. Most embolic events are associated with manipulation of the ascending aorta such as the clamping of the ascending aorta or the release of aortic crossclamping[9]. To reduce embolic complications, surgical treatments have changed, and there are several techniques, including AVR during hypothermic circulatory arrest (HCA)[10-12], complete thromboendarterectomy during HCA[13], endarterectomy or ascending aorta replacement during HCA[14], endoaortic balloon occlusion[15], and apicoaortic conduit[16]. Despite aggressive attempts to deal with the calcified ascending aorta, surgical outcomes such as the stroke rate, morbidity, and mortality have remained unsatisfactory. This paper describes our surgical strategy for patients with AS associated with a diseased calcified ascending aorta. Furthermore, meticulous techniques for atherosclerotic lesions designed to avoid perioperative morbidity are described in detail.

2. Patients and methods

2.1 Patients

Between May 2000 and December 2009, 705 patients underwent AVR due to AS (n=447) or aortic regurgitation (n=268). Of the patients with AS, 46 (11%) had a calcified ascending aorta. A calcified ascending aorta is defined on computed tomography (CT) as severe and extensive calcification, which would increase the risk of atheroembolic complications during operative procedures.

The patients were 25 males and 21 females, ranging between 44 and 93 years of age (mean, 73±10 years). Hemodialysis was required in 6 patients (13%) due to chronic renal failure. In this series, 10 patients (22%) had a porcelain aorta (a totally calcified aorta). Although preoperative imaging obtained by CT revealed the extent and thickness of calcification of the ascending aorta, operative procedures were determined by intra-operative findings.

2.2 Surgical technique

2.2.1 Preparation

Under general cardiac anesthesia and monitoring, an 8-mm, gelatin-impregnated, woven Dacron graft (Gelweave; VASCUTEK®, a TERUMO company, Renfrewshire, UK) was sewn to the right axillary artery[17]. After median sternotomy, cardiopulmonary bypass (CPB) was installed via the right axillary artery with single venous drainage. A pulmonary vein vent was used to prevent potentially damaging distension during ventricular fibrillation. The body was cooled to 28°C for internal inspection of the ascending aorta during brief circulatory arrest. Gentle palpation of the ascending aorta provided three-dimensional spatial imaging of the calcified aorta during cooling. Epiaortic echocardiography was also used to obtain intimal imaging of the ascending aorta along aortotomy.

2.2.2 Brief circulatory arrest for internal inspection of the ascending aorta

At a core body temperature of 28°C, brief circulatory arrest was initiated to observe the intimal condition of the ascending aorta. The ascending aorta was opened at the optimal site, which was determined by gentle palpation and epiaortic echocardiography. An oblique (J-shaped) incision is usually used for AVR. When severe calcification involves the sinus of Valsalva, a longitudinal (I-shaped) incision or transection would be indicated **(Fig. 1)**; a representative CT image of a calcified sinus of Valsalva is shown in **Fig. 2**. A severely calcified sinus of Valsalva prevents surgeons from obtaining a satisfactory surgical field around the aortic annulus, even if the anterior wall of the ascending aorta is retracted through the usual oblique incision. Moreover, prosthetic valves cannot be passed through a calcified sinus of Valsalva due to the limited diameter caused by nearly-circumferential calcification and the height of the prosthesis. For these reasons, it is very important to extend the I-shaped aortic incision to the sinus of Valsalva toward the commissure between the right and non-coronary cusps. After opening the ascending aorta, the intima was directly observed to confirm the existence of fragile debris. When the calcified ascending aorta was clampable at a safe site with just only calcification but no fragile debris, simple AVR was indicated. When there was severe calcification and no lesion for aortic crossclamping, both AVR and ascending aorta replacement were indicated during circulatory arrest with selective cerebral perfusion.

2.2.3 Simple AVR

The calcified ascending aorta was safely crossclamped after internal inspection of the ascending aorta during brief circulatory arrest at moderate hypothermia. Systemic perfusion was commenced via the right axillary artery after aortic crossclamping. Re-warming of the body was then started. Antegrade tepid blood cardioplegia was selectively delivered to obtain diastolic cardiac arrest. For maintenance, retrograde tepid blood cardioplegia was infused every 20 to 30 minutes. When remnant fragile debris was detected on the proximal ascending aorta, it was gently peeled as far as possible before AVR.

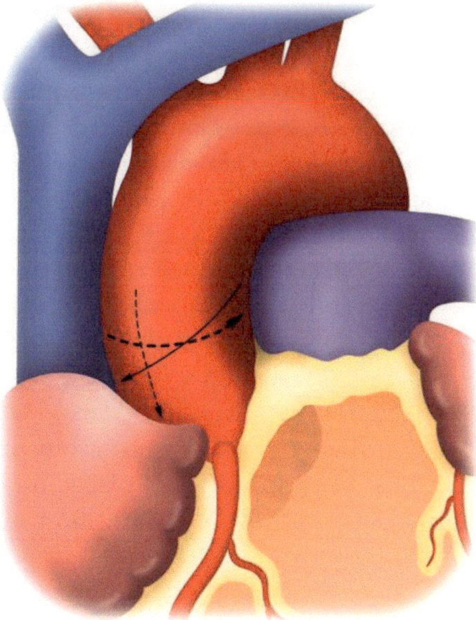

Fig. 1. A schema of the incisions of the ascending aorta for aortic valve replacement (AVR). There are three incision lines for aortotomy on the ascending aorta. The oblique (J-shaped) line for routine AVR is shown by the solid arrow. The horizontal or longitudinal (I-shaped) and transverse lines for patients with a calcified sinus of Valsalva are shown by dotted arrows. (Hirota et al.)

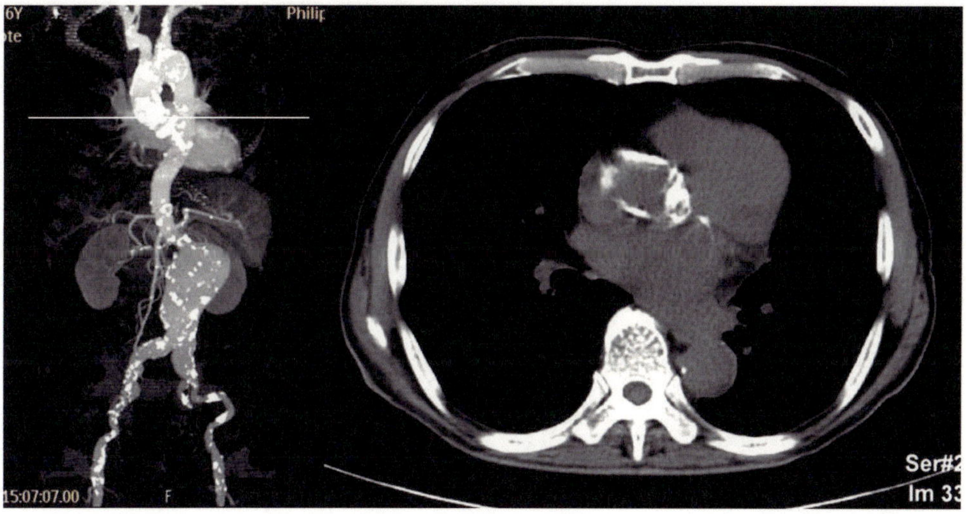

Fig. 2. On the left side, calcification of the aorta is shown by three-dimensional computed tomography (CT) images in a patient with a calcified sinus of Valsalva. On the right side, a representative image of a calcified sinus of Valsalva is obtained from the scanning level shown by a solid line on the three-dimensional CT. Nearly-circumferential calcification is detected on the sinus of Valsalva. (Hirota et al.)

Firstly, the aortic valves were sharply removed, and one-quarter of gauze was placed into the left ventricle (LV) to catch calcific debris. Decalcification was gently performed with Pean Hemostatic Forceps and Selman Tissue Forceps (Pilling®; Teleflex Medical, Tuttlingen, Germany) around the aortic annulus. The LV cavity was carefully irrigated with copious amounts of cold saline to reduce the risk of emboli. Secondly, a 2-0 polyfilament braided non-everting mattress suture with spaghetti (Matsuda-ika Kogyo, Tokyo, Japan) was placed for each commissure. Great attention is needed for commissural suturing between the right and non-coronary cusps. Deep stitches for the commissure would injure the conduction system, which would result in complete atrioventricular block. For patients with this complication, permanent pacemaker implantation would be necessary. Subsequently, sizing of the prosthetic valve was performed in accordance with each commercial sizer. When a bioprosthetic valve was selected, it was irrigated with saline for preparation. Thirdly, inter-commissural sutures were placed for each coronary cusp. Independent of the type of prosthetic valve, 15 sutures, one for each commissure and four for each coronary cusp, were usually placed **(Fig. 3)**. Then, a total of 15 sutures was placed on the prosthetic annulus, and the appropriate valve was seated in the supravalvular position.

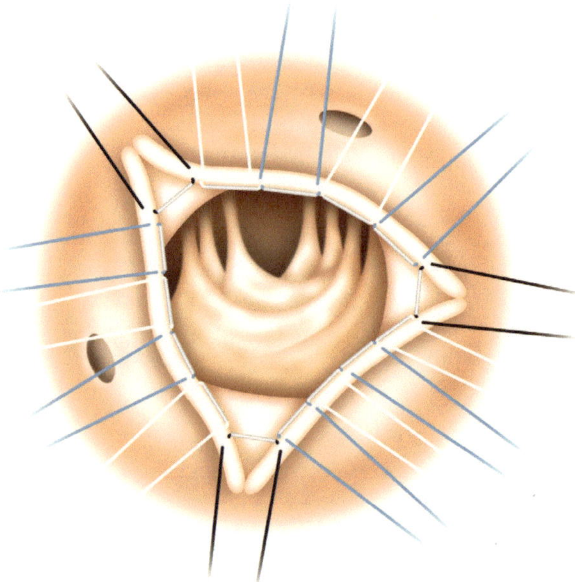

Fig. 3. Independent of the type of prosthetic valve, 15 2-0 polyfilament braided non-everting mattress sutures with spaghetti were usually placed for routine aortic valve replacement. Firstly, three black sutures were placed for each commissure. Secondly, four sutures, alternating white and blue, were placed for each coronary cusp. (Hirota et al.)

2.2.4 Closure of a calcified ascending aorta

For patients with a non-calcified aortic wall, the ascending aorta is usually closed with 5-0 polypropylene continuous horizontal mattress and over-and-over sutures. However, for patients with a fragile aortic wall, the aortotomy was closed with 4-0 polyfilament braided

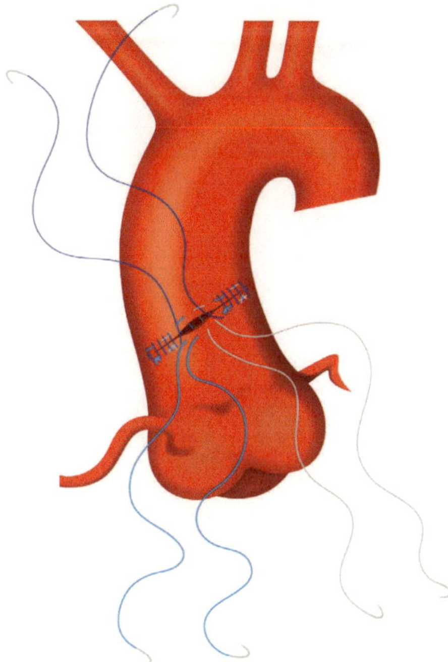

Fig. 4A. For patients with a fragile aortic wall, the aortotomy was closed with 4-0 polyfilament braided horizontal mattress and 5-0 polypropylene over-and-over sutures.

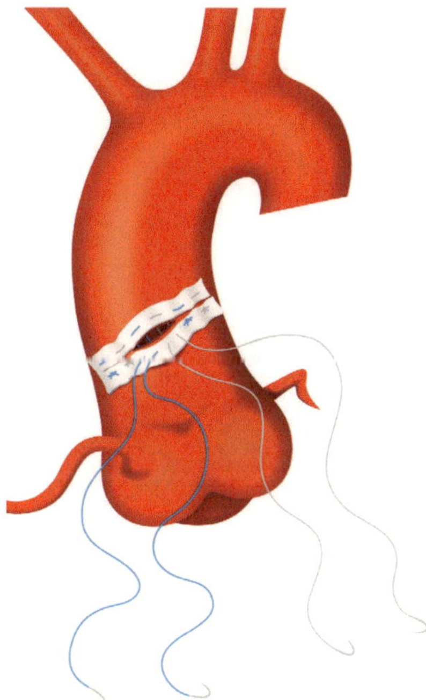

Fig. 4B. For patients with a severely calcified aorta, a knitted polyester strip of 2 cm in width was placed over the aortotomy. It was fixed with 4-0 polyfilament braided horizontal mattress sutures. Except for the two central sutures, all sutures were tied down.

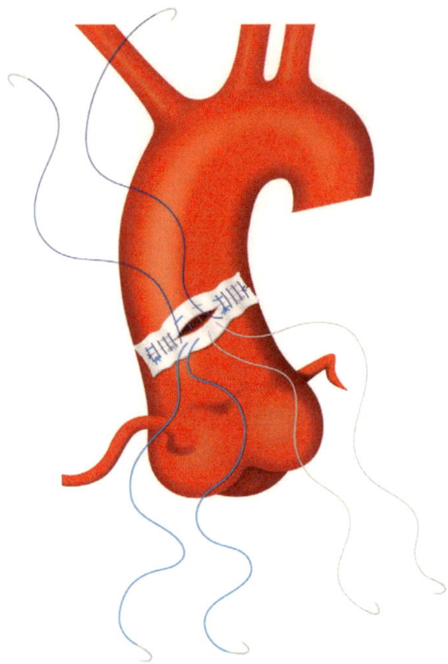

Fig. 4C. Closure of the aortotomy was started with 5-0 polypropylene over-and-over sutures from both edges toward the central untied sutures.

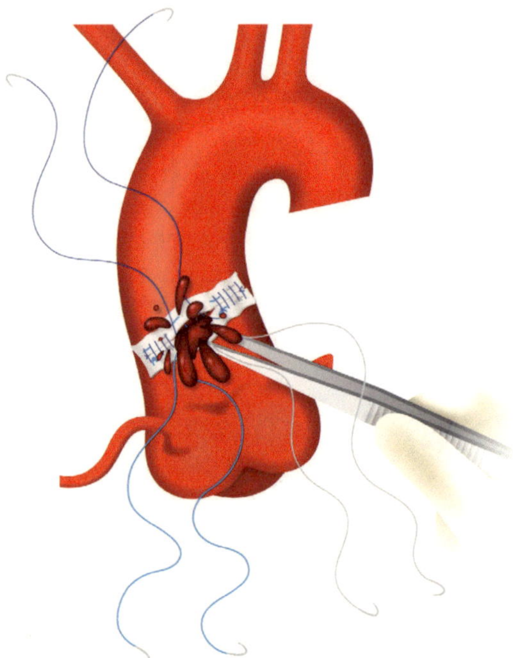

Fig. 4D. The aortotomy for the two untied sutures (about 2 cm in length) was kept open. Under low-flow cardiopulmonary bypass, the ascending aorta was carefully declamped to flush out remaining debris from the aortotomy for about 30 seconds.

horizontal mattress (Matsuda-ika Kogyo, Tokyo, Japan) and 5-0 polypropylene over-and-over sutures (Prolene®; Ethicon, Somerville, NJ, USA) **(Fig. 4A)**. When the edges of the aortotomy included calcification, an endarterectomy was performed to facilitate closure of the ascending aorta.

For patients with a severely calcified aorta, a knitted polyester strip of 2 cm in width (Sauvage Filamentous Fabric®; Bard Peripheral Vascular Inc., Tempe, AZ, USA) was used to prevent cutting and injury of the calcified ascending aorta. The left end of the strip was divided to place over the aortotomy. At first, 4-0 polyfilament braided horizontal mattress sutures were required for both ends to fix the trimmed strip. Other horizontal mattress sutures were placed along the aortotomy. Except for the two central sutures, all sutures were tied down **(Fig. 4B)**. Then, aortotomy closure was started with 5-0 polypropylene over-and-over sutures from both edges toward the central untied sutures **(Fig. 4C)**. The aortotomy between the two untied sutures (about 2 cm in length) was kept open to flush out the debris. Under low CPB flow, the ascending aorta was carefully declamped with manual occlusion of the neck vessels. A sufficient amount of blood was flushed out from the aortotomy for about 30 seconds **(Fig. 4D)**. Then, the two central sutures were tied down. The central portion of the aortotomy was reinforced with 5-0 polypropylene over-and-over suture.

2.2.5 AVR plus ascending aorta replacement

When simple AVR cannot be safely performed due to an unclampable ascending aorta, AVR plus ascending aorta replacement is selected for these patients. During circulatory arrest at a core body temperature of 28°C, cerebral perfusion was selectively initiated. Antegrade tepid blood cardioplegia was selectively delivered to obtain cardioplegic cardiac arrest. For maintenance, retrograde tepid blood cardioplegia was infused every 20 to 30 minutes.

The ascending aorta was transected above the level of the sinotubular junction and subsequently transected below the level of the innominate artery. The prosthetic aortic valve was seated in the supravalvular position. The technical details of the AVR were described above. After seating the prosthetic valve, localized endarterectomy for the distal anastomosis was performed if needed. The distal end of the ascending aorta was encircled by a 2-cm-wide felt strip. A gelatin-impregnated, woven Dacron graft (J Graft SEALED NEO®; JUNKEN-MEDICAL Co., Japan Lifeline, Saitama, Japan) with one side branch was implanted as open distal anastomosis. It was sewn to the distal end of the ascending aorta with 4-0 polyfilament braided sutures in a horizontal mattress fashion **(Fig. 5A)**. The distal end of the Dacron graft (1 cm in length) was gently fixed in an inverted form **(Fig. 5B)**. Then, the anastomosis was reinforced with additional 3-0 polypropylene over-and-over suture **(Fig. 5C)**. After completion of the distal anastomosis, cerebral perfusion was withdrawn, and antegrade systemic perfusion was started via the side branch of the Dacron graft **(Fig. 5D)**.

The proximal anastomosis was completed by single 3-0 polypropylene running sutures. Firstly, the proximal end of the graft was sewn to the posterior wall of the proximal aorta with 3-0 polypropylene running suture. Then, both ends of the suture were tied with other 3-0 polypropylene sutures to avoid relaxation of the posterior anastomosis. Thus, the posterior wall of the graft was fixed in an inverted form **(Fig. 6A)**. Secondly, one stay suture was placed at the toe for easy adjustment **(Fig. 6B)**. Thirdly, the anterior wall of the graft was sewn to the proximal aorta with 3-0 polypropylene running sutures from both ends **(Fig. 6C)**.

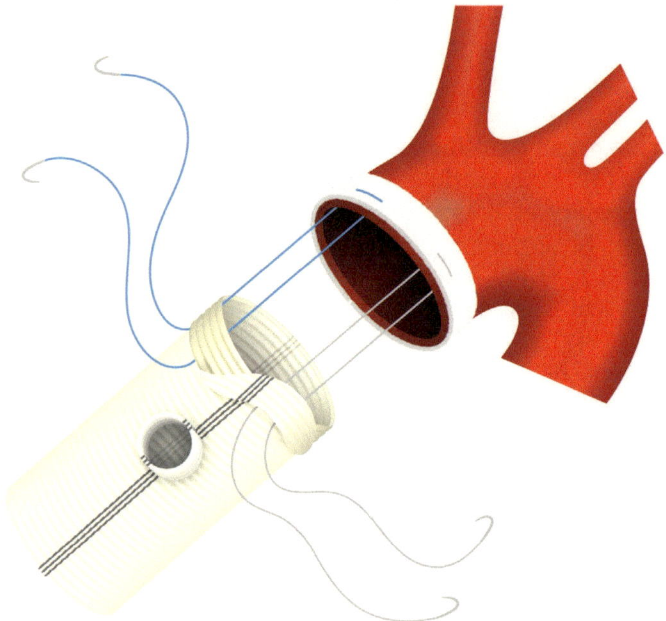

Fig. 5A. A Dacron graft with one side branch was sewn to the distal end of the ascending aorta with 4-0 polyfilament braided sutures in a horizontal mattress fashion.

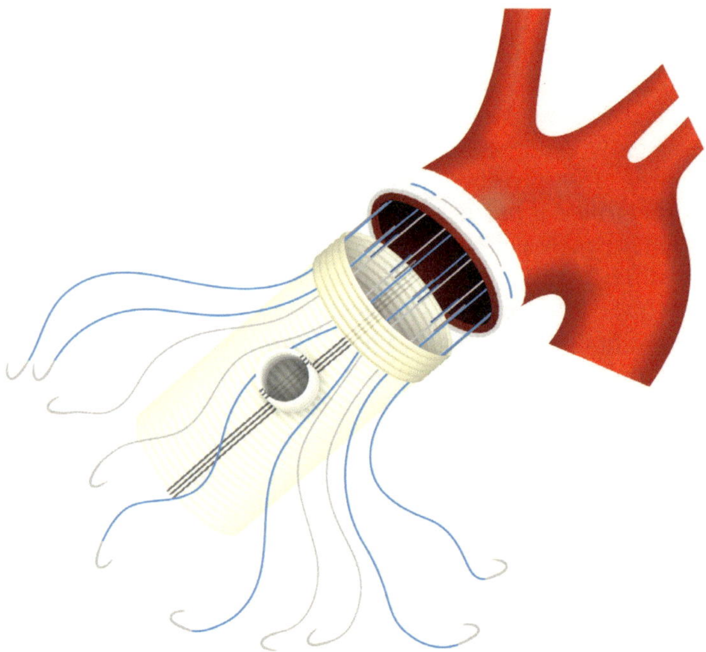

Fig. 5B. The distal end of the Dacron graft (1 cm in length) was gently fixed in an inverted form.

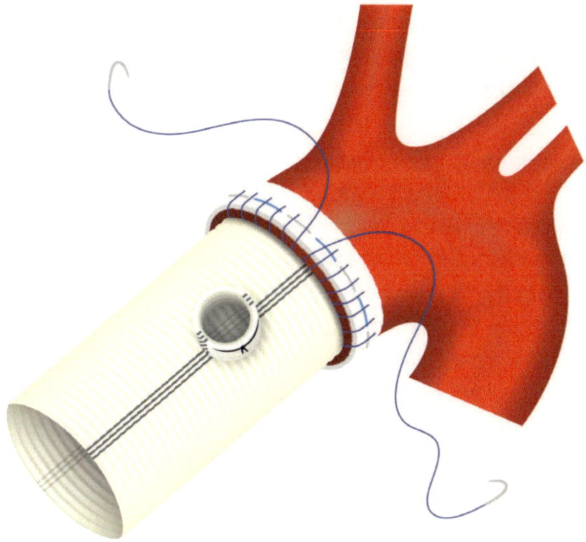

Fig. 5C. The anastomosis was reinforced with additional 3-0 polypropylene over-and-over suture.

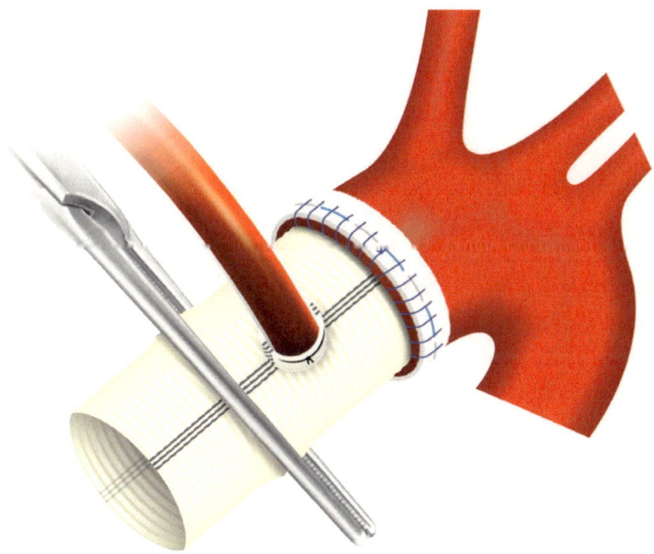

Fig. 5D. After completion of the distal anastomosis, cerebral perfusion was withdrawn, and antegrade systemic perfusion was started via the side branch of the Dacron graft. (Hirota et al.)

2.2.6 Concomitant procedure

In combined coronary artery bypass grafting (CABG) and AVR procedures, distal anastomoses were completed without crossclamping during cooling. For beating CABG procedures, a heart retracting system with the Tentacles Heart Positioner (Sumitomo Bakelite, Tokyo, Japan), which provides excellent exposure of target coronary arteries[18)], is usually used. Proximal anastomoses were performed during single crossclamping after AVR.

In combined mitral valve surgery and AVR, mitral valve plasty (MVP) or mitral valve replacement (MVR) was performed prior to AVR. For patients not requiring ascending aorta replacement, the ascending aorta was crossclamped after brief circulatory arrest. Subsequently, mitral valve surgery was initiated prior to AVR. For patients with ascending aorta replacement, the distal end of the ascending aorta was firstly sewn to a Dacron graft with one side branch during circulatory arrest **(Fig. 6A)**. After the distal anastomosis, systemic and cerebral perfusion was antegradely maintained via the side branch of the graft **(Fig. 6B)**. Then, mitral valve surgery was initiated prior to AVR. When the left side Maze procedure was indicated, it was performed via the right-sided left atriotomy during mitral valve surgery. After completion of mitral valve surgery, AVR was started as described above. Subsequently, the left atrium was closed and the proximal anastomosis of the ascending aorta was performed (**Fig. 6C**). Finally, the right side Maze procedure and/or tricuspid valve surgery was performed through the right atriotomy.

3. Results

Of a total of 705 patients having AVR, 46 patients (11%) with a calcified ascending aorta required brief circulatory arrest for internal inspection of the ascending aorta. Of these 46 patients, 42 (92%) underwent simple AVR after safe aortic crossclamping. The duration of circulatory arrest was less than 1 min in 40 patients and the longest duration was 3 min (mean 0.9±0.6 min). In 3 patients (7%), AVR plus ascending aorta replacement was performed due to an unclampable ascending aorta during circulatory arrest at moderate hypothermia (28°C). For 1 patient (1%), the Bentall operation was done due to a dilated sinus of Valsalva.

In this series, patients had AVR with a bioprosthetic (n=31; 67%) or a mechanical valve (n=15; 33%). Twenty-two patients (48%) had Carpentier-Edwards pericardial valves (Edwards Life Science Corporation, Irvine, CA, USA), 9 patients (20%) had CarboMedics Top Hat mechanical valves (CarboMedics, Inc., Austin, TX, USA), 6 patients (13%) had Sorin Bicarbon-Slim mechanical valves (Sorin Biomedica, Saluggia, Italy), 5 patients (11%) had Medtronic Mosaic valves (Medtronic Inc., Minneapolis, MN, USA), 1 patient had a Prima Plus Stentless valve (Edwards Life Science Corporation), and 1 patient had a Medtronic Freestyle valve (Medtronic Inc.).

Twenty-seven patients (59%) had concomitant procedures including CABG (n=18), MVR (n=6), MVP (n=2), the Maze procedure (n=4), and tricuspid annuloplasty (n=3). No intra-aortic balloon pumping was required postoperatively. Aortic crossclamping time was 76±18 min. CPB time was 148±29 min. Operative time was 330±69 min. The hospital mortality was 2.2% (1 of 46). One patient died of gastrointestinal bleeding. There was no cardiogenic death in this series. The postoperative morbidity was 2.2% (1 of 46). Cerebrovascular accident occurred in one patient.

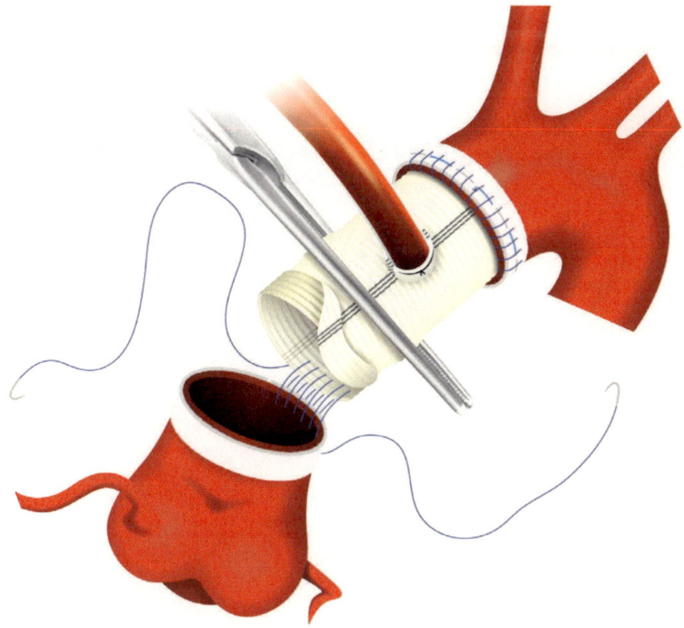

Fig. 6A. The proximal end of the graft was sewn to the posterior wall of the proximal aorta with 3-0 polypropylene running suture.

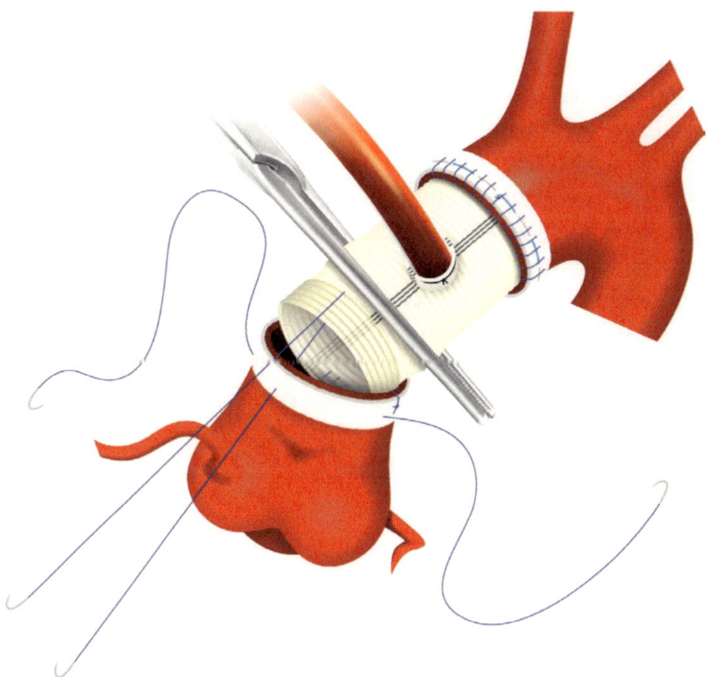

Fig. 6B. Both ends of the suture were tied with other 3-0 polypropylene sutures to avoid relaxation of the posterior anastomosis. Thus, the posterior wall of the graft was fixed in an inverted form. One stay suture was placed at the toe for easy adjustment.

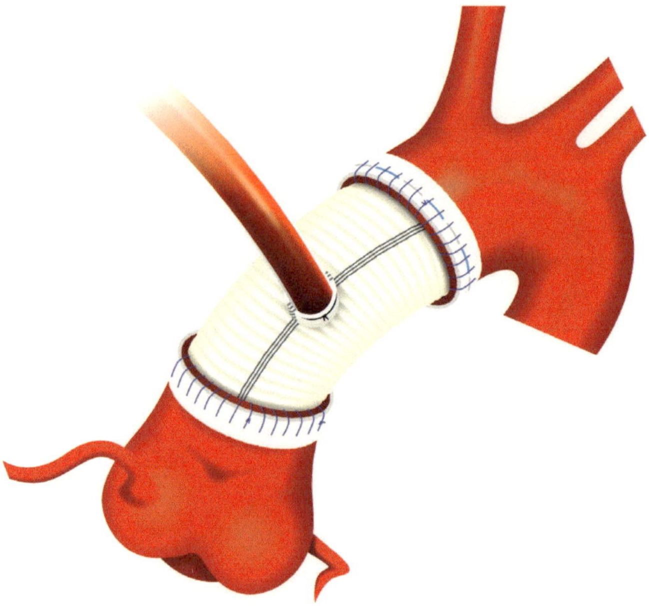

Fig. 6C. The anterior wall of the graft was sewn to the proximal aorta with 3-0 polypropylene running sutures from both ends.

4. Discussion

Patients with AS and a calcified ascending aorta were treated with meticulous techniques. Careful maneuvers for calcified lesions would reduce atheroembolic complications, contributing to better surgical outcomes.

The surgical challenge of dealing with patients with AS and calcified ascending aorta started in the 1980s[10,11]. With advances in medical technology, the surgical strategy has been modified in various ways. Theoretically, the simplest approach is supposed to be AVR without aortic crossclamping during HCA[10-12]. Although the no-touch technique to the calcified aorta effectively reduces the surgical risk of atheroembolic events, prolonged HCA time is a risk for stroke[19]. As a different strategy to facilitate AVR, endarterectomy during HCA has been reported to avoid embolic events[13,20]. No patients with postoperative stroke suggested a good early result, but there were no follow-up data relating to the long-term risks of aortic dissection or dilatation. Although HCA provides simple strategies for patients with AS and a calcified ascending aorta, technical modifications are needed to render the procedure less invasive.

Aortic crossclamping is one of the most technically difficult aspects for patients with a calcified ascending aorta. The release of aortic crossclamping is closely associated with embolic events during cardiac surgery[9]. As an alternative for aortic crossclamping, a method of internal occlusion of the ascending aorta was reported; i.e., endoaortic balloon occlusion[15]. According to that report, a Foley catheter was directly introduced via the usual aortotomy during a brief period of circulatory arrest at a nasopharyngeal temperature of 25°C. Although the advantages of endoaortic balloon occlusion include easy preparation and less invasive technique, a retrospective analysis demonstrated that it was frequently ineffective and was associated with a significantly higher risk of in-hospital death and a numerically higher risk of stroke[21].

We used brief circulatory arrest less than 1 min in most cases at moderate hypothermia (28°C) for internal inspection of calcified ascending aorta. The extent and severity of calcification is directly observed, and the firmness of the calcified ascending aorta is also palpable without wall stress caused by afterload. Thus, in this situation, it is easy to determine whether the calcified ascending aorta is clampable. When the calcified ascending aorta is clampable, simple AVR followed by aortic crossclamping is planned as a less invasive operation. However, ascending aorta replacement would be performed for patients with an unclampable calcified ascending aorta. At moderate hypothermia (28°C), simple AVR could be converted into ascending aorta replacement under circulatory arrest with selective cerebral perfusion. Thus, patients with AS and calcified ascending aorta are surgically repaired by our strategy without deep HCA.

A recent surgical report also demonstrated that short-term moderate hypothermic arrest is useful for safe aortic crossclamping after internal inspection of a bad ascending aorta[22]. Although this technique for safe crossclamping is almost the same as our strategy, all cases were treated with simple AVR followed by aortic crossclamping. The reason for this would include endarterectomy or debridement by the Cavitron ultrasonic surgical aspirator (CUSA)[23], which successfully achieves a safe aortic crossclamping site. Therefore, circulatory arrest time was slightly longer (3.4±1.5 min) compared to ours (less than 1 min). Although small calcific particles created by the CUSA are potential causes of postoperative stroke, all of them would be completely aspirated. As a result, the postoperative stroke rate remained low (2.5%), with no mortality. For patients with a calcified ascending aorta, the CUSA would also be useful for removing calcific debris during AVR.

As one of the alternatives for open heart surgery, transcatheter valve implantation (TAVI) had been newly developed for symptomatic patients at high risk or with contraindications for surgery[24]. A calcified ascending aorta would be a good indication for TAVI. Successful TAVI dramatically alleviates severe symptoms with a minimally-invasive method. However, TAVI involves major complications such as paravalvular leakage, valve malposition, coronary occlusion, annulus and aortic root rupture, atrioventricular block, and cerebrovascular events[25]. The 30-day all-cause mortality rate with the CoreValve Revalving System (Medtronic Inc.) ranges from 5.5% to 15.5%, while that with the Edwards Sapien prosthesis (Edwards Life Science Corporation) ranges from 6.3% to 10.3%[25]. Although the incidence of persistent neurological impairment was low (less than approximately 5%), the incidence of clinically silent peri-interventricular cerebral embolic lesions after TAVI was high[25,26]. The results of TAVI would be improved by further development of medical devices, but current results are not far superior to our surgical outcomes. Accordingly, there is no established treatment for AS and calcified ascending aorta at present.

In the future, prevalence of calcified lesions, including AS and calcified ascending aorta, is likely to increase as the average lifespan of populations increases. With the advances in medical technologies, new therapeutic technologies, such as TAVI, will be developed for safer strategies and to minimize invasiveness. However, TAVI is not the optimal treatment for all patients with AS, including patients requiring concomitant procedures such as CABG and mitral valve surgery. For these patients, conventional open heart surgery would be one of the therapeutic choices. Additionally, state-of-the-art technologies will not be available worldwide. Thus, cardiac surgeons should continue to modify their strategies by meticulous techniques and share their strategies for better outcomes. Addressing this surgical challenge would result in resolution for many more high-risk patients with complex calcified lesions.

5. Conclusion

Technical modifications such as right axillary artery cannulation and brief circulatory arrest at moderate hypothermia are useful for patients with AS associated with a calcified ascending aorta. The operative design would be important to minimize the surgical risk for such high-risk patients.

6. References

[1] Carabello BA, Paulus WJ. Aortic stenosis. Lancet. 2009 14; 373: 956-66

[2] Stewart BF, Siscovick D, Lind BK, Gardin JM, Gottdiener JS, Smith VE, Kitzman DW, Otto CM. Clinical factors associated with calcific aortic valve disease. Cardiovascular Health Study. J Am Coll Cardiol. 1997; 29: 630-4

[3] Otto CM, Lind BK, Kitzman DW, Gersh BJ, Siscovick DS. Association of aortic-valve sclerosis with cardiovascular mortality and morbidity in the elderly. N Engl J Med. 1999; 34: 142-7

[4] Vahanian A, Baumgartner H, Bax J, Butchart E, Dion R, Filippatos G, Flachskampf F, Hall R, Iung B, Kasprzak J, Nataf P, Tornos P, Torracca L, Wenink A; Task Force on the Management of Valvular Health Disease of the European Society of Cardiology; ESC Committee for Practice Guidelines. Guidelines on the management of valvular disease: The Task Force on the Management of Valvular Heart Disease of the European Society of Cardiology. Eur Heart J. 2007; 28: 230-68

[5] Varadarajan P, Kapoor N, Bansal RC, Pai RG. Survival in elderly patients with severe aortic stenosis is dramatically improved by aortic valve replacement: Results from a cohort of 277 patients aged > or =80 years. Euro J Cardiothorac Surg. 2006; 30: 722-7

[6] Bonow RO, Carabello BA, Chatterjee K, de Leon AC Jr, Faxon DP, Freed MD, Gaasch WH, Lytle BW, Nishimura RA, O'Gara PT, O'Rourke RA, Otto CM, Shah PM, Shanewise JS; American College of Cardiology/American Heart Association Task Force on Practice Guidelines. 2008 focused update incorporated into the ACC/AHA 2006 guidelines for the management of patients with valvular heart disease: a report of the American College of Cardiology/American Heart Association Task Force on Practice Guidelines (Writing Committee to revise the 1998 guidelines for the management of patients with valvular heart disease). Endorsed by the Society of Cardiovascular Anesthesiologists, Society for Cardiovascular Angiography and Interventions, and Society of Thoracic Surgeons. J Am Coll Cardiol. 2008; 52: e1-142

[7] van der Linden J, Hadjinikolaou L, Bergman P, Lindblom D. Postoperative stroke in cardiac surgery is related to the location and extent of atherosclerotic disease in the ascending aorta. J Am Coll Cardiol. 2001; 38: 131-5

[8] Gillinov AM, Lytle BW, Hoang V, Cosgrove DM, Banbury MK, McCarthy PM, Sabik JF, Pettersson GB, Smedira NG, Blackstone EH. The atherosclerotic aorta at aortic valve replacement: surgical strategies and results. J Thorac Cardiovasc Surg. 2000; 120: 957-63

[9] Barbut D, Hinton RB, Szatrowski TP, Hartman GS, Bruefach M, Williams-Russo P, Charlson E, Gold JP. Cerebral emboli detected during bypass surgery are associated with clamp removal. Stroke. 1994; 25: 2398-402
[10] Jacobowitz IJ, Rose DM, Shevede K, Cunningham JN. Use of profound hypothermia and circulatory arrest for the calcified aorta. Chest. 1984; 85: 288-9
[11] Coselli JS, Crawford ES. Aortic valve replacement in the patient with extensive calcification of the ascending aorta (the porcelain aorta). J Thorac Cardiovasc Surg. 1986; 91: 184-7
[12] Byrne JG, Aranki SF, Cohn LH. Aortic valve operations under deep hypothermic circulatory arrest for the porcelain aorta: "no-touch" technique. Ann Thorac Surg. 1998; 65: 1313-5
[13] Vogt PR, Hauser M, Schwarz U, Jenni R, Lachat ML, Zund G, Schupbach RW, Schmidlin D, Turina MI. Complete thromboendarterectomy of the calcified ascending aorta and aortic arch. Ann Thorac Surg. 1999; 67: 457-61
[14] Aranki SF, Nathan M, Shekar P, Couper G, Rizzo R, Cohn LH. Hypothermic circulatory arrest enables aortic valve replacement in patients with unclampable aorta. Ann Thorac Surg. 2005; 1679-86
[15] Cosgrove DM. Management of the calcified aorta: an alternative method of occlusion. Ann Thorac Surg. 1983; 36: 718-9
[16] Lockowandt U. Apicoaortic valved conduit: potential for progress? J Thorac Cardiovasc Surg. 2006; 132: 796-801
[17] Isomura T, Hisatomi K, Satoh T, Hayashida N, Aoyagi S. Axillary artery cannulation for cardiopulmonary bypass in the presence of diseased ascending aorta. Eur J Cardiothorac Surg. 1996; 10; 481
[18] Shimamura Y, Mochizuki Y, Yamada Y, Eda K, Shibasaki I, Inoue Y, Miyoshi S. Surgical technique of displacement and retraction of the heart with a pigtail shaped hook and Tentacles Heart Positioner. Kyobu Geka. 2007; 60: 547-9
[19] Svensson LG, Crawford ES, Hess KR, Coselli JS, Raskin S, Shenaq SA, Safi HJ. Deep hypothermia with circulatory arrest. Determinants of stroke and early mortality in 656 patients. J Thorac Cardiovac Surg. 1993; 106: 19-28
[20] Svensson LG, Sun J, Cruz HA, Shahian DM. Endarterectomy for calcified porcelain aorta associated with aortic valve stenosis. Ann Thorac Surg. 1996; 61: 149-52
[21] Zingone B, Gatti G, Rauber E, Pappalardo A, Benussi B, Dreas L. Surgical management of the atherosclerotic ascending aorta: is endoaortic balloon occlusion safe? Ann Thorac Surg. 2006; 82: 1709-4
[22] Takami Y, Tajima K, Terazawa S, Okada N, Fujii K, Sakai Y. Safer aortic crossclamping during short-term moderate hypothermic circulatory arrest for cardiac surgery in patients with a bad ascending aorta. J Thorac Cardiovasc Surg. 2009; 137: 875-80
[23] Kellner HJ, Pracki P, Hildebrandt A, Binner C, Eisele G, Struck E. Aortic valve debridement by ultrasonic surgical aspirator in degenerative, aortic valve stenosis: follow-up with Doppler echocardiography. Eur J Cardiothorac Surg. 1996; 10; 498-504
[24] Vahanian A, Alfirei O, Al-Attar N, Antunes M, Bax J, Cormier B, Cribier A, De Jaeqere P, Fournial G, Kappetein AP, Kovac J, Ludqate S, Maisano F, Moat N, Mohr F, Nataf P, Pierard L, Pomar JL, Schofer J, Tornos P, Tuzcu M, van Hout B, Von Seqesser LK, Walther T; European Association of Cardio-Thoracic Surgery;

European Society of Cardiology; European Association of Percutaneous Cardiovascular Interventions. Transcatheter valve implantation for patients with aortic stenosis: a position statement from the European Association of Cardio-Thoracic Surgery (EACTS) and the European Society of Cardiology (ESC), in collaboration with the European Association of Percutaneous Cardiovascular Interventions (EAPCI). Eur Heart J. 2008; 29: 1463-70

[25] Spaccarotella C, Mongiardo A, Indolfi C. Pathophysiology of aortic stenosis and approach to treatment with percutaneous valve implantation. Circ J. 24; 75: 11-19

[26] Ghanem A, Muller A, Nahle CP, Kocurek J, Werner N, Hammerstingl C, Schild HH, Schwab JO, Mellert F, Fimmers R, Nickenig G, Thomas D. Risk and fate of cerebral embolism after transfemoral aortic valve implantation: a prospective pilot study with diffusion-weighted magnetic resonance imaging. J Am Coll Cardiol. 2010; 55: 1427-32

9

Transcatheter Aortic Valve Implantation: New Hope for Inoperable and High-Risk Patients

Kentaro Hayashida and Thierry Lefèvre
Institut Cardiovasculaire Paris Sud, Massy, France

1. Introduction

Calcified aortic stenosis is the most frequently reported valvular disease in our industrialized countries. This pathology is mainly observed in elderly patients with 3% prevalence after the age of 70.

As a result of increasing life expectancy and the post war baby boom phenomenon, we can expect a "**granny and granddad boom**" in the years to come. Without surgical aortic valve replacement (SAVR), the prognosis of severe symptomatic aortic stenosis (AS) is poor and is associated with a short life expectancy after symptom onset (Bonow, Carabello et al. 2008). Although SAVR has been regarded as the gold standard treatment for severe AS for several decades (Bonow, Carabello et al. 2006; Vahanian, Baumgartner et al. 2007), many patients do not undergo surgical treatment as this therapeutic option is deemed to carry excessive risk by the patient's family or by his physician, cardiologist or even the surgeon because of advanced age and the presence of co-morbidities. Indeed, many studies have shown that 25% to 50% of symptomatic patients with severe AS do not receive surgical treatment. For instance, in the study by Iung et al. (Iung, Baron et al. 2003) 31.8% of eligible patients were not referred for SAVR.

Balloon valvuloplasty (BAV) was introduced by Cribier et al in 1986, to support the concept of mechanical dilatation of severely calcified aortic valve (Cribier, Savin et al. 1986) for inoperable patients. Despite initial improvement of symptoms observed immediately after the procedure (NHLBI Balloon Valvuloplasty Registry Participant. 1991), it was associated with high mortality, complication and recurrence rates (Safian, Berman et al. 1988). Because of its poor long term outcome (about 50% survival at 1 year and 20% at 3 years) (Otto, Mickel et al. 1994; Lieberman, Bashore et al. 1995), this procedure was performed in a dwindling number of cases, mainly as a bridge to SAVR in patients with poor hemodynamic status or in patients requiring urgent non cardiac surgery .

Percutaneous catheter-based systems for the treatment of aortic valve stenosis were assessed in experimental animal models (Andersen, Knudsen et al. 1992) for several years before Cribier et al successfully designed a percutaneous transcatheter implantation system for an aortic valve prosthesis. They reported their first human case in 2002 using an antegrade transseptal approach with local anesthesia and mild sedation (Cribier, Eltchaninoff et al. 2002). Subsequently, this system was developed by Edwards Lifesciences, for use via either a retrograde transfemoral approach (TF) with a new deflectable delivery system or a transapical approach (TA). In 2004, Grube et al carried out the first-in-man percutaneous implantation of the CoreValve self-expanding valve prosthesis for severe AS and the initial experience of 25 cases was reported in 2005 (Grube, Laborde et al. 2006). Transcatheter aortic valve implantation (TAVI) is no longer an emerging technology for the treatment of patients with severe AS who are at high risk or ineligible for conventional surgery. It has become a valid treatment option addressing an unmet clinical need (Figure 1). TAVI and aortic valvuloplasty are now integrated into the potential therapeutic strategies applicable to patients with severe aortic stenosis carrying a high surgical risk and a heart team approach has become essential to implementing this procedure (Figure 2).

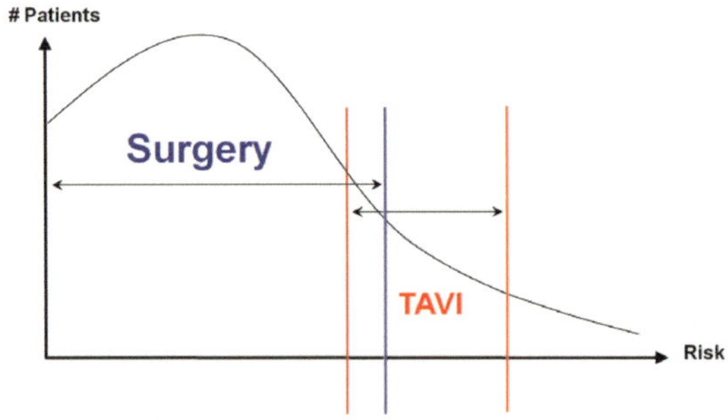

Fig. 1. TAVI addresses an unmet clinical need

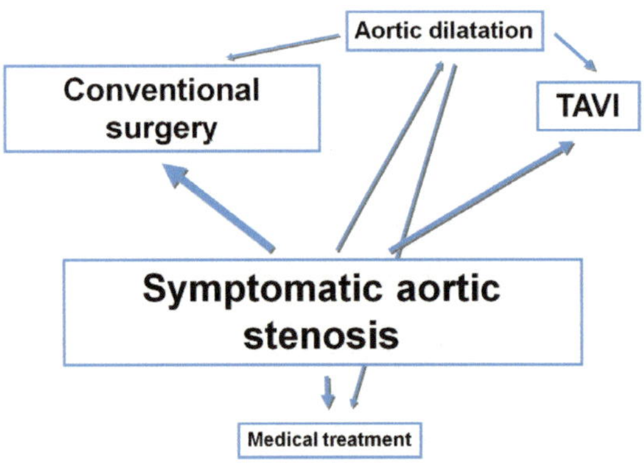

Fig. 2. Heart team approach is essential for TAVI

2. Clinical studies

2.1 Cribier-Edwards, Edwards-Sapien valve

The Edwards-Sapien (ES) valve is a trileaflet valve mounted on a balloon-expandable stent. The first-generation valve was made of polyurethane and the second-generation of bovine pericardium (Figure 3). After the pilot study involving six cases treated via the antegrade transvenous approach (Cribier, Eltchaninoff et al. 2004), initial feasibility studies (I-REVIVE and RECAST) were conducted in Rouen (Eltchaninoff, Tron et al. 2007) in 36 patients treated via both the antegrade and retrograde TF approaches. The retrograde delivery system was refined by Webb et al. and the results of the first 18 cases reported in 2006 showed improved procedural success and 30-day mortality (Webb, Chandavimol et al. 2006).

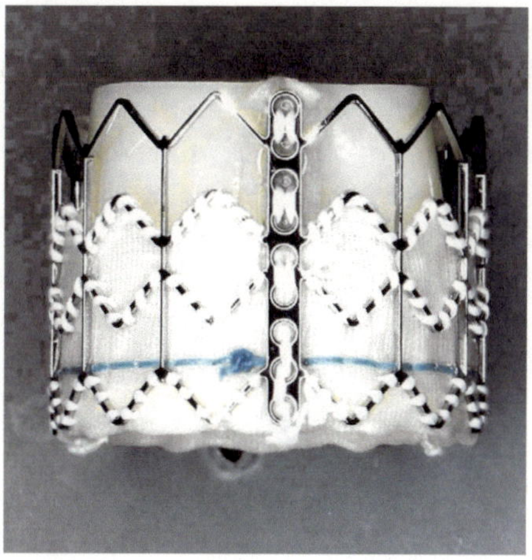

Fig. 3. The 1st generation Edwards valve
Balloon expandable bioprothesis
Stainless steel
23, 26 mm
Bovine pericardium
Thermafix preparation
Flex delivery system
Retrograde or Trans-apical approach
22 or 24 Fr femoral sheath

The first procedure via the TA approach was performed in 2005 and the initial clinical experience was reported in 2006 (Lichtenstein, Cheung et al. 2006). CE Mark for both TF and TA delivery systems with the same valve was obtained for this device in 2007. In total, 9 clinical trials and registries were completed from first-in-man to CE Mark. After CE Mark approval, a post-market registry (SOURCE) was conducted in Europe (Thomas, Schymik et al. 2010; Wendler, Schymik et al. 2010). In the United States, the PARTNER US trial (an FDA approved, two-cohort, four-arm multicenter trial with the second-generation Edwards valve) was initiated in 2007, and the results obtained in cohort B demonstrated that TF-TAVI not only reduces dramatically the risk of death from any cause compared to standard therapy (Leon, Smith et al. 2010), but also improves significantly the quality of life. The results of cohort A comparing TF / TA-TAVI with SAVR met the primary endpoint of the study, demonstrating the noninferiority of TAVI compared to conventional aortic valve replacement in terms of all-cause mortality (Smith and Leon 2011). At 30 days, deaths from any cause were numerically lower in the TAVI group by intention to treat (3.4% vs 6.5%), however, this was not statistically significant. At one-year follow-up, the mortality rate in both groups was nearly identical (24.2% vs 26.8%). The PARTNER 2 trial which has a similar design is currently assessing the third-generation Edwards valve. A comparable study evaluating the Corevalve is about to start in the United States.

2.2 Medtronic CoreValve revalving system

The Medtronic CoreValve revalving system (Medtronic Inc., Minneapolis, MN, USA) is a trileaflet porcine pericardium valve mounted on a self-expanding nitinol frame. The first-in-man clinical feasibility study (n = 14) was performed in 2004 with the first generation 25-Fr device. From 2005 to 2006, consecutive safety and efficacy studies (n = 65) were conducted using the second-generation 21-Fr device. The third-generation device (Figure 4) was developed in order to provide a lower profile system (18-Fr), which received CE Mark in 2007 (Grube, Schuler et al. 2007; Piazza, Grube et al. 2008).

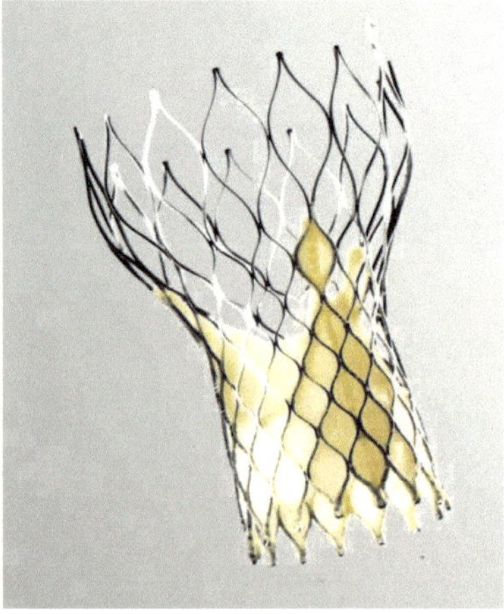

Fig. 4. The CoreValve Revalving™ System
Self-expandable bioprothesis
Nitinol
26 and 29 mm
Porcine Péricardium
Retrograde approach
18 Fr sheath

3. Current devices and procedures

3.1 Edwards Sapien XT valve

3.1.1 Design

The Edwards-Sapien valve has three bovine pericardium leaflets, mounted on a balloon-expandable tubular frame with high radial force in order to obtain uniform leaflet coaptation and to maintain an effective orifice area. As with all surgical Edwards bioprostheses, the leaflets are prepared using the Thermafix technology. The stent of the last generation, SAPIEN XT, is made of a cobalt-chromium alloy (Figure 5), and the delivery system (Novaflex) has been improved in order to reduce the profile to 18 Fr for the 23 mm valve and 19 Fr for the 26 mm valve (the former retroflex delivery system was 22 and 24 Fr, respectively). A 29 mm valve has been recently introduced (only for the TA approach in 2011) and a 20 mm valve will be available in the near future.

3.1.2 Procedures

The two main approaches for the Edwards Sapiens valve are the TF and TA routes. Careful screening of the ilio-femoral access by CT scan and/or selective ilio-femoral angiography from different orthogonal planes is crucial for optimal selection of the approach site. The decision to proceed with TF approach depends on minimal lumen diameter, calcification

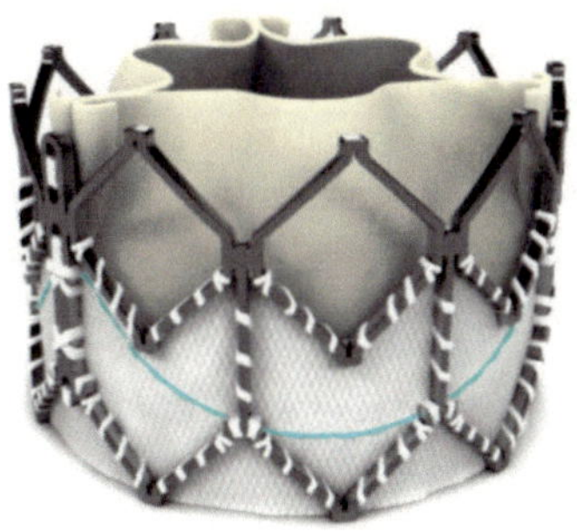

Figure 5: The 2nd Generation Edwards: Sapiens XT valve :
Balloon expandable bioprothesis
Cobalt chromium
23, 26, 29 mm
Bovine pericardium
Thermafix preparation
Novaflex delivery system
Retrograde and trans-apical approach
18 or 19 Fr femoral sheath

and tortuosity of ilio-femoral access, and presence of debris in the aorta. CT scan and/or transoesophagal echocardiography is an important part of the screening phase. The TA approach may be applied to patients with insufficient or risky vascular access. However, the presence of respiratory insufficiency or a hostile thorax must be taken into account. A novel, minimally invasive approach involving the direct puncture of the ascending aorta is currently being evaluated.

The TF approach requires arterial access via the femoral artery by insertion of the sheath using direct puncture or surgical cut-down of the common femoral artery. The Novaflex delivery system is advanced through the sheath into the aorta. The Sapien XT valve is then mounted on the balloon in the aorta, by pulling back the balloon underneath the valve. The system is advanced into the annulus position whilst avoiding direct contact with the aorta using the flex system. The valve position should subsequently be confirmed by aortography from perpendicular projection and the valve should be deployed under rapid pacing (180 to 240 beat/min.) in order to control blood pressure below 40 mmHg, and avoid migration of the valve during deployment. Closure of the femoral artery access is performed by ligation of the pre-deployed sutures of a Prostar XL device or two Proglide devices, or by surgical closure. In the early experience, surgical closure was adapted to the previously used 22- or 24-fr sheaths. Gradual sheath down-sizing contributed to the generalization of the "true percutaneous approach" using direct puncture of the femoral artery and closure with a suture-mediated device (Kahlert, Al-Rashid et al. 2009; Van Mieghem, Nuis et al. 2010; Hayashida, Lefevre et al. 2011) as well as the possibility of using local anesthesia.

TA-TAVI is performed using the current Ascendra 2 system inserted into the left ventricle (LV) via the apex. A double purse string is placed on the LV apex with mini anterior thoracotomy at the fifth or sixth intercostal space. The sheath is advanced into the LV cavity, followed by the insertion of the valve prosthesis after predilatation (Lichtenstein, Cheung et al. 2006). The valve is positioned under aortography guidance from a perpendicular projection and deployed with rapid pacing as in transfemoral procedures.

3.2 Medtronic CoreValve revalving system

3.2.1 Design

The CoreValve revalving system is a self-expanding multilevel support frame with a tri-leaflet porcine pericardial tissue valve. A multilevel self-expandable Nitinol frame retains the tissue valve in place with high hoop strength. This high strength frame serves to preserve the anatomy of the valve, and stabilize the orifice area. The device is anchored by the high radial force area in the aortic annulus and by the low radial force area in the ascending aorta.

This device is currently available in sizes of 26 mm for annuli of between 20 and 23 mm, 29 mm for annuli between 23 and 27 mm. In the near future, a 32 mm valve will be available for annuli between 27 and 29 mm.

The delivery system is an over-the-wire catheter system. The distal part of the catheter has an 18-fr housing capsule which contains the valve prosthesis, and both sizes of bioprostheses can be accommodated by this delivery system. "The Accutrak delivery system" has been recently developed to reduce friction between the metal frame and the delivery system, thus preventing valve migration into the LV, and ensuring more accurate positioning of the bioprosthesis.

3.2.2 Procedures

This device can be implanted via three potential approaches: the TF, the transsubclavian, and the transaortic approaches.

Like the Sapien valve, the Corevalve can be implanted via the TF approach using an ilio-femoral vascular access. The delivery system is advanced over a stiff wire into the LV cavity, with subsequent slow release of the bioprosthesis by turning the microknob under fluoroscopic guidance. Several aortographies should be performed to ensure that the valve is positioned correctly during deployment.

The transsubclavian route is a potential alternative in cases where the femoral access is not sufficient. Surgical cut-down is performed for subclavian access, followed by sheath insertion into the ascending aorta. The delivery system is advanced to the aortic annulus as with the TF approach. This approach has been shown to be at least as safe as the TF approach in registries conducted in Italy and the UK (Petronio, De Carlo et al. 2010; Moynagh, Scott et al. 2011).

The transaortic approach is implemented in patients in whom no other access options are available (Latsios, Gerckens et al. 2010). This approach requires a mini-sternotomy, and direct puncture of the ascending aorta under visual and fluoroscopic guidance (Latsios, Gerckens et al. 2010). The rest of the procedure is similar to the TF approach.

The advantage of this self-expandable system is that it avoids traumatic dilatation of the annulus. The full retrievability of the bioprosthesis into the sheath is also advantageous in cases of valve migration before disconnection of the metal anchor of the frame from the delivery system. The relatively smaller delivery system is also beneficial for patients with a >21mm annulus (18 Fr in CoreValve vs 19 Fr in Sapien valve) and borderline ilio-femoral access.

4. Optimal patient selection

Patients with symptomatic severe AS are considered candidates for TAVI if they have a high logistic EuroSCORE (European System for Cardiac Operative Risk Evaluation score) or STS score (the Society of Thoracic Surgeons Score), or if surgery is deemed to be of excessive risk due to significant comorbidities, or if other risk factors not captured by these scoring systems (eg, porcelain aorta, severe thoracic distortion, severe liver disease, pre-dialysis renal insufficiency etc…) are present.
The decision to proceed with TAVI should be discussed by a dedicated heart team including cardiologists, interventional cardiologists, cardiovascular surgeons, anesthesiologists, and specialists in cardiac imaging. The role of geriatricians is crucial in borderline cases. The main concerns for optimal patient selection are: 1) annulus diameter of the native valve, 2) arterial access, and 3) diameter of the ascending aorta (Wenaweser and Windecker 2010).

4.1 Annulus diameter

4.1.1 Annulus size to define a valve prosthesis size

Annulus size is a crucial parameter for selection of the appropriate type and size of valve. The annulus diameter criteria for Edwards valve are 18 to 21mm for the 23mm valve and 21 to 24.5mm for the 26mm device. In 2011, a 29mm valve covering 24.5 to 27mm annuli has been launched for the TA approach exclusively. The 20mm valve is currently being developed. For the CoreValve, a 26mm valve is used for 20 to 23mm annuli and a 29mm valve for 23 to 27mm annuli (Grube, Schuler et al. 2007). A 32mm valve should be available in the near future. All currently available valves can be used to treat most patients with annulus sizes ranging from 18 to 27 mm.

4.1.2 Imaging modalities for annulus diameter measurement

Four modalities are available for measuring the aortic annulus: Transesophageal echocardiography (TEE), transthoracic echocardiography (TTE), invasive aortography and cardiac computed tomography (CT) scan (Wenaweser and Windecker 2010). TEE has been considered as the gold standard method for measuring the annulus size (Hutter, Opitz et al. 2010), due to its better imaging quality compared to TTE and lower degree of inter-observer variability, however it represents only 1 dimension in the antero-posterior view. TTE is mainly

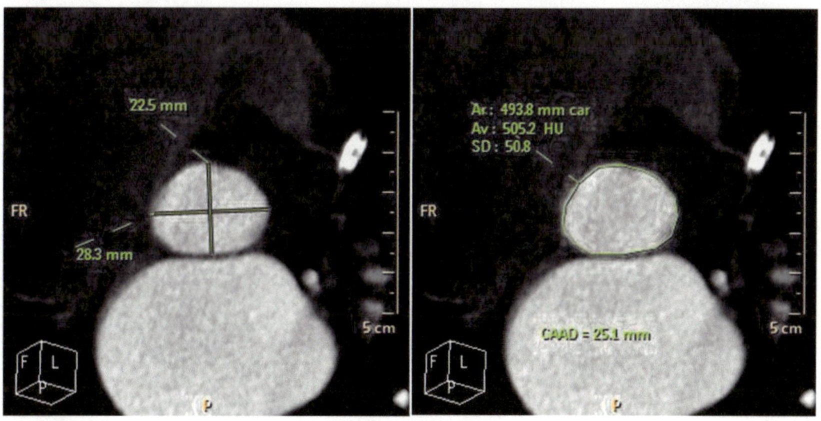

Fig. 6. MSCT and measurement of the annulus diameter

used for screening in order to exclude extremely small or large annuli or in instances where TEE is not applicable, due to its reduced imaging quality. Invasive aortography reflects the coronal view of the CT scan image. The fact that the aortic valve annulus is oval-shaped, rather than round-shaped must be taken into account when measuring the annulus size. CT scan is also a useful tool for measurement of the aortic annulus, providing appreciation of the oval shape of the annulus with high imaging quality. Due to its oval shape the annulus size measured by CT coronal view is larger than by sagital view (Schultz, Moelker et al. 2010).

One solution would be to measure the circumference or the surface of the annulus and use the theoretical diameter deducted from this measurement for selection of the valve (Figure 6). TEE (Figure 7) or MSCT (Figure 8) assessment of the patient is essential in order to detect potential aortic debris which could preclude the use of the transfemoral route.

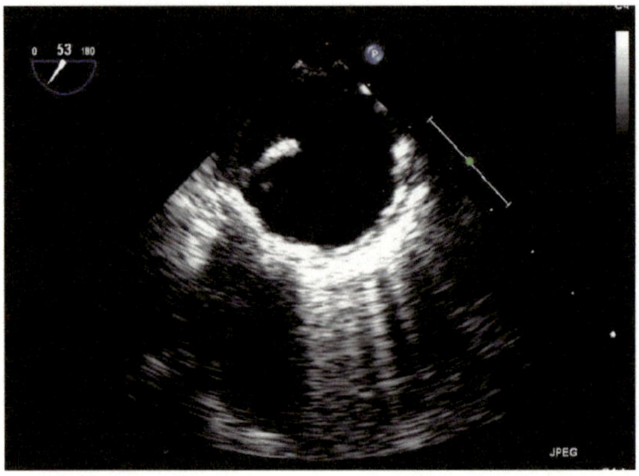

Fig. 7. Transoesophagal echocardiography and aortic debris

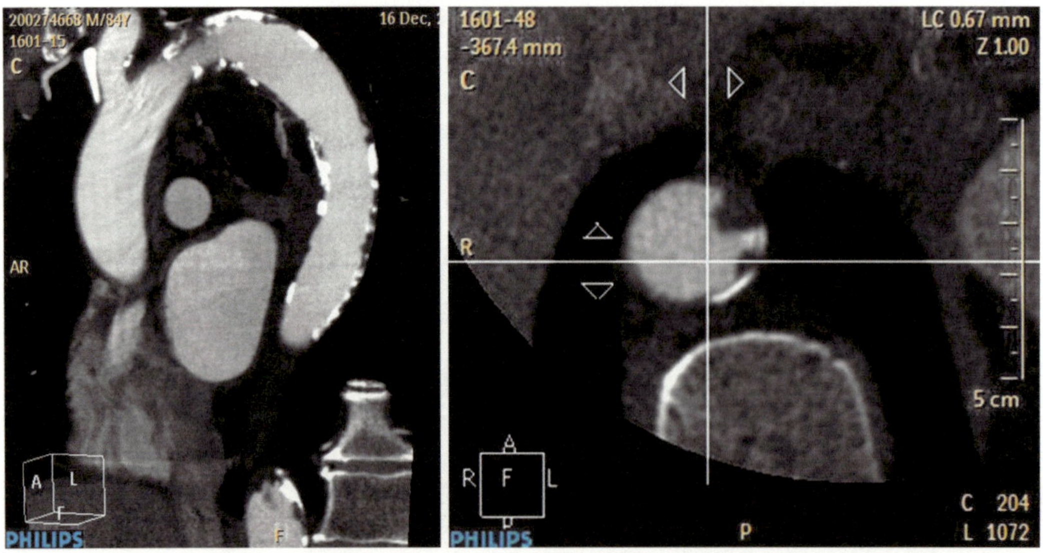

Fig. 8. MSCT and aortic debris

4.2 Arterial access

The assessment of the ilio-femoral vessels can be performed by selective ilio-femoral angiography from 2 orthogonal planes, or multislice computed tomography (MSCT). Renal dysfunction is frequent in these patients and it is important not to cumulate several explorations requiring contrast media over a short period of time. For this reason we perform a selective angiogram of the ilio-femoral axes during coronary angiography. The radial approach is used preferentially in order to preserve any future femoral access for TAVI. MSCT is a useful tool for appraising the anatomy of the arterial access site. Such criteria as minimal lumen diameter (MLD), degree of calcification and tortuosity of the ilio-femoral access are essential in determining patient eligibility for the TF approach. We established that the ratio between "sheath outer diameter" and "MLD of femoral artery" (SFAR) predicts the occurrence of major vascular complications and the cut-point of this ratio which best predicts vascular complications (Table 1) is 1.05 (Hayashida, Lefevre et al. 2011). In non-calcified ilio-femoral vessels, the SFAR may be increased to 1.10 and conversely decreased to 1.00 in calcified arteries. Using this SFAR threshold, the minimal femoral artery diameter necessary for the 19 and 18 Fr introducer sheaths was calculated to be 6.8 and 6.5 mm respectively in non-calcified ilio-femoral vessels, and 7.5 and 7.2 mm respectively in calcified ilio-femoral vessels (Hayashida, Lefevre et al. 2011). While these measurements represent more restrictive criteria than previously recommended (Eltchaninoff, Kerkeni et al. 2009; Ducrocq, Francis et al. 2010; Tchetche, Dumonteil et al. 2010; Thomas, Schymik et al. 2010), alternative approaches (TA, transthoracic, transsubclavian or retroperitoneal) should be considered in patients with borderline femoral artery diameters following careful vascular screening with selective ilio-femoral angiography or, if possible, MSCT.

Sheath/Femoral artery ratio (SFAR)	≥ 1.05 (n = 55)	< 1.05 (n = 72)	p value
Any vascular complication	**23 (41.8%)**	**12 (16.7%)**	**< 0.001**
VARC Major	**17 (30.9%)**	**5 (6.9%)**	**0.001**
VARC Minor	6 (10.9%)	7 (9.7%)	0.827
Femoral artery complication	15 (27.3%)	9 (12.5%)	0.035
Iliac artery complication	**11 (20.0%)**	**2 (2.8%)**	**0.002**
30-day mortality	**10 (18.2%)**	**3 (4.2%)**	**0.016**

Table 1. SFAR predict VARC major vascular complications

4.3 Others

Dimensions beyond 45 mm are considered to be an indication for replacement of the ascending aorta and constitute, therefore, a contraindication for CoreValve implantation, as the upper part of the frame supports the stability of the bioprosthesis. Recent myocardial infarction, severe pulmonary dysfunction (avoiding thoracotomy and intubation), and the presence of apical thrombus are considered contraindications for TA-TAVI. A bicuspid aortic valve is also considered a relative contraindication for TAVI. However, the annulus size and anatomy (eccentricity index) which can be accurately assessed by MSCT is more important than the bicuspidity itself and some patients have been successfully treated using the Edwards valve or Corevalve (Wijesinghe, Ye et al. 2010).

5. Complications, their management and avoidance

Complications of TAVI can be classified as cardiac or non-cardiac. Appropriate patient selection, thorough knowledge of each device and well-mastered technique based on adequate experience are important to avoid these complications.

5.1 Cardiac complications

5.1.1 Aortic regurgitation

Acute aortic regurgitation

It may occur after balloon dilatation. This relatively rare complication is poorly tolerated and may lead to cardiogenic shock within a few minutes, so it is crucial to identify the problem and implant the valve as soon as possible. For this reason, the valve should always be ready at the time of balloon predilatation.

Paravalular leak

Though of no clinical consequence, minor paravalvular regurgitation is a common occurrence with current transcatheter valve devices. However, significant paravalvular regurgitation has been reported as an independent predictor of mortality between 30-day and 1-year in the Italian multicenter study of the CoreValve bioprosthesis (Tamburino, Capodanno et al. 2011). In the initial experience, significant paravalvular leaks were observed in many cases after implantation of the first-generation balloon-expandable bioprosthesis (Cribier, Eltchaninoff et al. 2002; Cribier, Eltchaninoff et al. 2004). However, the incidence of moderate to severe aortic regurgitation has been reduced in recipients of the Sapien or CoreValve bioprosthesis (Grube, Schuler et al. 2007; Walther, Simon et al. 2007; Webb, Pasupati et al. 2007) mainly by better screening of the annulus size and selection of over-sized valves. Low aortic diastolic pressure (40-50 mmHg) is the initial sign of significant aortic regurgitation. The causes of significant aortic regurgitation are; 1) undersizing of the valve due to underestimation of the annulus size, 2) incorrect positioning of the bioprosthesis, and 3) underexpansion of the valve. Bioprosthesis/annulus discordance was reported as an independent predictor of significant aortic regurgitation (Detaint, Lepage et al. 2009) thus annulus measurements and prosthesis sizing are critical in order to avoid post procedure paravalvular leak. Correct positioning of the bioprosthesis can be achieved with increasing experience and technical enhancement of the device. Adequate long time inflation of the balloon (approximately 5 seconds) is recommended in order to avoid underexpansion of the balloon-expandable bioprosthesis. Optimal evaluation of paravalvular leak immediately after valve implantation is essential in order to address this issue during the procedure. In cases of significant paravalvular leak, post balloon dilatation using the same balloon with an extra 1 or 2 cc can be a useful option. However, the long-term outcome of this procedure in terms of prosthesis durability is currently unknown.

5.1.2 Valve malpositioning

Valve positioning is one of the most challenging steps of the procedure, even with all necessary precautions and substantial operator experience. Valve migration after deployment is generally the result of incorrect positioning or pacing failure leading to an effective ventricular contraction during deployment. In cases of valve migration into the aorta, the wire should be secured in order to keep the valve in a coaxial position and prevent it from flipping over and obstructing antegrade flow. The migrated valve can be positioned in the descending thoracic aorta by a partially inflated balloon or a goose-neck snare. However, care should be taken to avoid forceful repositioning of the valve as this may cause aortic dissection or rupture.

5.1.3 Coronary occlusion

Coronary occlusion may occur due to the shifting of the bulky calcified native leaflet toward the left main ostium. The main predictors are a short distance between the annulus and left main ostium, and small dimension of the sinus of Valsalva. It may also occur due to an excessively high implantation of the CoreValve, thouth this is a rare occurrence (<1%) in recipients of the Sapien as well as the CoreValve (Piazza, Grube et al. 2008; Lefevre, Kappetein et al. 2010). For the Sapien valve, preventive protection of the coronary ostium with a coronary guidewire and guiding catheter during TAVI may be effective in the presence of bulky calcified leaflets. Even though the presence of open cells over a coronary ostium is well-tolerated, selective coronary cannulation may prove difficult because of the stent struts jailing the coronary ostium. Preprocedural cardiac CT scan or aortography with simultaneous balloon valvuloplasty may help to detect any potential risk of coronary occlusion. A >10 mm distance between the annulus and the left main is recommended in order to avoid this complication (Wenaweser and Windecker 2010).

5.1.4 Annulus and aortic root rupture

Though rupture of the aortic annulus is an infrequently observed complication in TAVI (Himbert, Descoutures et al. 2009; Zajarias and Cribier 2009; Wendler, Schymik et al. 2010) as well as aortic valvuloplasty procedures (Hayes, Holmes et al. 1989), this complication (about 0.5%) can be fatal as it may rapidly result in cardiac tamponade and lead to catastrophic hemodynamic collapse in a few minutes. Excessive balloon dilatation, aggressive valve oversizing and extensive annular calcification may increase the incidence of this complication. Less aggressive balloon valvuloplasty and valve oversizing are recommended in the presence of markedly calcified annular and subannular tissues or an unusually small aortic root.

5.1.5 Heart block

Atrioventricular (AV) block is a known complication of surgical aortic valve replacement (Dawkins, Hobson et al. 2008) which occurs in 4 to 8% of cases. Heart block can also occur after TAVI, presumably due to continuous compression of the conduction system located in the LV outflow tract and interventricular septum. After Edwards valve implantation, AV block occurs in 2 to 7% of cases, usually immediately after the procedure (Piazza, Onuma et al. 2008; Vahanian, Alfieri et al. 2008). As the occurrence of AV block may be transient, it is recommended that pacemaker placement should not be considered until after 24 hours.

The lower "skirt" structure of the CoreValve lies within the left ventricular outflow tract and exerts continuous pressure on the left bundle branch (Khawaja, Rajani et al. 2011), leading to a subsequent new onset of left bundle branch block. The risk of AV block extends beyond the procedure duration up to day 4. Temporary pacemaker should be secured for at

least 48 hours and continuous monitoring for 4 days is recommended in patients who have not received a permanent pacemaker. When AV Block occurs during the procedure after Corevalve implantation, it is not necessary to wait for potential recovery as pacemaker implantation is a definite indication in such cases. Previous studies have reported a higher incidence of permanent pacemaker (PPM) implantation in recipients of the CoreValve (18% to 40%) (Jilaihawi, Chin et al. 2009; Khawaja, Rajani et al. 2011) compared to the Sapien valve (1.8% and 7.0%) (Sinhal, Altwegg et al. 2008; Godin, Eltchaninoff et al. 2010; Lefevre, Kappetein et al. 2010; Leon, Smith et al. 2010). Predictors of PPM requirement have been reported as periprocedural atrioventricular block, balloon predilatation, use of the larger (29 mm) CoreValve prosthesis, interventricular septum diameter, prolonged QRS duration in the UK collaborative study (Khawaja, Rajani et al. 2011) and pre-existing right bundle branch block (Piazza, Onuma et al. 2008; Roten, Wenaweser et al. 2011). The main predictor seems to be the level of implantation of the valve into the left ventricle.
Operators continue to endeavour to implant the valve in a relatively high position in order to reduce the risk of AVB. The new delivery system, Accutrak, should improve the accuracy of Corevalve deployment.

5.1.6 Specific complications of TA approach

Direct access to the left ventricle is obtained through an intercostal minithoracotomy and severe bleeding may occur at the end of the procedure. This seems to be related to technical problems during preparation of the access. Large deep stitches are recommended in order to avoid this problem. Apical pseudoaneurysm was reported as a specific complication of this approach (Masson, Kovac et al. 2009). Post procedural low-grade bleeding may result in cardiac tamponade and require further repair. Pleural effusion is also not uncommon. Mitral valve injury can also occur because of the nature of this procedure through the left ventricle. In some instances, the wire from the apex to the aorta can be pushed inadvertently behind the mitral chordae and create acute mitral regurgitation during manipulation of the introducer leading to cardiogenic shock. When identified, the problem is easily solved by pulling back the wire and rewiring the aorta whilst avoiding the mitral chordae.

5.2 Non-cardiac complications

5.2.1 Vascular complications

Vascular complications are among the most frequent and serious complications of TF-TAVI, and have been associated with significantly increased patient morbidity and mortality (Webb, Chandavimol et al. 2006; Piazza, Grube et al. 2008; Rodes-Cabau, Webb et al. 2010). To date, vascular complications have been described in 8%-30.7% of Edwards valve recipients (Webb, Altwegg et al. 2009; Ducrocq, Francis et al. 2010; Lefevre, Kappetein et al. 2010; Leon, Smith et al. 2010; Rodes-Cabau, Webb et al. 2010; Tchetche, Dumonteil et al. 2010; Thomas, Schymik et al. 2010), and 1.9%-16% of CoreValve patients (Piazza, Grube et al. 2008; Bleiziffer, Ruge et al. 2009; Tchetche, Dumonteil et al. 2010; Van Mieghem, Nuis et al. 2010). In an effort to standardize the reporting of TAVI data, the Valve Academic Research Consortium (VARC) has recently developed a consensus on TAVI-related endpoints (Leon, Piazza et al. 2011), including a uniform definition of vascular complications. In our prospective series of TF-TAVI patients (85% Edwards and 15% Corevalve), we observed a vascular complication rate of 27.6% (VARC definition), including major vascular complications in 17.3% (Hayashida, Lefevre et al. 2011). We also found that the occurrence of major vascular complications was a strong predictor of 30-day mortality (multiplying the risk of 30-day death by 4) and that major vascular complications were predicted by SFAR, center experience and the presence of femoral calcifications (Hayashida, Lefevre et al. 2011). Iliac perforation is a more severe potential vascular complication of TF-TAVI, because it may lead to retroperitoneal hemorrhage and hemodynamic collapse. In our study, all iliac complications were classified as VARC major complications (Hayashida, Lefevre et al. 2011). Careful screening of vascular access and multimodality approach is crucial for selection of vascular access for TAVI. With technological advances, down-sizing of the device should be associated with further reductions in the risk of vascular complications in the future.

5.2.2 Cerebro-vascular complications

The incidence of clinically apparent cerebrovascular embolism (CE) complicated by TAVI is reported to be between 1.7% and 6.9% (Grube, Schuler et al. 2007; Webb, Pasupati et al. 2007; Webb, Altwegg et al. 2009; Rodes-Cabau, Webb et al. 2010; Thomas, Schymik et al. 2010). Two reports described a lower incidence of clinically apparent stroke in patients undergoing TA-TAVI compared to those with TF-TAVI (Bleiziffer, Ruge et al. 2009; Himbert, Descoutures et al. 2009). However, these findings have not been confirmed by other large studies (Table 2) including both TF and TA approaches (Webb, Altwegg et al. 2009; Kahlert, Knipp et al. 2010; Rodes-Cabau, Webb et al. 2010; Thomas, Schymik et al. 2010).

Studies	Stroke rate (%)	Studies	Stroke rate (%)
PARTNER EU TF	3.2	FRANCE Corevalve	4.5
PARTNER EU TA	2.9	Belgian Registry Corevalve	3.4
SOURCE TF	2.4	German Registry Corevalve	2.6
SOURCE TA	2.6	UK Registry Corevalve	4.0
FRANCE TA	2.8	Italian Registry Corevalve	1.7
FRANCE TF	4.2	**AVR high-risk***	**2.8**
PARTNER US	6.9		
Belgian Registry Edwards	3.1		

Table 2. Risk of Stroke after TAVI procedures

In a study using diffusion-weighted magnetic resonance imaging (DW-MRI), TF-TAVI was associated with >70% incidence of new cerebral lesions following the procedure (Ghanem, Muller et al. 2010; Kahlert, Knipp et al. 2010) and there was also no difference between the TF and TA approaches (Rodes-Cabau, Webb et al. 2010). There are further data allowing comparison between TAVI and conventional SAVR (Kahlert, Knipp et al. 2010). Indeed, one report showed that despite a higher incidence of new foci of DW-MRI in the TAVI group (84% vs 48%, p = 0.011), the volumes of these lesions were significantly smaller after TAVI than after SAVR and no differences in clinically apparent stroke were evidenced. (Kahlert, Knipp et al. 2010). In the PARTNER US trial, a significant increase in any stroke was observed (5.5 vs 2.4%, p=0.04), but the combined endpoint of death or stroke at one year were similar (26.5 vs 28.0% respectively). The etiologies of procedural stroke are likely to be atheroembolism from the ascending aorta or the aortic arch, calcific embolism from the aortic valve, thromboembolism from catheters, air embolism from LV cannulation, and prolonged hypotension. Repeated or overly aggressive valvuloplasty may be associated with an increased risk of embolization of calcific material from the aortic valve (Isner 1991) and should be avoided.

5.2.3 Acute kidney injury

Renal function and the development of acute kidney injury (AKI) are important factors influencing the outcome of patients after invasive procedures, such as percutaneous coronary intervention or cardiac surgery (Chertow, Levy et al. 1998; Lok, Austin et al. 2004). AKI has been observed in 12% to 28% of patients undergoing TAVI and is associated with a 4-fold increase in post-procedural mortality (Aregger, Wenaweser et al. 2009; Bagur, Webb et al. 2010; Sinning, Ghanem et al. 2010). AKI after TAVI is related to an increased mortality risk in the short and mid-term, independent of whether renal function returns to baseline or not (Sinning, Ghanem et al. 2010). Although the mechanism of AKI after TAVI remains unknown, pre- and post-procedural impaired hemodynamics and hypotension caused by low ejection fraction, valvuloplasty and valve deployment, embolization of aortic debris during catheter manipulation, and amount of contrast media in these patients with poor renal function may be among the main causes.

6. Patient outcomes

Procedural success rates have steadily improved from 82% (Cribier, Eltchaninoff et al. 2006) in the initial antegrade approach to more than 95% in recent reports of both available bioprostheses (Coeytaux, Williams et al. 2010; Yan, Cao et al. 2010).

These data show that the procedure of TAVI is now reaching relative maturity.

A review of the literature involving 84 reports on both bioprostheses, showed an overall 30-day survival rate of 89% (Coeytaux, Williams et al. 2010). In the early reports of TAVI, 30-day survival was around 50-60% in recipients of the Edwards valve (Cribier, Eltchaninoff et al. 2004; Cribier, Eltchaninoff et al. 2006). Increased operator experience and device enhancement may account for the recent improvements in the outcome of TAVI patients. In patients implanted with the Sapien valve, 30-day survival is currently between 88 and 94% via the TF approach (Webb, Pasupati et al. 2007; Lefevre, Kappetein et al. 2010; Rodes-Cabau, Webb et al. 2010; Thomas, Schymik et al. 2010) and 81% to 92% via the TA route (Walther, Simon et al. 2007; Walther, Falk et al. 2008; Lefevre, Kappetein et al. 2010; Thomas, Schymik et al. 2010).

In recipients of the CoreValve via the TF approach, 30-day survival is 89 to 93% (Grube, Buellesfeld et al. 2008; Piazza, Grube et al. 2008; Piazza, van Gameren et al. 2009; Tamburino, Capodanno et al. 2011). It is noteworthy that the recent publication of 2 registries conducted in the UK and Italy in patients who underwent transsubclavian-TAVI using the CoreValve showed excellent short-term survival of 100% (Petronio, De Carlo et al. 2010; Moynagh, Scott et al. 2011). These results require further confirmation in large prospective and controlled registries.

The predictors of 30-day mortality are identified as logistic EuroSCORE, experience, low left ventricular ejection fraction, need for hemodynamic support during the procedure, conversion to open heart surgery, cardiac tamponade, major vascular complication, acute kidney injury and diabetes mellitus, (Wendler, Walther et al. 2010; Tamburino, Capodanno et al. 2011)

Survival rates at 1 year ranging from 69 to 85% have been reported (Webb, Altwegg et al. 2009; Coeytaux, Williams et al. 2010; Lefevre, Kappetein et al. 2010; Leon, Smith et al. 2010; Sinning, Ghanem et al. 2010; Yan, Cao et al. 2010). The predictors of late mortality are mainly related to comorbidities and reported as logistic EuroSCORE, STS score, age, severe mitral regurgitation, anemia, prior stroke, pulmonary disease, pulmonary hypertension, post procedural paravalvular leak ≥2, and chronic kidney disease (Walther, Simon et al. 2007; Piazza, Grube et al. 2008; Himbert, Descoutures et al. 2009; Leon, Smith et al. 2010; Rodes-Cabau, Webb et al. 2010; Sinning, Ghanem et al. 2010).

7. Valve performance

The hemodynamic performance of the valve is very promising and seems so be superior to surgical valves with a lower gradient and larger valve area. In the cohort A of the PARNTER US trial (21) the valve area was 1.4$\pm$0.5 in the SAVR group compared to 1.6$\pm$0.5 (p=0.004) in the TAVI group. Paravalvular leak remains a problem which should be solved in the future. Mild to moderate aortic regurgitation was observed in 12% of cases in this study.

8. Future perspectives

8.1 Wider application of TAVI

Until now, the indications for TAVI have been symptomatic severe AS with a EuroSCORE >20%, STS score >10% or instances where surgery is deemed to carry excessive risk due to significant comorbidities or contraindications. Recently, the results of the cohort B of the PARTNER US trial have demonstrated that, compared to standard medical therapy, TF-TAVI using the Sapien valve significantly reduces the rates of death from any cause and repeat hospitalization (Leon, Smith et al. 2010). In this landmark study, TAVI treatment of 5 patients resulted in one life being saved at one-year follow-up compared to medical treatment. The fact that one life was saved out of 5 patients treated is unparalleled in the history of medicine.

The benefit of TAVI in terms of mortality was observed in all predefined subgroups (Figure 9). Quality of life was also dramatically improved, as shown in Figure 10. Cohort A of this study comparing TF-TAVI vs conventional surgical aortic valve replacement (SAVR), and TA-TAVI vs SAVR has been recently published (Smith and Leon 2011) and demonstrated the noninferiority of TAVI compared to conventional aortic valve replacement in terms of all-cause mortality in high-risk patients. With respect to the CoreValve, SURTAVI, a multicenter, randomized clinical trial comparing the CoreValve with SAVR in patients with "intermediate" risk will start enrolling patients in Europe in 2011. PARTNER 2 will also explore the outcome of the third-generation Edwards valve in patients with intermediate risk in the United States.

8.2 Valve in valve technique

Percutaneous treatment of degenerated bioprostheses (Klaaborg, Egeblad et al. 2009; Webb, Wood et al. 2010) in patients at high risk for repeat surgery is currently being evaluated and seems very promising (Figure 11).

Subgroup	TAVI (%) n=179	Standard Rx (%) n=179	RR (95% CI)	RR (95% CI)	NNT	P interaction
Overall	30.7	49.7		0.62 (0.47, 0.81)	5	
Age < 85	29.2	51.1		0.57 (0.39, 0.83)	5	
Age > 85	32.5	48.3		0.67 (0.46, 0.98)	6	0.54
Female gender	30.9	48.4		0.64 (0.44, 0.92)	6	
Male gender	30.5	51.2		0.60 (0.40, 0.88)	5	0.80
Body-mass Index <25	38.6	52.9		0.73 (0.52, 1.02)	7	0.20
Body-mass index >25	24.0	46.7		0.51 (0.34, 0.78)	4	
STS score <11	23.7	42.1		0.56 (0.36, 0.88)	5	0.44
STS score >11	38.4	54.9		0.70 (0.51, 0.96)	6	
LV ejection fraction < 55	36.6	61.1		0.60 (0.43, 0.83)	4	0.50
LV ejection frcation >55	26.4	36.4		0.73 (0.46, 1.14)	10	
Pulmonary hypertension	26.1	45.5		0.57 (0.36, 0.92)	5	0.47
No pulmonary hypertension	35.4	49.4		0.72 (0.50, 1.03)	7	
Mitral regurgitation ≥3+	32.3	46.5		0.70 (0.51, 0.95)	7	0.09
Mitral regurgitation <3	23.7	60.5		0.39 (0.21, 0.73)	3	
Severe COPD	29.1	48.1		0.60 (0.44, 0.83)	5	0.70
No severe COPD	36.8	54.3		0.68 (0.41, 1.11)	6	
Prior CABG or PCI	27.8	47.1		0.59 (0.38, 0.93)	5	0.60
No prior CABG or PCI	27.4	54.3		0.50 (0.34, 0.75)	4	
Peripheral vascular disease	28.2	52.2		0.54 (0.39, 0.75)	4	0.10
No peripheral vasc. Disease	37.0	42.2		0.88 (0.54, 1.43)	19	

TAVI better | Standard Rx better

The consensus on TAVI-related endpoints published by the Valve Academic Research Consortium (VARC) (Leon, Piazza et al. 2011) should be useful for comparing new studies.

Fig. 9. All-cause mortality in PARTNER US (Subgroup Analysis)

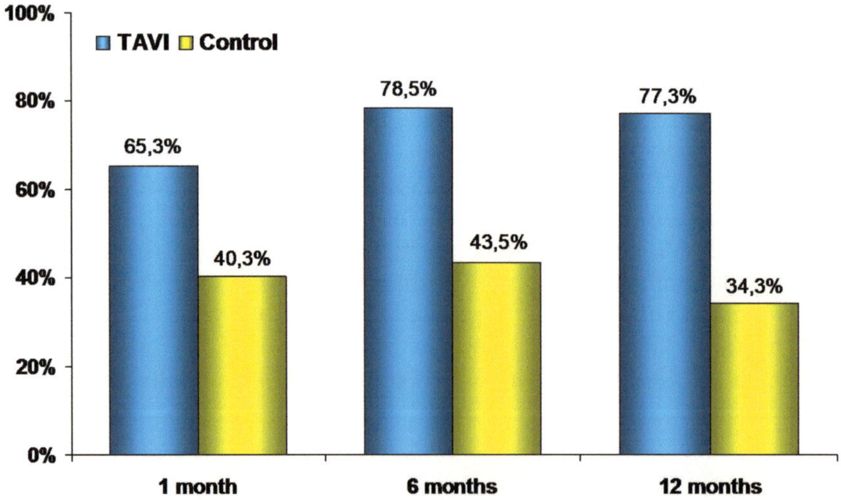

* Improvement ≥ 10 points vs. baseline using Kansas City Cardiomyopathy Questionaire

Fig. 10. Quality of life Improvement in PARTNER US*

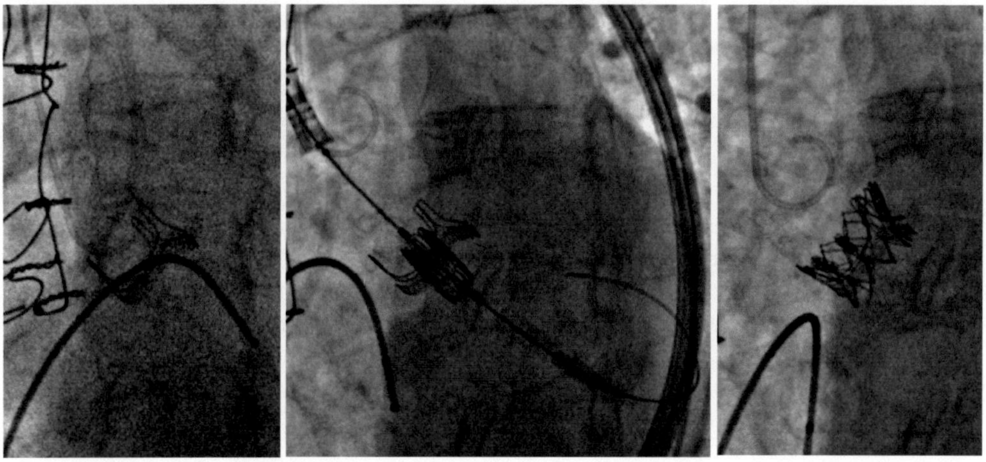

Fig. 11. Valve in valve technique

This new approach is likely to bring radical changes to the management of our patients in the years to come regarding which type of valve should be selected (mechanical or bioprosthesis) for conventional surgery. Indeed, the possibility of implanting a percutaneous valve in patients who have already received a surgical bioprosthesis may become a valid option. Currently, surgical bioprostheses have a 15- to 20-year durability.

8.3 New devices

A number of new devices are currently undergoing early clinical evaluation. The main improvement axes for enhancement of transcatheter valve technology are reduction in the delivery catheter size, a decrease in risks of paravalvular leaks, as well as facilitation of accurate positioning and retrieval (Low, Bolling et al. 2008; Schofer, Schluter et al. 2008; Falk, Schwammenthal et al. 2009; Treede, Tubler et al. 2010). The Sadra Lotus valve (Boston Scientific, USA), Direct Flow (Direct Flow Medical, USA), JenaClip (JenaValve, Germany), Engager (Medtronic, USA), St Jude (St Jude Medical, USA), Directflow and Symetis are examples of new valves. Although these valves have been the object of initial animal and even clinical studies, further evaluations in larger muticenter trials are needed.

9. Conclusion

The objective of this review was to describe state-of-the-art TAVI, as well as future perspectives. TAVI procedures are being carried out worldwide with encouraging results and reduced procedural risk and mortality. Although long-term data are required, short- and mid-term outcome of TAVI is comparable with that of conventional surgery in high-risk AS patients. As a result of increased experience and enhanced technology, TAVI is currently emerging as a new hope in our aging society for the growing number of elderly patients with severe AS.

10. Acknowledgments

The authors would like to thank Mrs. Catherine Dupic for her assistance in the preparation of this manuscript.

11. Disclosures

Dr T. Lefèvre is proctor for Edwards TAVI.

12. Reference

Andersen, H. R., L. L. Knudsen, et al. (1992). "Transluminal implantation of artificial heart valves. Description of a new expandable aortic valve and initial results with implantation by catheter technique in closed chest pigs." Eur Heart J 13(5): 704-8.

Aregger, F., P. Wenaweser, et al. (2009). "Risk of acute kidney injury in patients with severe aortic valve stenosis undergoing transcatheter valve replacement." Nephrol Dial Transplant 24(7): 2175-9.

Bagur, R., J. G. Webb, et al. (2010). "Acute kidney injury following transcatheter aortic valve implantation: predictive factors, prognostic value, and comparison with surgical aortic valve replacement." Eur Heart J 31(7): 865-74.

Bleiziffer, S., H. Ruge, et al. (2009). "Survival after transapical and transfemoral aortic valve implantation: talking about two different patient populations." J Thorac Cardiovasc Surg 138(5): 1073-80.

Bonow, R. O., B. A. Carabello, et al. (2008). "2008 focused update incorporated into the ACC/AHA 2006 guidelines for the management of patients with valvular heart disease: a report of the American College of Cardiology/American Heart Association Task Force on Practice Guidelines (Writing Committee to revise the 1998 guidelines for the management of patients with valvular heart disease). Endorsed by the Society of Cardiovascular Anesthesiologists, Society for Cardiovascular Angiography and Interventions, and Society of Thoracic Surgeons." J Am Coll Cardiol 52(13): e1-142.

Bonow, R. O., B. A. Carabello, et al. (2006). "ACC/AHA 2006 guidelines for the management of patients with valvular heart disease: a report of the American College of Cardiology/American Heart Association Task Force on Practice Guidelines (writing committee to revise the 1998 Guidelines for the Management of Patients With Valvular Heart Disease): developed in collaboration with the Society of Cardiovascular Anesthesiologists: endorsed by the Society for Cardiovascular Angiography and Interventions and the Society of Thoracic Surgeons." Circulation 114(5): e84-231.

Chertow, G. M., E. M. Levy, et al. (1998). "Independent association between acute renal failure and mortality following cardiac surgery." Am J Med 104(4): 343-8.

Coeytaux, R. R., J. W. Williams, Jr., et al. (2010). "Percutaneous heart valve replacement for aortic stenosis: state of the evidence." Ann Intern Med 153(5): 314-24.

Cribier, A., H. Eltchaninoff, et al. (2002). "Percutaneous transcatheter implantation of an aortic valve prosthesis for calcific aortic stenosis: first human case description." Circulation 106(24): 3006-8.

Cribier, A., H. Eltchaninoff, et al. (2006). "Treatment of calcific aortic stenosis with the percutaneous heart valve: mid-term follow-up from the initial feasibility studies: the French experience." J Am Coll Cardiol 47(6): 1214-23.

Cribier, A., H. Eltchaninoff, et al. (2004). "Early experience with percutaneous transcatheter implantation of heart valve prosthesis for the treatment of end-stage inoperable patients with calcific aortic stenosis." J Am Coll Cardiol 43(4): 698-703.

Cribier, A., T. Savin, et al. (1986). "Percutaneous transluminal valvuloplasty of acquired aortic stenosis in elderly patients: an alternative to valve replacement?" Lancet 1(8472): 63-7.

Dawkins, S., A. R. Hobson, et al. (2008). "Permanent pacemaker implantation after isolated aortic valve replacement: incidence, indications, and predictors." Ann Thorac Surg 85(1): 108-12.

Detaint, D., L. Lepage, et al. (2009). "Determinants of significant paravalvular regurgitation after transcatheter aortic valve: implantation impact of device and annulus discongruence." JACC Cardiovasc Interv 2(9): 821-7.

Ducrocq, G., F. Francis, et al. (2010). "Vascular complications of transfemoral aortic valve implantation with the Edwards SAPIEN prosthesis: incidence and impact on outcome." EuroIntervention 5(6): 666-72.

Eltchaninoff, H., M. Kerkeni, et al. (2009). "Aorto-iliac angiography as a screening tool in selecting patients for transfemoral aortic valve implantation with the Edwards SAPIEN bioprosthesis." EuroIntervention 5(4): 438-42.

Eltchaninoff, H., C. Tron, et al. (2007). "[Aortic bioprosthesis implanted percutaneously: three year follow up]." Arch Mal Coeur Vaiss 100(11): 901, 904-8.

Falk, V., E. E. Schwammenthal, et al. (2009). "New anatomically oriented transapical aortic valve implantation." Ann Thorac Surg 87(3): 925-6.

Ghanem, A., A. Muller, et al. (2010). "Risk and fate of cerebral embolism after transfemoral aortic valve implantation: a prospective pilot study with diffusion-weighted magnetic resonance imaging." J Am Coll Cardiol 55(14): 1427-32.

Godin, M., H. Eltchaninoff, et al. (2010). "Frequency of conduction disturbances after transcatheter implantation of an Edwards Sapien aortic valve prosthesis." Am J Cardiol 106(5): 707-12.

Grube, E., L. Buellesfeld, et al. (2008). "Progress and current status of percutaneous aortic valve replacement: results of three device generations of the CoreValve Revalving system." Circ Cardiovasc Interv 1(3): 167-75.

Grube, E., J. C. Laborde, et al. (2006). "Percutaneous implantation of the CoreValve self-expanding valve prosthesis in high-risk patients with aortic valve disease: the Siegburg first-in-man study." Circulation 114(15): 1616-24.

Grube, E., G. Schuler, et al. (2007). "Percutaneous aortic valve replacement for severe aortic stenosis in high-risk patients using the second- and current third-generation self-expanding CoreValve prosthesis: device success and 30-day clinical outcome." J Am Coll Cardiol 50(1): 69-76.

Hayashida, K., T. Lefevre, et al. (2011). "Transfemoral Aortic Valve Implantation: New Criteria to Predict Vascular Complications." J. Am. Coll. Cardiol. Intv. in press.

Hayes, S. N., D. R. Holmes, Jr., et al. (1989). "Palliative percutaneous aortic balloon valvuloplasty before noncardiac operations and invasive diagnostic procedures." Mayo Clin Proc 64(7): 753-7.

Himbert, D., F. Descoutures, et al. (2009). "Results of transfemoral or transapical aortic valve implantation following a uniform assessment in high-risk patients with aortic stenosis." J Am Coll Cardiol 54(4): 303-11.

Hutter, A., A. Opitz, et al. (2010). "Aortic annulus evaluation in transcatheter aortic valve implantation." Catheter Cardiovasc Interv 76(7): 1009-19.

Isner, J. M. (1991). "Acute catastrophic complications of balloon aortic valvuloplasty. The Mansfield Scientific Aortic Valvuloplasty Registry Investigators." J Am Coll Cardiol 17(6): 1436-44.

Iung, B., G. Baron, et al. (2003). "A prospective survey of patients with valvular heart disease in Europe: The Euro Heart Survey on Valvular Heart Disease." Eur Heart J 24(13): 1231-43.

Jilaihawi, H., D. Chin, et al. (2009). "Predictors for permanent pacemaker requirement after transcatheter aortic valve implantation with the CoreValve bioprosthesis." Am Heart J 157(5): 860-6.

Kahlert, P., F. Al-Rashid, et al. (2009). "Vascular access site complications after percutaneous transfemoral aortic valve implantation." Herz 34(5): 398-408.

Kahlert, P., S. C. Knipp, et al. (2010). "Silent and apparent cerebral ischemia after percutaneous transfemoral aortic valve implantation: a diffusion-weighted magnetic resonance imaging study." Circulation 121(7): 870-8.

Khawaja, M. Z., R. Rajani, et al. (2011). "Permanent Pacemaker Insertion After CoreValve Transcatheter Aortic Valve Implantation: Incidence and Contributing Factors (the UK CoreValve Collaborative)." Circulation 123(9): 951-60.

Klaaborg, K. E., H. Egeblad, et al. (2009). "Transapical transcatheter treatment of a stenosed aortic valve bioprosthesis using the Edwards SAPIEN Transcatheter Heart Valve." Ann Thorac Surg 87(6): 1943-6.

Latsios, G., U. Gerckens, et al. (2010). "Transaortic transcatheter aortic valve implantation: a novel approach for the truly "no-access option" patients." Catheter Cardiovasc Interv 75(7): 1129-36.

Lefevre, T., A. P. Kappetein, et al. (2010). "One year follow-up of the multi-centre European PARTNER transcatheter heart valve study." Eur Heart J 32(2): 148-57.

Lefevre, T., A. P. Kappetein, et al. (2010). "One year follow-up of the multi-centre European PARTNER transcatheter heart valve study." Eur Heart J.

Leon, M. B., N. Piazza, et al. (2011). "Standardized endpoint definitions for transcatheter aortic valve implantation clinical trials a consensus report from the valve academic research consortium." J Am Coll Cardiol 57(3): 253-69.

Leon, M. B., C. R. Smith, et al. (2010). "Transcatheter aortic-valve implantation for aortic stenosis in patients who cannot undergo surgery." N Engl J Med 363(17): 1597-607.

Lichtenstein, S. V., A. Cheung, et al. (2006). "Transapical transcatheter aortic valve implantation in humans: initial clinical experience." Circulation 114(6): 591-6.

Lieberman, E. B., T. M. Bashore, et al. (1995). "Balloon aortic valvuloplasty in adults: failure of procedure to improve long-term survival." J Am Coll Cardiol 26(6): 1522-8.

Lok, C. E., P. C. Austin, et al. (2004). "Impact of renal insufficiency on short- and long-term outcomes after cardiac surgery." Am Heart J 148(3): 430-8.

Low, R. I., S. F. Bolling, et al. (2008). "Direct flow medical percutaneous aortic valve: proof of concept." EuroIntervention 4(2): 256-61.

Masson, J. B., J. Kovac, et al. (2009). "Transcatheter aortic valve implantation: review of the nature, management, and avoidance of procedural complications." JACC Cardiovasc Interv 2(9): 811-20.

Moynagh, A. M., D. J. Scott, et al. (2011). "CoreValve transcatheter aortic valve implantation via the subclavian artery: comparison with the transfemoral approach." J Am Coll Cardiol 57(5): 634-5.

NHLBI Balloon Valvuloplasty Registry Participant (1991). "Percutaneous balloon aortic valvuloplasty. Acute and 30-day follow-up results in 674 patients from the NHLBI Balloon Valvuloplasty Registry." Circulation 84(6): 2383-97.

Otto, C. M., M. C. Mickel, et al. (1994). "Three-year outcome after balloon aortic valvuloplasty. Insights into prognosis of valvular aortic stenosis." Circulation 89(2): 642-50.

Petronio, A. S., M. De Carlo, et al. (2010). "Safety and efficacy of the subclavian approach for transcatheter aortic valve implantation with the CoreValve revalving system." Circ Cardiovasc Interv 3(4): 359-66.

Piazza, N., E. Grube, et al. (2008). "Procedural and 30-day outcomes following transcatheter aortic valve implantation using the third generation (18 Fr) corevalve revalving system: results from the multicentre, expanded evaluation registry 1-year following CE mark approval." EuroIntervention 4(2): 242-9.

Piazza, N., Y. Onuma, et al. (2008). "Early and persistent intraventricular conduction abnormalities and requirements for pacemaking after percutaneous replacement of the aortic valve." JACC Cardiovasc Interv 1(3): 310-6.

Piazza, N., M. van Gameren, et al. (2009). "A comparison of patient characteristics and 30-day mortality outcomes after transcatheter aortic valve implantation and surgical aortic valve replacement for the treatment of aortic stenosis: a two-centre study." EuroIntervention 5(5): 580-8.

Rodes-Cabau, J., J. G. Webb, et al. (2010). "Transcatheter aortic valve implantation for the treatment of severe symptomatic aortic stenosis in patients at very high or prohibitive surgical risk: acute and late outcomes of the multicenter Canadian experience." J Am Coll Cardiol 55(11): 1080-90.

Roten, L., P. Wenaweser, et al. (2011). "Incidence and predictors of atrioventricular conduction impairment after transcatheter aortic valve implantation." Am J Cardiol 106(10): 1473-80.

Safian, R. D., A. D. Berman, et al. (1988). "Balloon aortic valvuloplasty in 170 consecutive patients." N Engl J Med 319(3): 125-30.

Schofer, J., M. Schluter, et al. (2008). "Retrograde transarterial implantation of a nonmetallic aortic valve prosthesis in high-surgical-risk patients with severe aortic stenosis: a first-in-man feasibility and safety study." Circ Cardiovasc Interv 1(2): 126-33.

Schultz, C. J., A. D. Moelker, et al. (2010). "Cardiac CT: necessary for precise sizing for transcatheter aortic implantation." EuroIntervention 6 Suppl G: G6-G13.

Sinhal, A., L. Altwegg, et al. (2008). "Atrioventricular block after transcatheter balloon expandable aortic valve implantation." JACC Cardiovasc Interv 1(3): 305-9.

Sinning, J. M., A. Ghanem, et al. (2010). "Renal function as predictor of mortality in patients after percutaneous transcatheter aortic valve implantation." JACC Cardiovasc Interv 3(11): 1141-9.

Smith, C. R. and M. B. Leon, et al (2011). "Comparison of transcatheter and surgical aortic valve replacement for aortic stenosis in patients at high-risk for operation." N Engl J Med in press.

Tamburino, C., D. Capodanno, et al. (2011). "Incidence and predictors of early and late mortality after transcatheter aortic valve implantation in 663 patients with severe aortic stenosis." Circulation 123(3): 299-308.

Tchetche, D., N. Dumonteil, et al. (2010). "Thirty-day outcome and vascular complications after transarterial aortic valve implantation using both Edwards Sapien and Medtronic CoreValve bioprostheses in a mixed population." EuroIntervention 5(6): 659-65.

Thomas, M., G. Schymik, et al. (2010). "Thirty-day results of the SAPIEN aortic Bioprosthesis European Outcome (SOURCE) Registry: A European registry of transcatheter aortic valve implantation using the Edwards SAPIEN valve." Circulation 122(1): 62-9.

Treede, H., T. Tubler, et al. (2010). "Six-month results of a repositionable and retrievable pericardial valve for transcatheter aortic valve replacement: the Direct Flow Medical aortic valve." J Thorac Cardiovasc Surg 140(4): 897-903.

Vahanian, A., O. Alfieri, et al. (2008). "Transcatheter valve implantation for patients with aortic stenosis: a position statement from the European Association of Cardio-Thoracic Surgery (EACTS) and the European Society of Cardiology (ESC), in collaboration with the European Association of Percutaneous Cardiovascular Interventions (EAPCI)." Eur Heart J 29(11): 1463-70.

Vahanian, A., H. Baumgartner, et al. (2007). "Guidelines on the management of valvular heart disease: The Task Force on the Management of Valvular Heart Disease of the European Society of Cardiology." Eur Heart J 28(2): 230-68.

Van Mieghem, N. M., R. J. Nuis, et al. (2010). "Vascular complications with transcatheter aortic valve implantation using the 18 Fr Medtronic CoreValve System: the Rotterdam experience." EuroIntervention 5(6): 673-9.

Walther, T., V. Falk, et al. (2008). "Transapical minimally invasive aortic valve implantation; the initial 50 patients." Eur J Cardiothorac Surg 33(6): 983-8.

Walther, T., P. Simon, et al. (2007). "Transapical minimally invasive aortic valve implantation: multicenter experience." Circulation 116(11 Suppl): I240-5.

Webb, J. G., L. Altwegg, et al. (2009). "Transcatheter aortic valve implantation: impact on clinical and valve-related outcomes." Circulation 119(23): 3009-16.

Webb, J. G., M. Chandavimol, et al. (2006). "Percutaneous aortic valve implantation retrograde from the femoral artery." Circulation 113(6): 842-50.

Webb, J. G., S. Pasupati, et al. (2007). "Percutaneous transarterial aortic valve replacement in selected high-risk patients with aortic stenosis." Circulation 116(7): 755-63.

Webb, J. G., D. A. Wood, et al. (2010). "Transcatheter valve-in-valve implantation for failed bioprosthetic heart valves." Circulation 121(16): 1848-57.

Wenaweser, P. and S. Windecker (2010). "Anatomical suitability for transcatheter aortic valve implantation with complementary roles for 2 rivals." JACC Cardiovasc Interv 3(8): 867-9.

Wendler, O., G. Schymik, et al. (2010). "Development of a risk score for transcatheter aortic valve implantation. 1-year outcomes from over 1000 patients in the SOURCE registry." ESC Congress.

Wendler, O., T. Walther, et al. (2010). "Trans-apical aortic valve implantation: univariate and multivariate analyses of the early results from the SOURCE registry." Eur J Cardiothorac Surg 38(2): 119-27.

Wijesinghe, N., J. Ye, et al. (2010). "Transcatheter aortic valve implantation in patients with bicuspid aortic valve stenosis." JACC Cardiovasc Interv 3(11): 1122-5.

Yan, T. D., C. Cao, et al. (2010). "Transcatheter aortic valve implantation for high-risk patients with severe aortic stenosis: A systematic review." J Thorac Cardiovasc Surg 139(6): 1519-28.

Zajarias, A. and A. G. Cribier (2009). "Outcomes and safety of percutaneous aortic valve replacement." J Am Coll Cardiol 53(20): 1829-36.

10

Management of Congenital Aortic Stenosis by Catheter Techniques

Mehnaz Atiq
Aga Khan University Hospital, Karachi, Pakistan

1. Introduction

Aortic valve stenosis constitutes 3-6% of congenital heart diseases with an incidence of 1-4 per 10,000 live births (Khalid et al, 2006). The prevalence of aortic stenosis at birth is 0.03% (Mahle et al, 2010). If left untreated, it can lead to considerable morbidity and mortality in neonates, infants, children and adults.

Until three decades ago, the only treatment that could be offered to children with aortic stenosis was surgical valvotomy and valve replacement in adults. In 1983 balloon valvuloplasty was introduced as the initial palliation of choice for aortic valve stenosis in children and adolescents. Later in 1985, the procedure was extended to infants with critical aortic stenosis (Pass & Hellenbrand, 2002). Over the past 25 years advancement in technique and equipment has radically improved the safety and outcome of balloon valvuloplasty of aortic valve.

Pathologically the stenosed aortic valve may be tricuspid (trileaflet), bicuspid or unicuspid (Fernandes et al, 2007). The latter is the result of failure of separation of the three leaflets with stenosis being centrally located. Rarely the annulus may be hypoplastic or secondary calcification may develop in children and adolescents.

Bicuspid aortic valve is seen on 1-2% of general population (Bermudez, 2007). Natural history of bicuspid aortic valve is not well defined in children but has a spectrum ranging from critical stenosis to no stenosis or regurgitation (Han et al, 2007). After the fourth decade it can progress to aortic stenosis and regurgitation due to thickening, fibrosis and calcification, imparting rigidity to the fused cusps or due to infective endocarditis. There is associated aortopathy with bicuspid aortic valves, in adults as well as children, in which dilatation of ascending aorta is seen increasing the incidence of aortic dissection. Factors related to aortic dilatation are severity of aortic stenosis and regurgitation and jet angle of left ventricular ejection (Mahle et al, 2010).

2. Evaluation of aortic stenosis for intervention

Neonates with critical aortic stenosis present with a low cardiac output syndrome or cardiogenic shock. The stenosis in neonates is considered "severe" if there is no arterial duct dependent systemic circulation in which case it is "critical"(Magee et al, 1997). In older children, pertinent clinical evaluation of severity of aortic stenosis includes presence of symptoms and signs of congestive cardiac failure, pulsus alternans, carotid shudder, reversed splitting of second heart sound and intensity of the ejection systolic murmur. Electrocardiogram is useful in noting the degree of left ventricular hypertrophy and strain.

Echocardiography offers the most reliable way of assessing suitability for catheter intervention and also to predict its outcome. Aortic valve morphology can be identified as tricuspid, bicuspid or unicuspid. In evaluating bicuspid aortic valve, echocardiographic appearance of vertical or horizontal commissural orientation is noted in parasternal short axis view in diastole which makes the cusps either left-right or anterior-posterior in location respectively. It would be worthwhile noting the raphe which denotes fusion of two leaflets in bicuspid aortic valve (Bermudez et al, 2007). The fusion is categorized as right-left fusion, right-non coronary fusion or left-non coronary fusion. Fusion of right and non-coronary cusp has a two fold increase in the probability of requiring intervention.
Thick leaflets are characteristic of dysplastic aortic valve. 2-D measurements include left ventricular size in length, diameter, systole and diastole, functional assessment of left ventricle and aortic annulus diameter. The latter is measured at the hinge point in the parasternal long axis view. It is important to note the presence and severity of aortic regurgitation before patient selection for balloon valvuloplasty. Aortic regurgitation can be graded as mild, moderate or severe according to criteria mentioned elsewhere (Bonow et al, 2008). Mitral valve disease and incompetence should be assessed. Doppler gradients across aortic valve, peak and mean, have to be measured. Previously exercise testing was used to grade severity of aortic valve stenosis. But the accuracy of echocardiography in evaluating severity has limited its use (Khalid et al, 2006).

3. Indications for intervention

According to AHA/ACC guidelines, aortic stenosis is graded as mild, moderate and severe on basis of hemodynamic and natural history data using basis of aortic jet velocity, mean pressure gradient and valve area (in adolescents and adults). Severe aortic stenosis is when the area is <1 cm^2, MPG is $>$ 40mmHg and jet velocity is greater than 4 m/sec. Intervention should be done if the peak to peak gradient is 50 mmHg in symptomatic and 60mmHg in the asymptomatic patients (Bonow et al, 2008). Additional indications include strain on electrocardiogram, presence of symptoms or LV dysfunction irrespective of gradients. Moderate or severe aortic regurgitation is a contraindication to valvuloplasty.

4. Pre-catheterization stabilization

In critically sick neonates and infants, stabilization should begin in the intensive care unit. All neonates, infants and children should be mechanically ventilated, controlled on temperature with warming mattress, optimized on acid-base and electrolyte balance, calcium and magnesium status, blood pressures and cardiac output. The latter is done with intravenous inotrope and prostaglandin infusion to maintain ductal patency in neonates. An arterial blood gas should be analyzed prior to the procedure. Blood products should be made available in case of complications. Antiarrhythmic drugs and defibrillator should be ready in case ventricular arrhythmias occur, as these patients are at a high risk for such complications due to catheter and wire manipulation particularly in a failing left ventricle (Pass & Hellenbrand, 2002).

5. Balloon aortic valvuloplasty

In neonates and children, balloon aortic valvuloplasty has become the palliative procedure of choice, preferred over open aortic valvotomy (Weber et al, 2006; Egito et al, 1997; Knirsch et al, 2008).The aim of balloon valvuloplasty is to relieve left ventricular outflow tract obstruction thereby improving cardiac output, myocardial hypertrophy and function (Bonow et al, 2008). Monitoring during the procedure includes hemodynamic non-invasive pulse oximetry, blood pressures and many clinicians advocate transesophageal echocardiography for guidance as well as hemodynamic monitoring. This would avoid over dilation of aortic valve and also provide a reliable noninvasive way of assessing aortic insufficiency without having to perform frequent ascending aortogram.

5.1 Approach for valvuloplasty

Historically, over the last 25 years, various approaches have been used for balloon valvuloplasty. These different catheter techniques have their own advantages and disadvantages and there is no consensus as to which is the optimal approach, particularly in neonates with critical aortic stenosis. Some of these have historical importance only.

5.1.1 Retrograde umbilical artery approach

Umbilical arterial approach was advocated by Beekman in 1991 in neonates with critical aortic stenosis. They found this method technically easier than transvenous antegrade approach particularly in cases with hypertrophied small left ventricle. This route also avoided injury to the femoral artery by large catheters available in those days (Beekman et al, 1988).

The procedure involves canulating both the umbilical arteries with 4 or 5 French catheters and a transvenous catheter for gaining antegrade access to the left ventricle. The umbilical arteries were used for balloon dilation through one and monitor aortic pressure with the other. The transvenous catheter was used to perform left ventriculogram and monitor left ventricular pressures during the procedure. Egito et al reported their series of 33 cases with a 91% success with this route (Egito et al, 1997). Despite these successful studies, no recent reports are found with this technique presumably due to availability of better alternatives.

5.1.2 Right scapular artery approach

Reported in 1995 by Alekyan et al in a cohort of 21 infants, this procedure involves surgical exposure of the right axillary and subscapular artery with introduction of sheaths and balloon catheters. This route can accommodate larger catheters. Post procedure the incision is closed with sutures. Success rate was reported to be 68% by these authors with failures attributed to aberrant right subclavian artery or to technical difficulties caused by anatomy in small infants (Alekyan et al,1995).

5.1.3 Transcarotid approach

This approach was introduced by Fischer et al in 1990 as an alternate to retrograde femoral approach in critically ill neonates (Fischer et al, 1990; Maeno et al, 1997). The right carotid was surgically cut down and balloon catheter introduced. An 80-97% success rate was reported with complications occurring in 10% of patients (Weber et al). These included significant blood loss, ventricular fibrillation and ventricular perforation. The carotid artery on follow up was found occluded in 3%, stenotic in 8% and patent in the remaining 89%. The approach has the advantage of ease of crossing the aortic valve and avoiding injury to femoral artery.

5.1.4 Transvenous antegrade approach

This is favored by many clinicians because of the sparing effect on femoral artery and avoiding inadvertent perforation of aortic valve cusp. It was first introduced by Hausdorf in 1993 (Hausdorf et al, 1993) and then endorsed by several workers (Magee et al, 1997; Han et al 2007). The approach involves crossing of foramen ovale and entering the left ventricle. A loop is then formed using balloon tipped catheter to avoid mitral valve apparatus. The aortic valve is crossed antegradely over a wire thus avoiding injury to its cusps. This approach also ensures a relative stable position of the balloon during inflation without being forced out due to contractions. Risks involved include jeopardy of mitral valve apparatus producing mitral regurgitation, inherent risks of trans-septal puncture in a small infant or neonate if it has to be done, difficulty in directing the flow guided catheter towards the aortic valve in a small and hypertrophied left ventricle, and the threat of ventricular arrhythmias and perforation.

5.1.5 Transfemoral retrograde approach

This is the most commonly used method having the obvious advantage of easy access and straight catheter course. Balloons used initially were of high profile requiring large sheaths. There was a high risk of cusp perforation with the use of stiffer guide wires to cross the aortic valve (Weber et al, 2006). However with the improvement in technology, low profile balloons have significantly reduced the frequency of femoral arterial injury. The incidence of cusps perforation has also diminished with the use of floppy tipped guide wires.

5.1.6 Double balloon technique:

Use of double balloon is a modification of single balloon, originally proposed by Beekman et al in 1988. It is applicable when balloon valvuloplasty is performed in older children and young adults where the big size of single balloon would endanger the femoral artery. Both the femoral arteries are accessed and aortic valve is crossed twice from both sides in a retrograde fashion. Two balloons of the same size are chosen, the sum of their diameters amounting to 1.3 times the size of the aortic annulus. The two balloons are inflated simultaneously. The advantages are not only less injury to the two femoral arteries but also the crevice between two balloons avoids complete left ventricular outflow obstruction during balloon inflation. (Beekman et al, 1988) .

5.2 Technical considerations

Percutaneous technique for retrograde balloon aortic valvuloplasty involves femoral arterial and venous access. The bottleneck is access in neonates with critical aortic stenosis. Ultrasound guided percutaneous access is a good way to deal with such difficulties. The other option is to expose the artery through a surgical cut down. The femoral venous access is for insertion of a temporary pacemaker. A 3-4 Fr sheath initially for the artery and a 5Fr sheath for the vein are inserted using the modified Seldinger technique (Randolph et al). A temporary pacemaker is inserted in the right ventricle and the rate, output and sensitivities are determined before commencing the procedure for balloon dilation. The desired paced heart rate is the one that would reduce the systemic blood pressure by half. The concept of pacing to achieve tachycardia is to temporarily reduce the cardiac output in order to stabilize the balloon position during inflation (Leon et al, 2010; Marshall et al, 2005; Gupta et al, 2010). Another method of reducing cardiac output, very popular a decade ago, was to inject intravenous adenosine rapidly to produce cardiac standstill (by inducing sinoatrial and atrioventricular block) to allow unproblematic balloon inflation (Karago et al, 2008). Many clinicians would not pace neonates particularly if the left ventricular function is decreased.

With a pigtail catheter, an ascending aortogram is done. This helps in identifying and grading aortic regurgitation as well as measuring the aortic valve annulus diameter and jet width and direction. The thickness of valve leaflet is measured and classified on anteroposterior or lateral cineangiograms as thin (< 2mm) or thick (>2mm) (Egito et al, 1997). The major impediment is crossing the stenosed, invariably eccentric orifice of the aortic valve. The catheter used for this purpose is usually pediatric right Judkin's catheter or any other suitable catheter that would align itself to the jet direction. The aortic valve orifice is traversed with a floppy tipped guide wire. This would avoid valve perforation and crossing through the valve leaflet which was a problem encountered in early years. The initial guide wire to cross the aortic valve could either be a 0.014-in. coronary wire (C.R. Bard Inc.), a 0.035-in. flexible tipped wire (Wholey, Mallinckrodt Medical), a 0.035- or 0.018-in. hydrophilic wire (Terumo Corp., Tokyo, Japan) or a 0.025-in. Teflon-coated wire (Cook Inc.) (Magee, 1997).

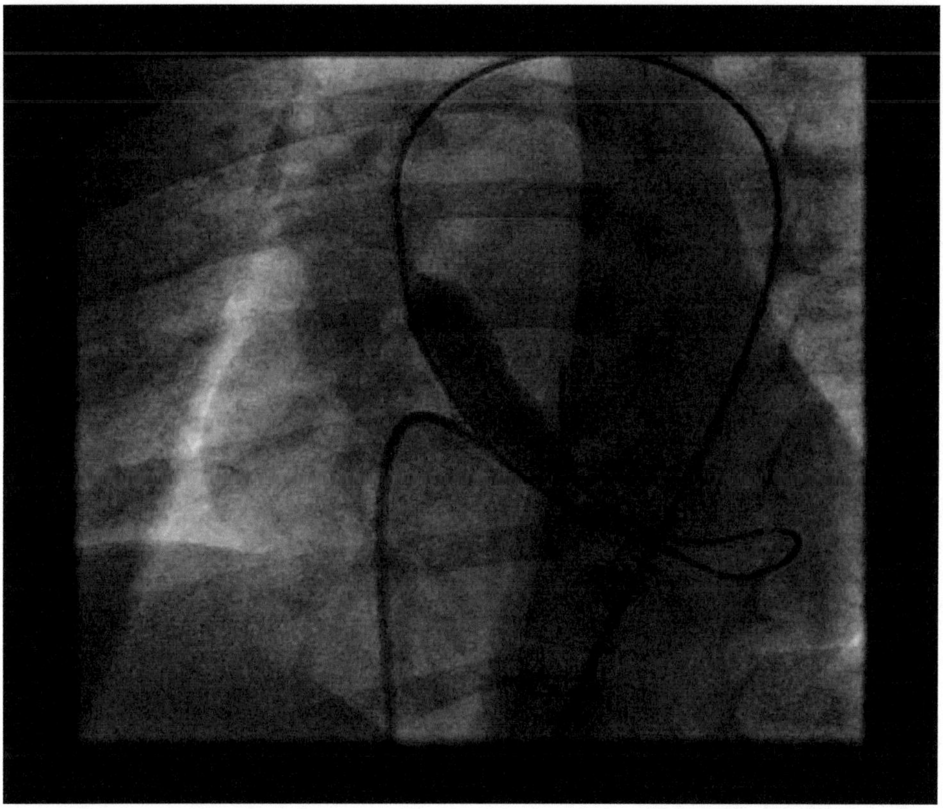

Fig. 1. Retrograde balloon aortic valvuloplasty in an infant with a temporary pacemaker wire in place

Once across, depending upon the severity of stenosis and patient stability, the floppy guide wire is exchanged for a stiffer wire whose end has been shaped manually to make it curl inside the left ventricle. A left ventriculogram is done which would further define the aortic valve anatomy, degree of mitral regurgitation and left ventricular function. A low profile balloon whose size should be 80-90% of the aortic valve annulus diameter and 2-3 cm in length is selected and advanced across the aortic valve annulus. Rapid pacing is ensued and balloon inflated using 1/3rd to 1/4th diluted contrast, preferably with the help of an inflation device. This is a crucial part in which a controlled inflation is aimed at, looking for the appearance and disappearance of the waist, to avoid over dilation and producing aortic valve regurgitation (Figure 1). Some newer balloons have been designed with a double step dilation (example first 15mm and then 20 mm) (Berland et al, 1989) and may be of use in adolescents.

Post dilation, catheters are changed and pressures measured again in the left ventricle and aorta, preferably with a multi-track catheter. If the left ventricular pressures are unacceptably high, re-dilation is done with the same balloon or sometimes with another balloon 1mm larger in size. A left ventriculogram is performed to relook at the aortic valve mobility, mitral regurgitation and left ventricular function (Magee et al, 1997). A post dilation aortogram is done to look at aortic regurgitation and jet width.

5.3 Difficulties and complications

Balloon aortic valvuloplasty like most interventional procedures is semi-blind. The major hindrance is crossing the aortic valve, particularly to be anticipated in neonates with critical or severe aortic stenosis. At times the guide wire crosses but the catheter or balloon catheter may not cross. In such a situation, pre-dilation with a small coronary balloon catheter is done.

There is a risk of ventricular tachycardia and fibrillation due to irritation produced by guide wires and catheters placed in an ischemic left ventricle. Cardiac perforation can occur particularly if soft wires are not used. Femoral artery access, particularly in neonates, carries the risk of damage to the vessel, resulting in thrombosis and potential limb complications up to 39% (Pass & Hellenrand,2002; Magee et al, 1997; Egito et al !997). Aortic arch dissection flaps are seen during or post procedure and are related to use of stiffer wires or balloons with larger internal diameter lumen than the wire. This problem can be overcome to some extent by pre-shaping the guide wire.

Mitral regurgitation is a complication after balloon valvuloplasty particularly with the antegrade approach, less commonly with the retrograde approach. This is mainly due to the catheter, guide wire and/or balloon catching on the mitral valve. In many patients the myomatous nature of the mitral valve and the small left ventricular cavity are compounding factors for this complication. Mitral and acute aortic regurgitation can lead to acute pulmonary edema.

5.4 Poor outcome

The results of balloon aortic valvuloplasty are considered suboptimal is the valve fails to dilate and there are residual Doppler gradients of more than 50 mmHg, moderate or severe aortic valve regurgitation, moderate or severe mitral valve regurgitation and worsening left ventricular function (Rao et al, 1989).

Risk factors for poor results (residual gradients of >50mmHg) include older or neonatal age group, symptomatic patient (Knirsch et al. 2008), dysplastic aortic valves and left ventricular dysfunction. The procedure is contraindicated in patients with associated moderate aortic regurgitation or hypoplastic left ventricle. Additional risk factors for poor outcome in a neonate include ductal dependency, mitral valve disease, notably stenosis, non-apex forming left ventricle, and hypoplastic aortic valve annulus (<6mm in diameter)(Knirsch et al, 2008).

Mortality related to the procedure has been reported to be around 12% mainly due to cusp perforation and avulsion producing severe regurgitation, and left ventricular perforation with guide wire. One study reported 46% mortality due to ventricular fibrillation, avulsion of aortic valve cusp and severe aortic regurgitation (Magee et al, 1997). This would lead to a sudden volume overload, together with reduced coronary perfusion of a poorly functioning or hypertrophied left ventricle can rapidly lead to hypotension and acidosis which can prove fatal.

5.5 Aortic regurgitation

The single complication to be avoided during balloon valvuloplasty is development or worsening of aortic regurgitation. Aortic regurgitation was caused by a combination of commissural avulsion, cusp dehiscence with retraction, cusp tear, central incompetence, perforated cusp, cusp prolapse, or cusp adhesion to the aortic wall (Bacha et al, 2001; Balmer et al, 2004). There is a relationship of this complication to the use of oversized balloons. The dilemma faced in the catheterization laboratory is the decision on when to upsize (or not to upsize) the balloon, if residual gradients of 30 to 40 mm Hg are found. In older patients if residual gradients are high and the degree of aortic regurgitation is only mild or trivial, one can afford to upsize the balloon. However if residual gradients are <30 mm Hg, there is very little to be gained in upsizing the balloon as aortic regurgitation would be produced. Furthermore, balloons usually are only available in 1- to 2-mm increments, making upsizing very risky. Holzer et al found that freedom from aortic valve replacement was not any worse (and potentially better) in patients with residual gradients of <35 mm Hg and moderate or severe aortic regurgitation compared with patients with residual gradients of >35 mm Hg and mild aortic regurgitation. This report should help in persuading operators to upsize the balloon if the gradient is 35 to 40 mm Hg with just mild aortic regurgitation, rather than a more conservative approach for fear of creating more aortic regurgitation (Holzer et al, 2010).

It should be noted that even if the degree of aortic regurgitation is minimal immediately after balloon valvuloplasty, it does not remain so in the medium and long term follow up, it is usually progressive. Explanation for this phenomenon is that blood flow through the aortic valve leads to constant hemodynamic trauma to the valve tissue resulting in progressive tearing, scarring, retraction, and calcification of the valve (Balmer et al, 2004).

5.6 Balloon aortic valvuloplasty in adults

In symptomatic adolescents and adults with aortic stenosis, the procedure of choice is surgical therapy with either valve replacement or Ross procedure. Balloon aortic valvuloplasty may be offered to pregnant females to reduce the risks of pregnancy. It can also be offered to young adults with pliable valves who are not considered candidates for surgical therapy. Another group is adults who need stabilization before undergoing valve replacement. These are patients with severe aortic stenosis and poor left ventricular function who have symptoms of congestive heart failure. If not operated upon, they have a mortality rate of 60% at 1 year. Although the exact place of the valvuloplasty procedure in the treatment of aortic stenosis in adults is yet to be determined, there is immediate clinical improvement in most of the patients with poor left ventricular function for whom surgery is not definitely contraindicated. It is therefore to be considered as a bridge to surgery in hemodynamically unstable patients to improve their operative risks (Berland et al, 1989; Singh et al, 2008).

5.7 Balloon aortic valvuloplasty in special circumstances

Balloon aortic valvuloplasty is done in all patients undergoing percutaneous valve implantation to allow the balloon- valve assembly to cross the aortic valve (Leon et al, 2010). Balloon aortic valvuloplasty has been attempted in stenosed surgical bioprostheses with mixed results in literature. Majority admit it has limited application with great caution in some instances and disappointment in others (Kirwan et al, 2004; Waller et al, 1991). The reason is that the bioprosthetic valve leaflets are at relatively high risk of tearing resulting in dehiscence, regurgitation or embolism. Lasting significant benefit has not been documented because of high incidence of restenosis (Webb J, 2011). Therefore repeat surgery or supportive medical therapy is advocated in such patients. It may be possible that the growing experience with percutaneous valve implantation may make the future of patients with failed bioprosthetic valves bright by "valve in valve" implantation.

Balloon valvuloplasty can be done as a hybrid procedure with a trans-apical access in premature infants in whom peripheral vascular access may not be possible (Maschiettom et al, 2011).

5.8 Balloon valvuloplasty for aortic stenosis in the fetus

This is an evolving field with successful reports from several workers. The main idea is to improve left ventricular growth in cases of suspected hypoplasia of left ventricle (Marshall et al, 2005). Aortic stenosis is identified by fetal echocardiography. Noted are the thickness of the aortic valve leaflets, marked turbulence across the aortic valve and left ventricular dysfunction. Mothers undergo general anesthesia and are placed in an optimal position to obtain good ultrasound images. This position may be supine with required uterine displacement with external manipulation. Poor position may result in technical failure. In that case sometimes a mini laprotomy may be helpful and ultrasound being done directly per-uterine. The fetus is then given intramuscular anesthetic agent and muscle relaxant.

Balloon size is determined by the aortic valve annulus and a balloon size can go up to 120%. A low profile coronary balloon catheter is chosen and mounted over a floppy tipped guide wire. The introducer is advanced through the fetal chest into the left ventricular cavity. The trocar is removed and intra ventricular position confirmed by the back flow of blood.

The wire catheter assembly is passed through the canula until the wire is identified in the ascending aorta. The balloon is advanced and inflation done gently with an inflation device to achieve the required pressure. One or more inflations can be done, each not being for more than 5 seconds. The whole wire and catheter assembly is then withdrawn.

The results are usually good with relief of gradient. It is difficult to determine the ideal balloon size. There is no way to measure decrease in gradient. Waist produced during inflation is not seen. One can appreciate improved flow across the aortic valve and appearance of new aortic regurgitation. In experimental animals, fetal aortic regurgitation occurring post balloon valvuloplasty led to hydrops fetalis. This complication has not been reported in human subjects. In fact aortic regurgitation can improve due to the remodeling capacity of fetal aortic valve leaflets. Thus fetal aortic valvuloplasty has promising future for severe aortic stenosis.

6. Clinical outcome of balloon aortic valvuloplasty at intermediate and long term follow up

Intermediate and long term results of aortic valvuloplasty of congenital aortic valve stenosis in preventing or postponing aortic valve surgery are very good (Fratz et al, 2008). Survival after successful balloon valvuloplasty without significant residual stenosis or regurgitation has been reported to be 86% at 1 year and continues to remain the same until 10 years (Han et al, 2007). Left ventricular dysfunction improved in 87% on follow up (Egito et al, 1997). Incidence of re-intervention is variable and depends on the age of intervention and conservative interventional strategy used at the time of dilation. Pass et al reported a 64% freedom from re-intervention at 8 years follow up. A second re-dilation is usually required in neonates 1 month to 6 years after the initial procedure. Criteria for re-dilation would be the same as stated previously. Presence moderate or severe aortic regurgitation should preclude further balloon valvuloplasty (Khalid et al, 2006)[1].

Special reference must be made to neonatal severe or critical aortic stenosis which may be a different disease from congenital aortic stenosis treated later in life (Brown et al, 2010). The risk for both mortality and re-dilatation is higher in newborns with symptomatic aortic stenosis than in older infants, children, and adolescents or adults. Prime aim of dilating these frail neonates is to provide some relief of obstruction to allow the left ventricle to recover and at the same time avoid regurgitation. Therefore acceptable residual gradients may be higher in this group with an understanding that they may have recurrent aortic stenosis much earlier due to their rapid growth phase.

Surgical intervention is required as a subsequent procedure when the aortic regurgitation is moderate to severe, or the valve is dysplastic and could not be dilated. In neonates and young children, surgical valvotomy for stenosis and repair for regurgitation are standard procedure. Aortic regurgitation is a complication of aortic valvotomy as well. Other surgical options are Ross operation or aortic valve replacement in older children. A significant number of patients after both aortic valvuloplasty and aortic valve surgery may require aortic valve replacement for progressive aortic regurgitation. Many non randomized comparisons have been made between results of aortic valvuloplasty and aortic valve surgery. The two were found comparable in terms of gradient relief, procedural mortality and long term survival. Therefore both procedures are essentially palliative. Consequently proponents of aortic valvuloplasty as an initial procedure can argue that with it the patient can benefit from one less surgery in their life (Knirsch et al, 2008). In one follow up data the freedom from aortic valve replacement was 79% at 10 years and 55% at 20 years (Brown et al, 2010 a). This becomes an important part of patient counseling while committing to care of patients with aortic valve stenosis. Those with severe left ventricular dysfunction and endocardial fibrosis may be candidates for cardiac transplant.

The risk for late sudden cardiovascular death after balloon aortic valvuloplasty is not associated with acute post-procedural hemodynamic status. However, there are some significant predictors for the same, notably the presence of multiple left-heart obstructive lesions. Patients undergoing balloon valvuloplasty in the neonatal period also have a higher risk for sudden cardiovascular death after balloon valvuloplasty, which may be a marker of more severe or progressive disease (Brown et al, 2010 b).

7. Percutaneous aortic valve implantation

Calcific aortic stenosis is the most common valvular heart disease, affecting 2% to 4% of adults over age 65 in the United States. The prevalence of degenerative aortic stenosis increases with advancing age. It has a long asymptomatic phase, but when symptoms finally occur, clinical deterioration can be rapid with 50% mortality within two years of developing symptoms (Leon e al, 2010). Surgical aortic valve replacement is the gold standard therapy for adult patients with symptomatic severe aortic stenosis, be it congenital or degenerative in etiology.

The steady increase in the number of patients requiring aortic valve replacement and the high surgical risk in patients with multiple co-morbidities have been driving the development of percutaneous techniques for the treatment of aortic stenosis. Other perceived advantages include less trauma, often faster recovery and fewer hospital days. There is a reluctance of some patients to undergo the trauma and pain associated with open heart surgery via sternotomy.

It is estimated that for each two patients with severe symptomatic aortic stenosis undergoing surgical valve replacement, there is at least one patient who will never undergo surgery because of the perceived high risk. A recent study showed that 33% of patients over age 75 were deemed too high-risk for open heart surgery and thus were left untreated (Spargias et el, 2008).

In 2002, Cribier al reported the first successful human percutaneous aortic valve implantation done antegradely via femoral vein. The approach had an inherent risk of mitral valve damage, ventricular perforation and tamponade. Thereafter the retrograde approach has become popular. Indications for percutaneous valve implantation are severe aortic stenosis with an aortic valve area of <0.8 cm2, MPG of>49 mmHg or a peak flow velocity of >4m/s (28). Pertinent exclusion criteria are bicuspid aortic valve, acute myocardial infarction, significant coronary artery disease, left ventricular ejection fraction less than 20%, diameter of aortic valve annulus less than 18mm or more than 25mm, severe aortic or mitral regurgitation and severe renal failure (Leon et al, 2008).

Details of the technique and its application are described elsewhere.

8. Conclusion

Transcatheter treatment of congenital aortic valve stenosis is the intervention of choice in neonates, infants, children and also adolescents with good results. Valvuloplasty has a limited role in adults. Percutaneous aortic valve replacement has emerged as a therapeutic option in the elderly who are not candidates for surgical aortic valve replacement.

9. References

Alekyan BG, Petrosyan YS, Coulson JD, Danilov YY, Vinokurov AV. Right scapular artery catheterization for balloon valvuloplasty for critical aortic stenosis in infants. Am L Cardiol 1995; 76: 1049-52.

Bacha EA, Satou GM, Moran AM, et al. Valve-sparing operation for balloon induced aortic regurgitation in congenital aortic stenosis. J Thorac Cardiovasc Surg 2001; 122:162–8.

Balmer C, Beghetti M, Fasnacht M, Friedli B, Arbenz U. Balloon aortic valvuloplasty in paediatric patients: progressive aortic regurgitation is common. Heart 2004; 90(1): 77-81.

Beekman RH, Rocchini AP, Crowlely DC, Snider AR, Serwer GA, Dick M, Rosenthal A. Comparison of single and double balloon valvuloplasty in children with aortic stenosis. J Am Coll Cardiol 1988; 12:480-5.

Berland J, Cribier A, Savin T, Lefebvre E, Koning R, Letac B. Percutaneous balloon aortic valvuloplasty in patients with severe aortic stenosis and low ejection fraction: Immediate results and intermediate follow up. Circulation1989; 79: 1189-96.

Bermudez EA. Echocardiographic assessment of aortic stenosis, Chapter 11 in Contemporary Cardiology: Essential Echocardiography: A practical handbook. Editor Solomon SD. Humana Press, Totowa, NJ. 1st Edition, 2007, 209-21.

Bonow RO, Carabello AB Chatterjee K, de Leon AC et al.AHA/ACC 2008 Guidelines for the management of patients with valvular heart disease. Circulation 2008; 118; 523-661.

Brown DW, Dipilato AE, Chong EC, Lock JE, McElhinneyDB. Aortic valve reintervention after balloon aortic valvuloplasty for congenital aortic stenosis: Intermediate and late follow up. J Am Coll Cardiol 2010; 56 (21): 1740-9.

Brown DW, Dipilato AE, Chong EC, Gauvreau K, McElhinney DB, Colan SD, Lock JE.Sudden unexpected death after balloon valvuloplasty for congenital aortic stenosis. J Am Coll Cardiol. 2010; 56(23):1939-46.

Egito EST et al. Transvascular balloon dilation for neonatal critical aortic stenosis: Early and midterm results. J Am Coll Cardiol 1997; 29 (2): 442-7.

Fernandes SM, Khairy P, Sanders SP, Colan SD. Bicuspid aortic valve: morphology and interventions in the young. J Am Coll Cardiol 2007; 49 (22):2211-4.

Fischer DR, Ettedgui JA, Park SC, Siewers RD, Del Nido PJ. Carotid artery approach for balloon dilation of aortic valve stenosis in the neonate: A preliminary report. J Am Coll Cardiol 1990; 15:1633-36.

Fratz S, Gildein P, Balling G, Sebening W, Genz T, Eicken A, Hess J. Aortic valvuloplasty in pediatric patients substantially postpones the need for aortic valve surgery. Circulation 2008; 117:1201-6.

Gupta SD, Das S, Ghose T, Sarkar A, Goswami A, Kundu S. Controlled transient respiratory arrest along with rapid right ventricular pacing for improving balloon stability during balloon valvuloplasty in pediatric patients with congenital aortic stenosis--a retrospective case series analysis. Ann Card Anaesth 2010, 13 (3). 236-40.

Han RK, Gurofsky RC, Lee KJ, Dipchand AI, Williams WG, Smallhorn JF, et al. Outcome and growth potential of left heart structures after neonatal intervention for aortic valve stenosis. J Am Coll Cardiol 2007; 50: 2406-14.

Hausdorf G, Schneider M, Schirmer KR, Schulze-Neick I, Lange PE, antegrade balloon valvuloplasty of aortic stenosis in children. Am J Cardiol 1993; 71: 460-3.

Holzer RJ, Cheatham JP. Shifting the balance between aortic insufficiency and residual gradients after balloon aortic valvuloplasty. J Am Coll Cardiol 2010; 56 (21): 1750-1.

Karago T, Aypar E, Erdog I, Sahin M, Ozer S, Celiker A. Congenital aortic stenosis: A novel technique for ventricualr pacing during valvuloplasty.Catheter Cardiovasc Interv 2008; 72:527–530.

Khalid O, Luxenberg DM, Sable C, Benavidex O, Geva T. Hanna B, Abdulla R. Aortic stenosis: The spectrum of practice. Pediatr Cardiol 2006; 27 (6): 661-9.

Kirwan C, Richardson G, Rothman MT. Is there a role for balloon valvuloplasty in patients with stenotic aortic bioprosthetic valves? Catheter Cardiovasc Interv. 2004 Oct; 63(2): 251-3.

Knirsch W, Berger F, Harpes P, Kretschmar O. Balloon valvuloplasty of aortic valve stenosis in childhood: early and medium term results. Clin Res Cardiol 2008; 97 (9): 587-93

Leon MB et al. Transcatheter aortic-valve implantation for aortic stenosis in patients who cannot undergo surgery. N Eng J Med 2010; 363: 1597-1607.

Maeno Y, Agaki T, Hashino K, Ishi M, Sugimura T, Takagi J, Suzuki K, Kato H. Carotid artery approach to balloon aortic valvuloplasty in infants with critical aortic stenosis. Pediatr Cardiol 1997; 18:288-91.

Magee AG. Balloon dilation of severe aortic stenosis in the neonate: Comparison of anteograde and retrograde catheter approaches. J Am Coll Cardiol 1997; 30: 1061-6.

Mahle WT, Sutherland JL, Frias PA. Outcome of isolated bicuspid aortic valve in childhood. J Pediatr 2010; 157: 445-9.

Marshall Ac et al. Aortic Valvuloplasty in the fetus: Technical characteristics of successful balloon dilation. J Pediatr 2005; 147: 535-9.

Maschiettom N, Vidam V, Milanesi O. Transapical aortic balloon valvuloplasty in a 890 gram infany: hybrid is better! Catheter Cariovasc nterv 2011; 77(1): 112-4.doi 10.1002/ccd.22754.

Mehta C, Desai T, Shebani S, Stickley J, DE Giovanni J. Rapid ventricular pacing for catheter interventions in congenital aortic stenosis and coarctation: effectiveness, safety, and rate titration for optimal results. J Interv Cardiol. 2010; 23 (1):7-13.

Pass RH, Hellenbrand WE. Catheter Intervention for critical aortic stenosis in the neonate. Cath Cardiovasc Interv 2002; 55: 88-92.

Randolph AD, Cook DJ, Gonzales CA, et al: Ultrasound guidance for placement of central venous catheters: A meta-analysis of the literature. Crit Care Med 1996; 24:2053-2058.

Rao PS, Thapar MK, Wilson AD, Levy JM, Chopra PS. Intermediate term follow-up results of balloon aortic valvuloplasty in infants and children with special reference to causes of restenosis. Am J Cardiol 1989; 64:1356–60.

Singh IM, Shishehbor MH, Christofferson RD, Tuzcu EM, Kapadia SR. Percutaneous treatment of aortic valve stenosis. Cleve Clin J Med. 2008 Nov; 75(11):805-12.

Spargias K, Manginas A, Pavlides G, et al. Transcatheter aortic valve implantation: first Greek experience. Hellenic J Cardiol 2008; 49:397-407.

Waller BF, Mckay C, Van Tassel J, Allen M. Catheter balloon valvuloplasty of stenotic porcine bioprosthetic valves: Part II: Mechanisms, complications and recommendation for clinical use. Clin Cardiol 1991; 14 (9): 764-72.

Webb J. Balloon valvuloplasty for stenotic bioprosthetic aortic valves. Catheter Cardiovasc Interv 2011; 77(4):593. doi: 10.1002/ccd.22986.

Part 5

Molecular Considerations in Aortic Stenosis

11

Proteomics - A Powerful Tool to Deepen the Molecular Mechanisms of Aortic Stenosis Disease

Felix Gil-Dones[1], Fernando de la Cuesta[1], Gloria Alvarez-Llamas[2], Luis R. Padial[3], Luis F. López-Almodovar[5], Tatiana Martín-Rojas[1], Fernando Vivanco[2,4] and Maria G. Barderas[1]
[1]*Department of Vascular Physiopathology. Hospital Nacional de Paraplejicos, SESCAM, Toledo,*
[2]*Department of Immunology, IIS- Fundacion Jimenez Diaz, Madrid,*
[3]*Department of Cardiology, Hospital Virgen de la Salud, SESCAM, Toledo,*
[4]*Department of Biochemistry and Molecular Biology, Universidad Complutense, Madrid,*
[5]*Cardiac Surgery, Hospital Virgen de la Salud, Toledo*
Spain

1. Introduction

Valvular aortic stenosis (AS) produces a slowly progressive obstruction in left ventricular outflow track. Aortic valve replacement is warranted when symptoms or left ventricular dysfunction develop, which happen when the valvular stenosis is hemodynamically significant. Among the three main causes of valvular AS (congenital, rheumatic or degenerative), degenerative AS is the most prevalent in the older population, and due to the aging population it is the most frequent cause of valve replacement in western countries. Currently it is responsible for most valve replacements performed in Europe, and there is a steady increase of this disease and its social significance (Iun *et al.*, 2003).

Degenerative or calcific aortic valve disease is characterized by aortic valve leaflet thickening and calcification of the aortic valve, usually in an anatomically normal trileaflet valve. Several studies have demonstrated an association between degenerative AS and cardiovascular risk factors for atherosclerosis, such as hypercholesterolemia, hypertension, tobacco, the metabolic syndrome, etc, and as a consequence a similar pathobiologic process has been suggested for degenerative AS and atherosclerosis (Stewart *et al.*, 1997; Agmon *et al.*, 2001). But although there are many similarities between these two diseases, the differences are also significant.

The pathobiology of aortic valve calcification comprises three main processes: lipid accumulation, inflammation and calcification. Accumulation and oxidation of LDL-cholesterol particles, T-lymphocytes, macrophages, and production of inflammatory mediators such as interleukin-1-beta and transforming growth factors beta-1 have been observed at tissue level in the aortic leaflets of patients with degenerative AS. Angiotensin converting enzyme production has also been detected at valvular level in these patients. In later stages of the disease, active cartilage and bone formation have also been reported (Mohler *et al.*, 2001; Freeman *et al.*, 2005). All these findings suggest that degenerative AS is an active process instead of a passive "wear and tear" phenomenon as it has been considered for decades.

Although hypercholesterolemia has been pointed out as a risk factor for degenerative AS, its relationship with this disease is far from being clear. The similarities between the pathobiology of degenerative AS and atherosclerosis suggested that statins could decrease the progression of degenerative AS and help avoiding its clinical consequences as has been demonstrated in coronary artery disease. However, the last trials that analysed moderate-to-severe degenerative AS have failed to demonstrate any benefit of statins in the clinical evolution of this disease (Cowell *et al.*, 2005; Chan *et al.*, 2010), despite having demonstrated, in the SEAS trial (Rossed *et al.*, 2008), a reduction of some coronary events with the reduction in LDL cholesterol. Therefore, once significant degenerative AS has progressed cholesterol does not appear to be longer related with the process, which is opposed to what has been observed in atherosclerosis. This has also been suggested by the only trial performed in patients with mild degenerative AS, the RAAVE trial, in which rosuvastatin showed a mild positive impact of cholesterol reduction on the progression of degenerative AS as assessed by echocardiography (Moura *et al.*, 2001). Taken together, this suggests that some risk factors can play a role only in the early stages of the disease, but once the calcification process starts to develop, the role played by the classical risk factors appears to wane, although the information so far available is somewhat contradictory (Walter *et al.*, 2010).

The conflicting information available makes it necessary to further study the pathophysiologic process of degenerative AS in order to unveil the basic mechanisms of the disease, a needed step in the process of developing reliable biomarkers of the disease as well as preventive therapies for it. Proteomics, a science aimed at discovering the proteins involved in the pathogenic process of diseases in an unbiased way, appears especially suited for studying the pathogenic processes involved in the development of degenerative AS. This chapter provides information about the different proteomics techniques for the AS study. We have begun to apply these methodologies to examine the physiological changes that accompany this pathology in a comprehensive manner. The techniques described in this chapter were optimized in our laboratory for the analysis of different kind of human samples. Data reported by our lab as well as by other authors will be presented to give the reader a wide perspective of the information available about the pathogenesis of this prevalent and clinically significant disease.

2. AS plasma proteome

At present, it is possible to perform a differential proteomic approach on a variety of biological samples, including cells, tissues or biological fluids (plasma, urine). In the context of biomarker discovery, biological fluids such as plasma or urine, represent the most logical compartment for investigation.

Plasma is the best clinical sample in terms of diagnosis and prognosis, due to several advantages including its low cost, not invasive and easy access (Veenstra TD *et al.*, 2005). Human plasma is a rich source of proteins and other metabolites which reflect the physiological or clinical status of patients. Since blood circulates throughout every organ and tissue of the body, it is expected to contain valuable information about the real physiological state of the organism. The protein concentration in plasma is tightly controlled and, thus, variations can be considered as an indicator of the current state of health. Numerous biomedical/clinical proteomic studies have demonstrated that plasma protein levels reflect human physiological and pathological states and can be used for disease diagnosis and prognosis (Anderson NL *et al.*, 2002).

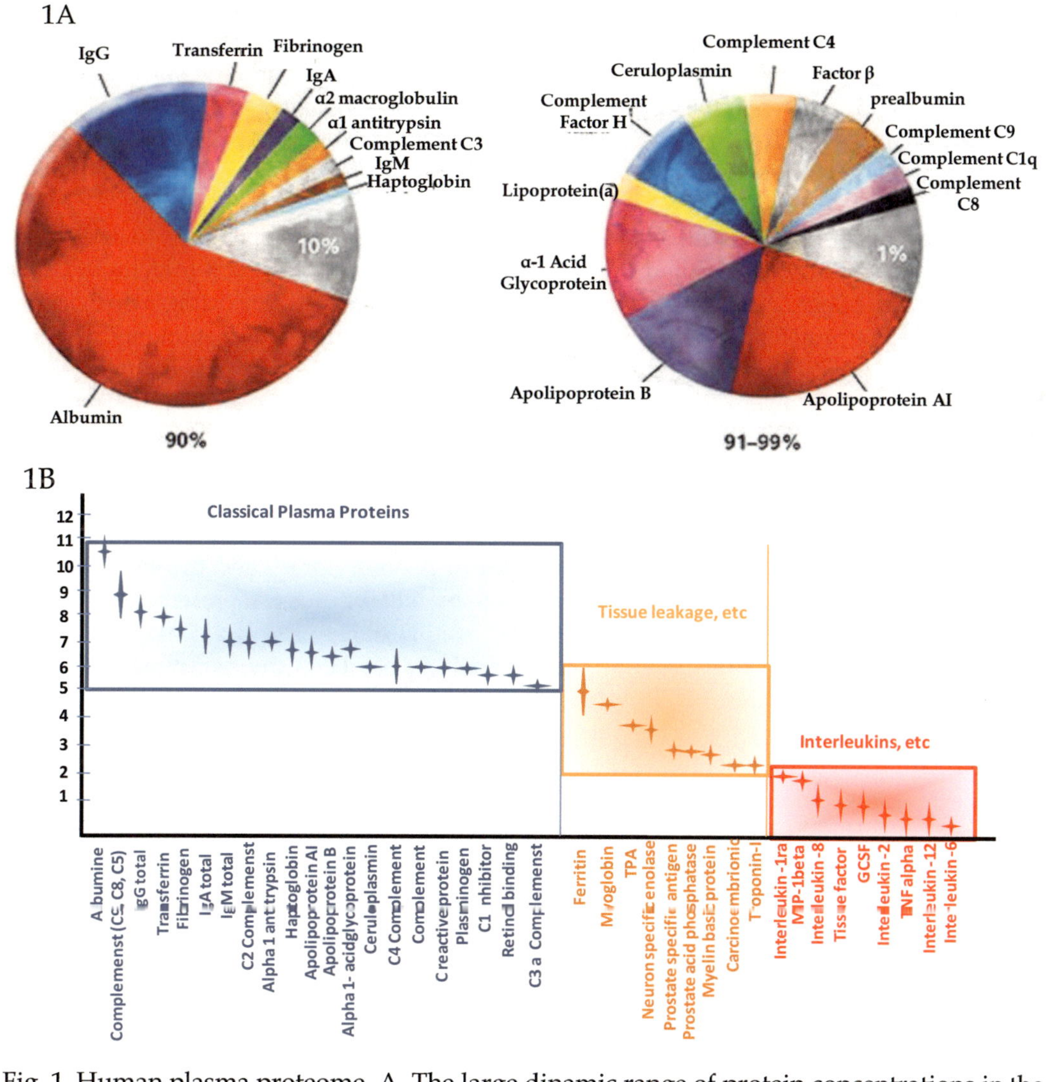

Fig. 1. Human plasma proteome. A, The large dinamic range of protein concentrations in the human proteome represents a significant experimental challenge as technologies must be sensitive across nearly 12 orders of magnitude (a 1 trillionfold range) for comprehensive analysis and the development of biomarkers. B, Estimated concentration of plasma proteins (based in Anderson and Anderson, 2002 Molecular and cellular proteomics)

However, the plasma proteome is very complex and presents a wide dynamic range of proteins (more than 10 magnitude orders) what makes its proteomic analysis very challenging, because high-abundance proteins tend to mask those of lower abundance

(Anderson NL *et al.*, 2005). In other words, only 20 major proteins comprise 99% of the plasma proteome and the rest of the proteins making up 1% of the plasma content (Figure 1). Potential disease biomarkers could be present in low concentrations, and not be detected by the current proteomic techniques (Darde VM *et al.*, 2010). Hence, it is essential to perform a pre-fractionation method. Cibacron Blue Dye and protein A/G columns have been used to effectively remove serum albumin and immunoglobulins from serum, allowing detection of proteins present at very low concentrations. Nowadays, the most common technique is the immunodepletion, which has been extensively used for the specific removal of the most abundant proteins, based on the action of specific antibodies (Zolotarjova N. *et al.*, 2005 and Wang YY *et al.*, 2003). Among these, Multiple Affinity Removal Columns (MARC) is the most effective method because it simultaneously removes multiple abundant proteins (Bjorhall K, *et al.*, 2005 and Seam N *et al.*, 2007).

There are several affinity columns as MARS-6 or MARS-14 (Agilent Tecnologies) to deplete the 6 or 14 more abundant proteins and even to deplete the 20 more abundant proteins with the Top-20 column (Sigma). In any case, there has been concerned regarding whether less abundant plasma proteins are removed jointly with albumin and other commonly depleted proteins by "nonspecific" binding (albuminome) (Yocum AK, *et al.*, 2005 and Granger J *et al.*, 2005). To save this problem, the combinatorial peptide ligand libraries (CPLL) have been proposed as an alternative method (Righetti PG *et al.*, 2006 and Sihlbom C *et al.*, 2008). This methodology was designed for sample equalization and it is used to analyze the "low-abundance proteome" in association with mass spectrometry (MS). CPLL have been recently used in plasma analysis to reduce their complexity, hence the most abundant plasma proteins would saturate all its corresponding hexapeptides in peptide library and the excess will be eliminated, while the less abundant plasma proteins will be more represented and more accessible to the differential analysis of protein expression (Righetti P G *et al.*, 2006).

Until now, the main approximation to plasma analysis has been the two-dimensional gel electrophoresis (2-DE), although it presents several limitations, since highly acidic or hydrophobic proteins and those with the highest or the smallest molecular weight in the sample may not be represented. However, 2-DE allows detecting changes in specific isoforms and, in general, approximately 1000-2000 protein spots can be visualized on a gel (Tannu NS and Hemby SE. 2006). Gel based approaches have enabled important advances in measurement of protein expression alterations in normal and diseases states. Moreover, new more sensitive fluorescence probes (Sipro Ruby, Cy2, Cy3 and Cy5) have been designed to improve spots detection and identification from 2-DE gels, improving hugely the "classical" silver stain. A methodological advance in 2-DE has been the 2-D Fluorescence Difference Gel Electrophoresis (2D-DIGE) (GE Healthcare). 2D-DIGE is based on direct labeling of lysine groups on proteins with cyanine CyDye DIGE Fluor minimal dyes before isoelectric focusing, enabling the labeling of 2-3 samples per gel with different dyes. This capability minimizes spot pattern variability and the number of gels by experiment providing a simple, accurate and reproducible spot matching. This is achieved by inclusion of an internal standard for every spot in every 2-DE gel, providing with experimental reproducibility and the highest accuracy in protein ratio measurements. In this way, the individual protein data from the control and diseased samples (Cy3 or Cy5) are normalized against the internal standard sample (Cy2 dye-labeled), Cy5:Cy2 and Cy3:Cy2.

To avoid 2-DE limitations, new alternatives have been developed, the most successful is based on multidimensional liquid chromatography coupled to MS (LC-MS/MS).

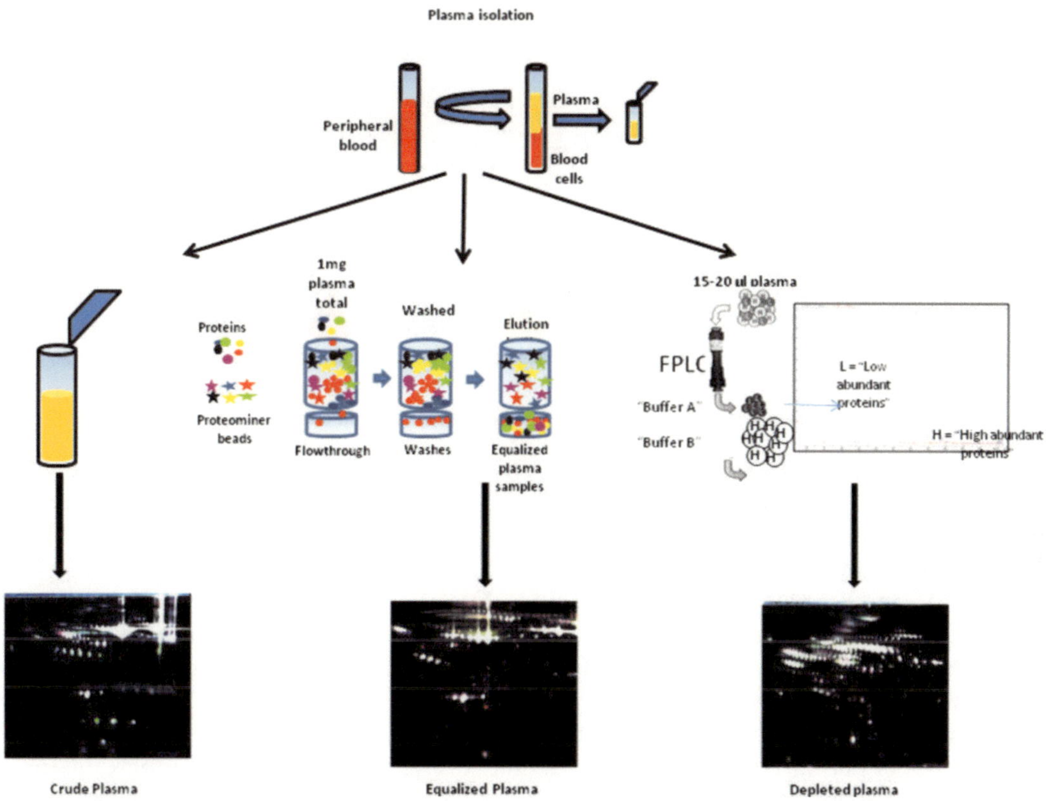

Fig. 2. Schematic workflow in 2D-DIGE plasma analysis. Isolation and processing of plasma samples 2D-DIGE analysis (left). 2D-DIGE of processed plasma samples using the combinatorial peptide ligand libraries (CPLL) (proteominer) (center) and depletion of most abundant plasma protein with affinity columns (right).

Electrospray ionization (ESI) development and recent advances in mass spectrometry (MS) provided the second-generation of proteomics technology based on LC-MS/MS. This approach is nowadays referred to as shotgun proteomics or MudPIT (Chen EI *et al.*, 2006 and MacCoss MJ *et al.*, 2002). To perform differential expression analysis , several probes have been designed for labeling both at protein and peptide levels (ICAT (isotope-coded affinity tagging), SILAC (stable isotope-labeling with amino acids in cell culture) or iTRAQ (stable isotope-tagged amine-reactive Reagents)) (Wu WW et al., 2006 and Graumann J *et al.*, 2008).
iTRAQ is an LC-based methodology which is gradually gaining in popularity. iTRAQ reagents have permitted relative expression measurements of large sets of proteins with a high grade of automation. The isobaric nature of the tags allows the peptide samples to be pooled postlabeling, without increasing the complexity of MS analysis. Identical peptides labeled with the different iTRAQ reagents exhibit the same parent ion in MS. Upon MS/MS fragmentation of parent ion, unique signature ions are generated which distinguish the individual samples and, hence, the relative abundance among the samples can be determined (Figure 3).

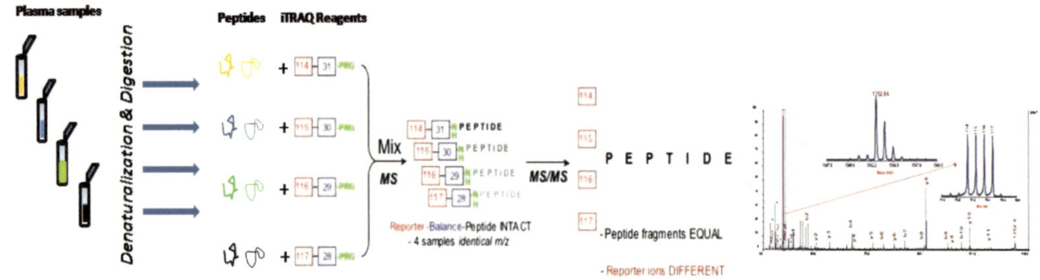

Fig. 3. Schematic workflow of iTRAQ labeling: After denaturation, reduction, alkylation, and digestion, each protein sample is modified with a distinct iTRAQ ® reagent. The iTRAQ ®-modified samples are then mixed to be analyzed by mass spectrometry. The MS/MS spectra of the individual peptides show signals reflecting amino acid sequences and also show reporter ions reflecting the protein contents of the samples.

In a different approach, the low molecular weight fraction can be investigated (plasma peptidome) by LC-MS/MS or by Matrix-Assisted Laser Desorption/Ionization-mass Spectrometry (MALDI-MS). The peptidome has been described as all peptides that have been expressed in any cell, tissue, or biofluid at any given time (Schulte I *et al.*, 2005 and Schrader M and Schulz-Knappe P, 2001). Peptidomics holds considerable promise for the discovery of new bioactive molecules and for elucidating biochemical regulatory networks. Endogenous peptides have already been established as messengers, hormones or cytokines in many physiological processes. Alterations in peptide levels under disease conditions implicate this class of molecules as potential biomarkers.

Ultrafiltrates of plasma have been recognized for several years to contain complex mixtures of thousands of peptides that are smaller than apolipoprotein C-I, the smallest major plasma protein. The complete set of small peptides from plasma has been termed the plasma peptidome, or the fragmentome (Tirumalai R S *et al.*, 2003) because it has been recognized that most small peptide components of plasma are derived from proteolytic degradation of larger proteins. Peptide fragments of many major plasma proteins, such as fibrinogen, apolipoproteins, transthyretin, and complement factors, have been detected (Adkins JN et al., 2002, Tirumalai RS et al., 2003). To obtain the plasma peptidome some authors have applied molecular weight filters (ranging 10-3,5kDa) to isolate small proteins and whole peptidome. With the focus on peptides rather than proteins, a hydrophobic-based capture technique, which removes salts and other hydrophilic compounds in a single step, is more compatible with direct LC-MS analysis (Zhou H *et al.*, 2006 and Tian R *et al.*, 2007).

Some biochemical studies in AS plasma samples using the ELISA technique have reported alterations in their proteins levels. Most of these studies were focused in proteins implicated in cardiovascular diseases outstanding the natriuretic peptide (Yandle TG *et al.*, 1986; Yandle TG *et al.*, 1993 and Hunt PJ. *et al.*, 1997) whose levels are prognostic of cardiovascular outcomes independently (26, Tsutamoto T. *et al* 1997). Recently, Qi W *et al.*, 2001, Prasad N *et al.*, 1997 and Talwar S et al., 2001. published that plasma natriuretic peptide levels were related to disease severity in AS. In addition, they also reported that cardiothrophin-1 (CT-1) levels were increased in AS patients and these results correlated with the trans-valvular aortic pressure gradient (TVPG) and could potentially be used to monitor progression of disease in a non-invasively manner. Ferrari G. et al have recently shown that individuals with severe AS exhibited higher plasma levels of NT-proBNP, BNP fragment, and

osteopontin compared with controls. Fetuin-A levels were lower in individuals with AS than in healthy controls. Asymmetric dimethylarginine (ADMA) were lower while homocysteine levels were higher in theAS patients.
Despite the potential offered by proteomics, plasma from AS patients has not been studied, until now. Taking into account the studies performed with one protein or with a small number of proteins, a proteomic plasma analysis, without bias, could give us a more complete sight at molecular level of this pathology and its possible relation with atherosclerosis. The HUPO Plasma Proteome consortium has identified a group of 345 cardiovascular-related proteins that could constitute a baseline proteomic blueprint for the future development of biosignatures for cardiovascular diseases (Vivanco, F. *et al.* 2007). Hence, new studies focusing in plasma from AS patients will be necessary to deepen in this pathology, in order to find new biomarkers and therapies.

3. Tissue, isolated cells and secretome

Protein tissue biomarkers offer a great promise to provide a clinical diagnosis and prognosis information that cannot be obtained from genomics or serum biomarkers. In the past, the discovery phase has been delayed by several hurdles including tissue heterogeneity and the lack of sensitive technology to identify and measure protein in small volumes of human biopsy tissue (Espina *et al.*, 2009). These hurdles have been largely overcome by the wide availability of laser microdissection technology, protein microarrays, and advances in mass spectrometry (Emmert-Buck *et al.*, 1996; Petricoin *et al.*, 2005). Under such considerations, the tools and methodology of proteomics are becoming increasingly important and, we could postulate that tissue proteomics studies provide us two main information data sets: 1) potential biomarkers of disease directly released from tissue lesions, which should be validated in wider cohorts before being applied to clinics; 2) discovery of action mechanisms and pathways involved in the formation and development of AS by direct "in-situ" proteomics (Alvarez-Llamas et al., 2007).

3.1 Stability in tissue: pre-analitycal variability

Today, there is an important need to develop standardized protocols and novel technologies that can be used in the routine clinical settings for seamless collection and immediate preservation of tissue in the search for biomarker proteins. In this sense, both clinicians and researcher are implicated. The fidelity of the data obtained from a diagnostic assay applied to the tissue must be monitored and quality controlled. Under the current standard of care, AS tissue is procured by AS replacement in a hospital-based operating room. The instant a tissue biopsy is removed from a patient, the cells within the tissue react and adapt to the absence of vascular perfusion, ischemia, hypoxia, acidosis, accumulation of cellular waste, absence of electrolytes and temperature changes (Espina *et al.*, 2008). Normally tissue is frozen in dry ice or liquid nitrogen or fixed to avoid degradation and to preserve for later proteomics analysis. Otherwise, the tissue is maintained in physiological serum if we want to develop secretome analysis. A multitude of known and unknown variables can influence the stability of AS tissue molecules: temperature, pH, hypoxia, dehydration, RNAses activity, proteinases activity, *ex-vivo* stress (Espina *et al.*, 2008) etc. For these reasons the protocol to follow must be the strictest as possible: The recommended maximum elapsed time ranges between 20 minutes to 2 hours from surgery to stabilization (freezing, tissue culture, fixation, etc.). Finally, the study of tissue can be addressed according to three main sample sources: a) whole tissue proteomics, by which total proteins extracts obtained from areas of interest are studied; b) tissue sub-proteomes, i.e. specific aortic valve layers and cells isolated directly from tissue (apart from those studies based on cultured cells); c) tissue secretome, which is a media enriched in proteins that derive from diseased tissue and, therefore, one of the best sources for biomarker discovery.

3.2 Whole tissue

Different techniques were applied to human samples from shotgun proteomics or 2-DE to antibody arrays and MS Imaging. In the case of AS valves tissue proteomics analysis, the main tools employed until now are the 2-DE and the 2D-DIGE. Focus on the aim of maximizing the number of extracted proteins, AS valves must be processed following a "strong" and sequential extraction protocol (Gil-Dones *et al.*, 2010). The first step relies on a strong lysis buffer in which most of the soluble proteins are extracted, and the second was designed to extract the membrane and hydrophobic proteins. It is important to note that one of the most important problems associated with proteomic analyses of AS valves is the high concentration of calcium that interferes with further analyses. For this reason the extracts must be desalting (Gil- Dones *et al.*, 2010). Our group found that approximately 500 spots were well resolved in IPG strip of pH4-7 when compared with the 350 spots evident from the pH 3-10 strip, by 2-DE. Attending to 2D-DIGE, 1346 spots were detected. Significantly, the protein extraction protocol was compatible with both methods. The improvement in sensitivity associated with the 2D-DIGE technology with respect to 2-DE was clearly evident. We conclude that the use of fluorescent labeling and Decyder analysis software considerably increases the number of protein spots that can be detected in the analysis when compared to more traditional methods (Gil-Dones *et al.*, 2010).

In this sense, Matt P et al, 2007 studied aortic aneurysm associated with bicuspid (BAV) and tricuspid aortic valve (TAV) using 2-DE and mass spectrometry (MS). Few proteins showed significant differences, among these a phosphorilated form of HSP27 with significantly lower expression in BAV compared to TAV aortic samples. The phosphoprotein tracing revealed four different phosphoproteins including Rho GDP dissociation inhibitor, calponin 3, myosin regulatory light chain 2 and 4 phosphorilated forms of HSP27. Western blot analyses were made to validate the results obtained by proteomics analysis.

Following the same approach, mitral valves of chronic rheumatic heart disease (RHD) patients were studied by Fae KC et al., 2008, identifying three proteins recognized by heart infiltrating and peripheral T cells as protein disulfide isomerase ER-60 precursor, 78kDa glucose-regulated protein precursor and vimentin. These proteins were recognized in a proliferation assay by peripheral and heart infiltrating T cells from RHD patiens suggesting that they may involved in the autoimmune (Fae *et al.* 2008).

In a different approach, antibody array technology has experienced an important advance in the latest times. Commercially pre-arrayed platforms in diverse research areas are nowadays available, but only one study has been recently reported applying commercial antibody arrays to atherome plaque extracts (Slevin *et al.*, 2006).

3.3 Aortic stenosis sub-proteomes

Within the stenotic aortic valve coexists several cell types, mainly valvular fibroblasts or interstitial cells (VICs), endothelial cells (ECs), macrophages/foam cells and T-lymphocytes. Aortic valve tissue studies constitute a very valuable tool in the search for alterations and

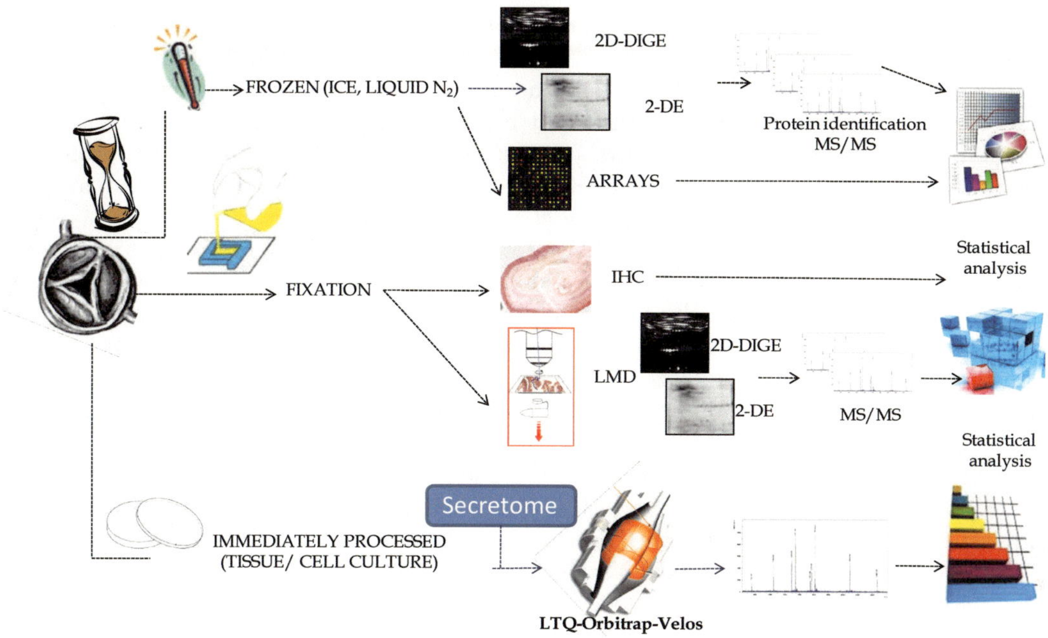

Fig. 4. Schematic diagram illustrating the methodology used for the proteomics analysis of aortic valve tissue.

disease specific biomarkers which would shed light on the understanding of AS and contribute to its early diagnosis. However, sub-fractionation of the aortic valve tissue in its structures or cellular components seems to be a complementary strategy to whole tissue analysis, in order to determine the specific contribution of those cells/structures in the pathogenesis of AS. Concretely, in the field of Proteomics, protein alterations observed in whole tissue samples may benefit from complementary assays involving localization of these proteins in the tissue, such as immunostaining techniques. Although the proteomic analysis of the different sub-fractions from the aortic valve tissue may represent a noteworthy strategy for AS research, this field remains almost unexplored. Strategies involving the combination of aortic valve tissue sub-fractionation and proteomic analysis of these sub-proteomes will be therefore discussed.

3.3.1 Laser microdissection

The different structures from a histology section of a tissue can be isolated by means of microscopical dissection. In this case, manual microdissection may be applied with the use of a microscopical needle under an optical microscope. However, laser microdissection (LMD), first described in 1996 (Emmert-Buck *et al.*, 1996), is a more accurate technique for the isolation of tissue regions, cells or even subcellular fractions. This first method, called laser capture microdissection (LCM), involved irradiation with a laser beam of a thermoplastic membrane in contact with the tissue. Since the heating of the tissue during microdisecction contributes to protein degradation, newly developed laser cutting techniques may be more adequate to implement in a proteomic workflow.

Even though laser microdissection is an outcoming methodology which has been applied in several cardiovascular studies, involving cardiac (De Souza *et al.*, 2004; Chimenti *et al.*, 2004;

Kuhn *et al.*, 2006, 2007; Roy *et al.* 2006; Grube *et al.*, 2006; Pan *et al.*, 2008) and arterial tissue (Stolle *et al.*, 2004; Chimenti *et al.*, 2010; Kwapiszewska *et al.*, 2005; Bagnato *et al.*, 2007; Ciervo *et al.*, 2008; Okami *et al.*, 2009; De la Cuesta *et al.*, 2009, 2011), it has been only used to date for the analysis of valvular tissue in a rat model of pharmacologically-induced valvulopathy (Elangbam *et al.*, 2008). Furthermore, its combination with proteomic methodologies may yield interesting results, in the same way that has been proven in other cardiovascular tissue samples (De Souza *et al.*, 2004; Bagnato *et al.*, 2007; De la Cuesta *et al.*, 2009, 2011). The principal challenge in the combination of LMD with Proteomics, is the scarce amount of protein that can be obtained from laser-microdissected tissue, since no long microdissection periods should be applied in order to avoid protein degradation. Nowadays, mass spectrometers can deal with scarce amounts of sample due to an exponential improvement in their sensitivity, therefore facilitating the analysis by LC-MS/MS of laser-microdissected tissue. On the other hand, the use of fluorescent labels such as the CyDyes from the *DIGE Fluor Labeling Kit for Scarce Samples* (GE Healthcare) allowed analyzing protein extracts from LMD-isolated structures/cells by means of two-dimensional electrophoresis. These dyes label through saturation the cystein residues from the proteins in the mixture and allow running 2-DE gels with less than 5μg of total protein (Sitek *et al.*, 2005). Since protein identification by MS of the spots in such gels is only possible with most abundant spots, these identifications can be performed using pooled samples from LMD or a reference proteome, which may be the one from the whole tissue microdissected (Kondo & Hirohashi, 2007).

The application of LMD to the analysis of the aortic valve tissue could provide specific data from the different layers/structures in the tissue, as well as from the behavior of the different cells in the stenotic milieu. In addition, its combination with a proteomic workflow may constitute a step forward in the understanding of the role played by the different cells involved in AS pathogenesis and in the search for novel tissue biomarkers of this pathology.

3.3.2 Living cells isolation

An alternative methodology to simplify tissue complexity and to study its cellular components is to enzymatically digest the tissue and separate the cells for subsequent analysis. This can be done by cell sorting methodologies or by specific explant culturing. In the first one, specific cell populations can be separated in a flow-cytometer and directly analyzed by proteomic techniques. The main problem in this workflow would be the high amount of tissue necessary to obtain enough cells for a proteomic analysis, which sometimes is impossible to extract, especially when dealing with biopsy material. Culturing sorted cells is an option, but constitutes a more complicated approach than explants culturing, since sorted cells may be damaged in the cytometer, which involves lesser sub-culturing capacity. In contrast, non-sorted cell suspensions should be cultured under specific conditions to favor a certain cell type, which sometimes may imply contamination by other cells. The main drawback of sub-culturing methodologies is that the cells may lose its *in vivo* phenotype within the culture, since the environmental conditions are completely altered in the *in vitro* situation. Nevertheless, cell cultures allow setting very strictly experimental parameters in order to diminish variation between replicates, and analyzing cells responses to different stimuli, which turns them into a very useful tool for proteomic analysis. For such purposes, the methodology called *stable isotope labeling with aminoacids in cell culture* (SILAC) (Ong *et al.*, 2002), constitutes a valuable approach to analyze both proteome and secretome of the different subset of aortic valve cells by means of differential LC-MS/MS.

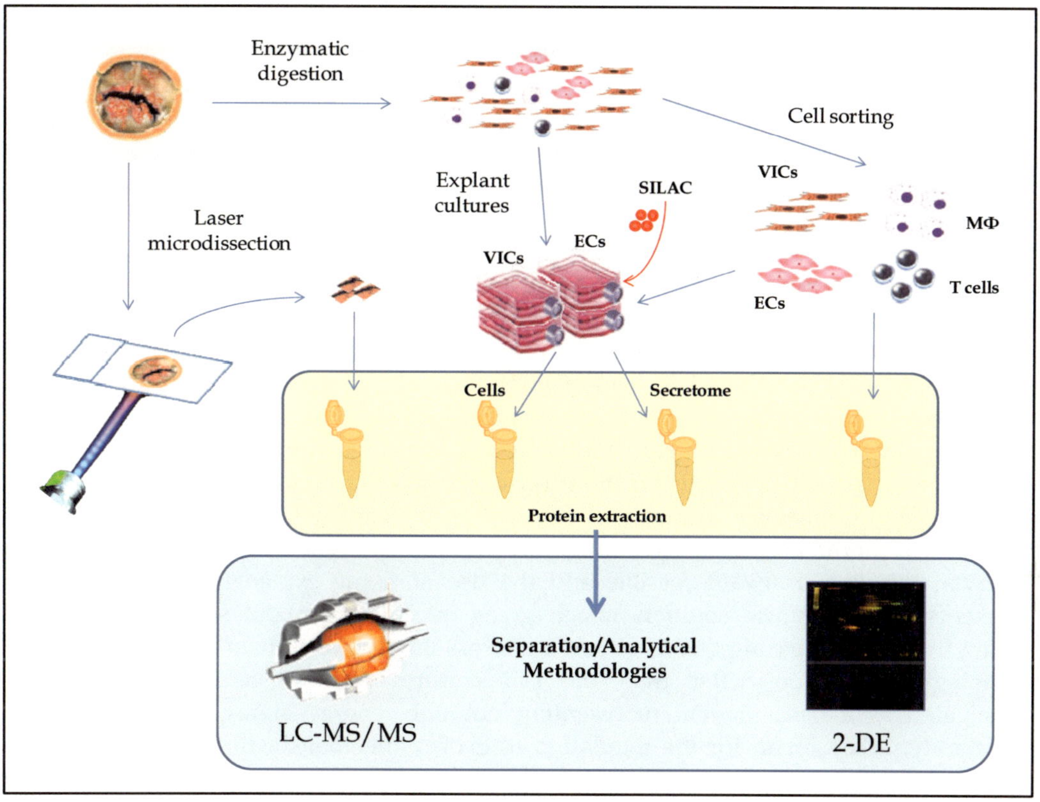

Fig. 5. Scheme of a proteomic workflow for the analysis of AS valve tissue sub-proteomes.

An additional step in the sub-fractionation of the tissue would be to isolate cell structures/organelles. Conventional ultracentrifugation can be applied to separate membranes, nuclei and cytosolic fractions for subsequent proteomic analysis (Huber *et al.* 2003). Using this approach, membrane and cytosolic proteins from Pro-calcific VICs after lipopolysaccharide (LPS) treatment were compared to non-treated ones by 2-DE (Bertacco *et al.*, 2010), in which constitutes the first proteomic study performed with cells isolated from aortic valves. On the other hand, cellular organelles and vesicles, like mithocondrias, Golgi stacks and vesicles or endosomes, are efficiently separated by density gradient centrifugation (Huber *et al.* 2003). Concerning secreted vesicles (microparticles, exosomes…), ultracentrifugation, either under density gradient or not (Van der Pol *et al.*, 2010), constitutes the easiest methodology to set up and to combine with proteomic analysis.
As far as we step forward in sub-fractionating cells proteome, the further the decrease on protein recovery will go. For this reason, while designing the strategy of a proteomic study, we should take into account the balance between the number of sub-fractionation steps and the amount of protein recovered.

3.3.3 Secretome

The term secretome comprises the sub-set of proteins that are actively released by cells or tissue in the extracellular compartment as consequence of the normal metabolism or in response to some stimuli. As such, it is a powerful source of key molecules involved in pathogenesis development, individual response to pharmacological intervention or recovery status. Secretome studies are increasing in the last years as it provides an accurate model of the *in vivo* situation and it represents a sub-proteome of serum/plasma, showing a much narrower proteins concentrations dynamic range which enormously facilitates detection of minor proteins whose identification is otherwise obscured by high-abundance plasma proteins. Plasma, serum and urine are traditional sample sources for biomarker discovery, as they are easily and commonly obtained in clinical practice; however, secretome-based research will favor the detection of novel proteins or, at least, known molecules with new implications in the disease under study. Most studies are focused on the secretome obtained from in vitro cell cultures, assuming that such cells' behavior well simulates the *in vivo* condition *(Roelofsen et al.,* 2009). In particular, the cancer secretome, namely the whole collection of proteins secreted by cancer cells through various secretory pathways, has recently been shown to have significant potential, as secreted proteins might represent putative tumor biomarkers or therapeutic targets (Karagiannis *et al.,* 2010). The most perfect approximation to the real situation is the study of the *in vivo* secretome. In this research line, one of the few proteomics studies was carried out by implanting capillary ultrafiltration probes into tumor masses induced in mice (Alvarez-Llamas *et al.,* 2007; Hocking et al., 2010). However, this is not always feasible and the use of tissue explants (*ex vivo* approach) represents a compromise solution which gives information about secretory molecules coming from all tissue components as result of cross-talk between them and approaches the physiological situation better than the cell culture. Adipose tissue secretome was investigated as a tissue model representing not only energy storage depot but, more importantly, a key organ for the regulation of energy metabolism through secretion of a variety of adipokines involved in the regulation of energy metabolism (Roelofsen *et al.,* 2009; Hocking *et al.,* 2010). Two key points to consider when working directly with tissue in culture are: a) the need to ensure that all detected proteins are truly coming from the tissue and not "contaminants" derived from plasma and b) validation of identified proteins as secreted. A metabolic labelling approach allows differentiation between proteins synthesized by the tissue (labelled) and contaminating proteins from blood which remain unlabelled (Alvarez-Llamas *et al.,* 2007). In this sense, an optimized culture protocol should be developed to maximize label incorporation into proteins including a series of medium changes during the initial hours of culture, followed by an extended step of tissue culture. In any case, label incorporation is influenced by the rate of synthesis of each particular protein, which may condition the number of labelled proteins that can be detected at a particular time point. Incorporation of the label by a protein validates tissue origin but does not necessarily imply "intentional" secretion. Once synthesized by the tissue, the release of a protein into the media could be attributed to damage-induced tissue leakage and results in detection of intracellular proteins. One can assume that it is very challenging to totally avoid the presence of intracellular proteins, as cell lysis always takes place during cell/tissue culture. However, optimum culture conditions may favor secreted proteins enrichment. Classification of identified proteins as secreted ones is usually done by computational methods: classically secreted proteins (via the ER-Golgi pathway) can be predicted as containing a signal peptide by SignalP (Bensten JD, *et al.,* 2004) or being classified as extracellular via Gene Ontology analysis; non-classically secreted proteins, which do not contain N-terminal signal peptide, can be predicted by SecretomeP (Bendsten JD, *et al.,* 2004) and more recently by SecretP (Yu et al., 2010).

The aortic valve secretome is therefore an attractive target to further understand the AS pathogenic process, while revealing mechanisms in common to atherosclerosis. The study of atherosclerotic plaque secretome in the search of potential biomarkers of atherosclerosis has been reported (Duran *et al.*, 2007; Duran *et al.*, 2007), finding that HSP-27 release was decreased in atherosclerotic plaques and barely detectable in complicated plaques supernatants. Further validation and feasible detection in biological fluids should follow prior to the use of discovered proteins as markers of diagnosis or prognosis. In this case, circulating concentrations of HSP27 were found to be decreased in subjects with atherosclerosis compared to healthy subjects, which confirms the hypothesis that plasma content can reflect arterial wall secretion (Martin-Ventura *et al.*, 2004). Effects of atorvastatin treatment on atherosclerotic plaque secretion was also investigated, finding that 66% of the proteins differentially released by atherosclerotic plaques reverted to control values after administration, in particular, cathepsin D which becomes a potential target for therapeutical treatment (Duran *et al.*, 2007). Recent studies carried out in our laboratory point to a sub-set of proteins which are differentially released by healthy arteries in comparison to atherosclerotic coronary ones [submitted for publication] and whose role in AS development is currently ongoing. In Figure 4 a proposal for AS secretome obtention and proteomic analysis is shown.

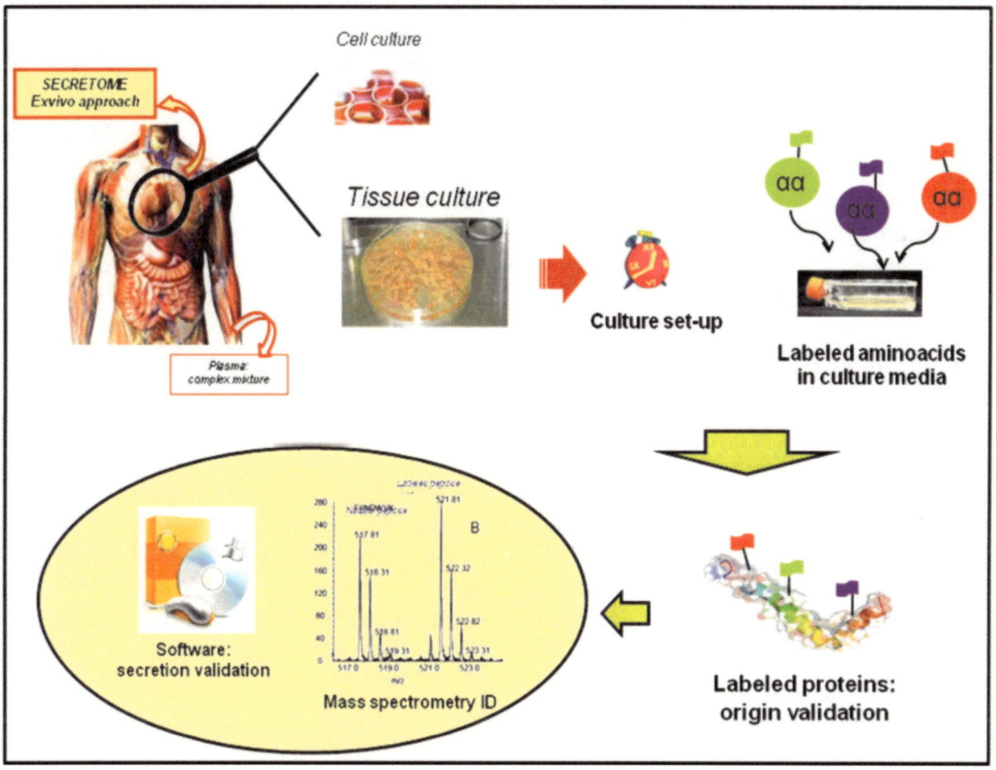

Fig. 6. Secretome from tissue explants is an ex-vivo approach with enormous potential as biomarkers source. It is key to validate proteins origin by i.e. label inclusion at protein level and secretion patterns by available softwares.

4. Conclusions

Recently, cardiovascular proteomics has experienced an impressive development. At present, hundreds of proteins have been associated with cardiovascular diseases using proteomic approaches and different kinds of biological samples. The proteomic approaches allow to explore the expression of multiple proteins at once, giving us the opportunity to know which proteins are involved in pathophysiologic process of degenerative aortic stenosis in order to unveil the basic mechanisms of this disease. Most probably, these novel approaches will facilitate the study of this pathology and disclose diagnostic markers and multiple potential targets for the design of more powerful and personalized therapies.

5. Acknowledgment

We thank the grants from the Instituto de Salud Carlos III (FIS PI070537), Fondo de Investigación Sanitaria de Castilla la Mancha (FISCAM, PI2008/08), Fondo de Investigación Sanitaria de Castilla la Mancha (FISCAM PI2008/28) and Redes Temáticas de Investigación Cooperativa, FONDOS FEDER (RD06/0014/1015).

6. References

Adkins J.N., Varnum, S. M., Auberry, K. J., Moore, R. J., Angell, N. H., Smith, R. D., Springer, D. L. & Pounds, J. G. (2002) Toward a Human Blood Serum Proteome: ANALYSIS BY MULTIDIMENSIONAL SEPARATION COUPLED WITH MASS SPECTROMETRY. *Mol. Cell. Proteomics*, Vol. 1, pp. 947–955.

Agmon Y, Khandheria BK, Meissner I, Sicks JR, O'Fallon WM, Wiebers DO, Whisnant JP, Seward JB, Tajik AJ.2001. Aortic valve sclerosis and aortic atherosclerosis: different manifestations of the same disease? Insights from a population-based study. *J Am Coll Cardiol,*Vol. 38, pp. 827-34.

Alvarez-Llamas G, Szalowska E, de Vries MP, Weening D, Landman K, Hoek A, Wolffenbuttel BH, Roelofsen H, Vonk RJ. Characterization of the human visceral adipose tissue secretome. *Mol Cell Proteomics*, 6:589-600

Anderson NL & Anderson NG. (2002) The Human Plasma Proteome: History, Character, and Diagnostic Prospects. *Molecular & Cellular Proteomics.* Vol. 1, No. 11, pp. 845-867.

Anderson NL. (2005) Candidate-based proteomics in the search for biomarkers of cardiovascular disease. *J Physiol.* Vol. 563, pp. 23-60.

Bagnato C., Thumar J., Mayya V., Hwang S.I., Zebroski H., Claffey K.P., Haudenschild C., Eng J.K., Lundgren D.H. & Han D.K. Proteomics analysis of human coronary atherosclerotic plaque: a feasibility study of direct tissue proteomics by liquid chromatography and tandem mass spectrometry. *Mol Cell Proteomics.* Vol.6, No. 6, (June 2007), pp. 1088-102.

Bendtsen JD, Nielsen H, von Heijne G, Brunak S. (2004) Improved prediction of signal peptides: SignalP 3.0. *J. Mol. Biol,* Vol. 340, pp. 783-795.

Bendtsen JD, Jensen LJ, Blom N, von Heijne G, Brunak S. (2004) Feature based prediction of non-classical and leaderless protein secretion. *Protein Eng. Des. Sel.* Vol. 17, pp. 349-356.

Bertacco E., Millioni R., Arrigoni G., Faggin E., Iop L., Puato M., Pinna L.A., Tessari P., Pauletto P., Rattazzi M. (2010) Proteomic analysis of clonal interstitial aortic valve cells acquiring a pro-calcific profile. *J Proteome Res*. Vol. 9, No. 11, (November 2010), pp. 5913-21.

Bjorhall K Miliotis T & Davidsson P. (2005) Interest of major serum protein removal for Surface-Enhanced Laser Desorption/Ionization - Time Of Flight (SELDI-TOF) proteomic blood profiling. *Proteomics*, Vol. 5, pp. 307-317.

Chan KL, Teo K, Dumesnil JG, Ni A, Tam J. (2010) Effect of Lipid lowering with rosuvastatin on progression of aortic stenosis: results of the aortic stenosis progression observation: measuring effects of rosuvastatin (ASTRONOMER) trial. *Circulation*, Vol. 121, pp. 306-14.

Chen E.I., Hewel J., Felding-Habermann B. & Yates J.R. III. (2006) Large Scale Protein Profiling by Combination of Protein Fractionation and Multidimensional Protein Identification Technology (MudPIT)*. *Molecular & Cellular Proteomics*, Vol. 5, pp. 53–5.

Chimenti C., Sale P., Verardo R., Cicalini S., Petrosillo N., Russo M.A., Fedele F. & Frustaci A. (2010) High prevalence of intramural coronary infection in patients with drug-resistant cardiac syndrome X: comparison with chronic stable angina and normal controls. *Heart*. Vol. 96, No. 23, (December 2010), pp. 1926-31.

Chimenti C., Russo A., Pieroni M., Calabrese F., Verardo R., Thiene G., Russo M.A., Maseri A. & Frustaci A. Intramyocyte detection of Epstein-Barr virus genome by laser capture microdissection in patients with inflammatory cardiomyopathy. *Circulation*. Vol. 110, No. 23, (December 2004), pp. 3534-9.

Ciervo A., Mancini F., Sale P., Russo A. & Cassone A. (2008) Real-time polymerase chain reaction and laser capture microdissection: an efficient combination tool for Chlamydophila pneumoniae DNA quantification and localization of infection in atherosclerotic lesions. *Int J Immunopathol Pharmacol*. 2008 Vol. 21, No. 2, (June 2005), pp. 421-8.

Cowell SJ, Newby DE, Prescott RJ, Bloomfield P, Reid J, Northridge DB, Boon. A. 2005. A randomized trial of intensive lipid-lowering therapy in calcific aortic stenosis. N *Engl J Med*. Vol. 352, pp. 2389-97.

Dardé V.M., de la Cuesta F., Dones F.G., Alvarez-Llamas G., Barderas M.G. & Vivanco F. (2010). Analysis of the plasma proteome associated with acute coronary syndrome: does a permanent protein signature exist in the plasma of ACS patients? *J Proteome Res*. Vol. 9, No. 9, (September 2010), pp. 4420-32.

De la Cuesta F., Alvarez-Llamas G., Maroto A.S., Donado A., Juarez-Tosina R., Rodriguez-Padial L., Pinto A.G., Barderas M.G.& Vivanco F. (2009) An optimum method designed for 2-D DIGE analysis of human arterial intima and media layers isolated by laser microdissection. *Proteomics Clin Appl*. Vol. 3, No. 10, (October 2009), pp. 1174-84.

De la Cuesta F, Alvarez-Llamas G, Maroto A.S., Donado A, Zubiri I, Posada M, Padial L.R., Pinto A.G., Barderas M.G. & Vivanco F. (2011) A proteomic focus on the molecular mechanisms occurring at the atherosclerotic coronary intima. *Mol Cell Proteomics*. Vol. 10, No. 4, (April 2011), pp. M110.003517.

De Souza AI., McGregor E., Dunn MJ. & Rose ML. (2004) Preparation of human heart for laser microdissection and proteomics. *Proteomics*. Vol. 4, No. 3, (March 2004), pp. 578-86.

Durán M.C., Martín-Ventura J.L., Mas S., Barderas M.G., Dardé V.M., Jensen O.N., Egido J. & Vivanco F. (2007) Characterization of the human atheroma plaque secretome by proteomic analysis. *Methods Mol Biol*, 357:141-50.

Durán M.C., Boeri-Erba E., Mohammed S., Martín-Ventura J.L., Egido J., Vivanco F., Jensen O.N. (2007) Characterization of HSP27 phosphorylation sites in human atherosclerotic plaque secretome. *Methods Mol Biol*, 357:151-63.

Durán M.C., Martín-Ventura J.L., Mohammed S., Barderas M.G., Blanco-Colio L.M., Mas S., Moral V., Ortega L., Tuñón J., Jensen O.N., Vivanco F. & Egido J. (2007) Atorvastatin modulates the profile of proteins released by human atherosclerotic plaques. *Eur J Pharmacol*, Vol. 562, No. 1-2, (May 2007), pp. 119-29.

Elangbam C.S., Job L.E., Zadrozny L.M., Barton J.C., Yoon L.W., Gates L.D. & Slocum N. 5-hydroxytryptamine (5HT)-induced valvulopathy: compositional valvular alterations are associated with 5HT2B receptor and 5HT transporter transcript changes in Sprague-Dawley rats. *Exp Toxicol Pathol*. Vol. 60, No. 4-5, (Aug 2008), pp. 253-62.

Emmert-Buck M.R., Bonner R.F., Smith P.D., Chuaqui R.F., Zhuang Z., Goldstein S.R., Weiss R.A. & Liotta L.A. (1996) Laser capture microdissection. *Science*. Vol. 274, No. 5289, (November 1996) pp. 998-1001.

Espina V, Mueller C, Edmiston K, Sciro M, Petricoin EF, Liotta LA. (2009). Tissue i salive: New technologies are needed to addresss the problems of protein biomarker pre-analytical variability. *Proteomics Clin Appl.*, August 1; 3(8), pp. 874-882.

Espina V, Edmiston KH, Heiby M, Pierobon M, Sciro M, Merritt B, Banks S, Deng J, VanMeter AJ, Geho DH, Pastore L, Sennesh J, Petricoin EF 3rd, Liotta LA. 2008. A portrait of tissue phosphoprotein stability in the clinical tissue procurement process. *Mol Cell Proteomics*, 7, pp. 1998-2018.

Freeman, RV, Otto, CM. (2005) Spectrum of calcific aortic valve disease: pathogenesis, disease progression, and treatment strategies. *Circulation*, 111:3316.

Fae KC, da Silva DD, Bilate AMB, Tanaka AC, Pomerantzeff PMA, Kiss MH, Silva CAA, Cunha.Neto E, Kalil J, Guilherme L. 2008. PDIA3, HSPA5, vimentin, proteins identified by 2DE in the valvular tissue, are target antigens of peripheral and heart infiltrating T cells from chronic rheumatic heart disease patients. *Journal of Anutoimmunity*, pp. 136-141

Ferrrari G. 2010. Validation of plasma biomarkers in degenerative Calcified Aortic Stenosis. *J Surgical Res*, 163, pp. 12-17.

Gil-Dones F, Martin-Rojas T, Lopez-Almodovar LF, Juarez-Tosina R, de la Cuesta F, Alvarez-Lamas G, Alonso Orgaz S, Vivanco F, Padila LR, Barderas MG. 2010. Development of an Optimal Protocol for the Proteomic Analysis of Stenotic and Healthy Aortic Valves. *Rev Esp Cardiol*, 63(1),pp. 46-53

Gil-Dones F, Martin-Rojas T, Lopez-Almodovar LF, de la Cuesta F, Darde VM, Alvarez-Llamas G, Juarez-Tosina R, Barroso G, Vivanco F, Padila LR, Barderas MG. 2010. Valvular Aortic Stenosis: A proteomic insight. *Clinical Medicine Insights: cardiology*, 4; pp. 1-7

Granger J., Siddiqui J., Copeland S. & Remick D. (2005) Albumin depletion of human plasma also removes low abundance proteins including the cytokines. *Proteomics*. Vol. 5, pp. 4713-4718.

Graumann J., Hubner N.C., Kim J.B., Ko K., Moser M., Kumar C., Cox J., Scholer H. and Mann M. (2008) Stable Isotope Labeling by Amino Acids in Cell Culture (SILAC) and Proteome Quantitation of Mouse Embryonic Stem Cells to a Depth of 5,111 Proteins. *Mol Cell Proteomics*. Vol. 7, No. 4, pp. 672-83.

Grube M., Meyer zu Schwabedissen H.E., Präger D., Haney J., Möritz K.U., Meissner K., Rosskopf D., Eckel L., Böhm M., Jedlitschky G. & Kroemer H.K (2006). Uptake of cardiovascular drugs into the human heart: expression, regulation, and function of the carnitine transporter OCTN2 (SLC22A5). *Circulation*. 2006 Vol. 113, No. 8, (February 2006):1114-22.

Hocking SL, Wu LE, Guilhaus M, Chisholm DJ, James DE. 2010. Intrinsic depot-specific differences in the secretome of adipose tissue, preadipocytes, and adipose tissue-derived microvascular endothelial cells. *Diabetes*.,59:3008-16.

Huber L.A., Pfaller K. & Vietor I. (2003) Organelle Proteomics: Implications for Subcellular Fractionation in Proteomics. *Circ. Res*. Vol. 92, (May 2003), pp. 962-968.

Hunt PJ, et al. 1997. Immunoreactive aminoterminal pro-brain natriuretic peptide (NT-PROBNP): a new marker of cardiac impairment. *Clin Endocrinol (Oxforfd9,* 47, 287–296.

Iung B, Baron G, Butchart EG, Delahaye F, Gohlke-B?rwolf C, Levang OW, Tornos P, Vanoverschelde JL, Vermeer F, Boersma E, Ravaud P, Vahanian A . 2003. A prospective survey of patients with valvular heart disease in Europe: The Euro Heart Survey on Valvular Heart Disease. *Eur Heart J*, 24, pp. 1231-43.

Karagiannis GS, Pavlou MP, Diamandis EP. 2010. Cancer secretomics reveal pathophysiological pathways in cancer molecular oncology. *Mol Oncol*. 4, pp. 496-510.

Kondo T & Hirohashi S. (2007) Application of highly sensitive fluorescent dyes (CyDye DIGE Fluor saturation dyes) to laser microdissection and two-dimensional difference gel electrophoresis (2D-DIGE) for cancer proteomics. *Nat Protoc*. Vol. 1, No. 6, (February 2007), pp. 2940-56.

Kuhn D.E., Roy S., Radtke J., Gupta S & Sen C.K (2006). Laser microdissection and pressure-catapulting technique to study gene expression in the reoxygenated myocardium. *Am J Physiol Heart Circ Physiol*. 2006 Vol. 290, No. 6, (June 2006), pp. H2625-32.

Kuhn D.E, Roy S., Radtke J., Khanna S. & Sen C.K (2007). Laser microdissection and capture of pure cardiomyocytes and fibroblasts from infarcted heart regions: perceived hyperoxia induces p21 in peri-infarct myocytes. *Am J Physiol Heart Circ Physiol*. Vol. 292, No. 3, (March 2007), pp. H1245-53.

Kwapiszewska G., Wilhelm J., Wolff S., Laumanns I., Koenig I.R., Ziegler A., Seeger W., Bohle R.M., Weissmann N. & Fink L. (2005) Expression profiling of laser-microdissected intrapulmonary arteries in hypoxia-induced pulmonary hypertension. *Respir Res*. Vol. 19, No. 6, (September 2005), pp. 109.

MacCoss M.J., McDonald W.H., Saraf A., Sadygov R., Clark J.M., Tasto J.J., Gould K.L., Wolters D., Washburn M., Weiss A., Clark J.I. & Yates J.R. III. 2002. Shotgun identification of protein modifications from protein complexes and lens tissue. *PNAS* , 99, 12, 7900-7905

Martin-Ventura JL, Duran MC, Blanco-Colio LM, Meilhac O, Leclercq A, Michel JB, Jensen ON, Hernandez-Merida S, Tuñón J, Vivanco F, Egido J. 2004. Identification by a differential proteomic approach of heat shock protein 27 as a potential marker of atherosclerosis. *Circulation*, 110, pp. 2216-2219.

Matt P, Fu Z, Carrel T, Huso DL, Dirnhofer S, Lefkovits I, Zerkowski HR, Van Eyk JE. Proteomic alterations in heat shock protein 27 and identification of phosphoproteins in ascending aortic aneurys associated with bicuspid and tricuspid aortic valve. *Journal of Molecular and Cellular Cardiology*. 43, pp. 792-801.

Mohler ER 3rd, Gannon F, Reynolds C, Zimmerman R, Keane MG, Kaplan FS. 2001. Bone formation and inflammation in cardiac valves. Circulation, 103, pp. 1522-8.

Moura LM, Ramos SF, Zamorano JL, Barros IM, Azevedo LF, Rocha-Gon?alves F, Rajamannan NM 2007. Rosuvastatin affecting aortic valve endothelium to slow the progression of aortic stenosis. *J Am Coll Cardiol*, 49:554-61.

O'Brien KD, Shavelle DM, Caulfield MT, McDonald TO, Olin-Lewis K, Otto CM, Probstfield JL. . Association of angiotensin- converting enzyme with low-density lipoprotein in aortic valvular lesions and in human plasma. *Circulation*. 106, pp. 2224–2230.

Okami N., Kawamata T., Yamamoto G., Okada Y., Hori T. & Tachikawa T. Laser microdissection-based analysis of hypoxia- and thioredoxin-related genes in human stable carotid plaques. *Cardiovasc Pathol*. 2009 Vol. 18, No. 5, (October 2009), pp. 294-300.

Ong S.E., Blagoev B., Kratchmarova I., Kristensen D.B., Steen H., Pandey A. & Mann M. (2002) Stable isotope labeling by amino acids in cell culture, SILAC, as a simple and accurate approach to expression proteomics. *Mol Cell Proteomics*. Vol. 1, No. 5, (May 2002), pp. 376-86.

Pan P., Guo Y. & Gu J. (2008) Expression of cystic fibrosis transmembrane conductance regulator in ganglion cells of the hearts. *Neurosci Lett*. Vol. 441, No. 1. (August 2008), pp. 35-8.

Petricoin EF 3rd, Bichsel VE, Calvert VS, Espina V, Winters M, Young L, Belluco C, Trock BJ, Lippman M, Fishman DA, Sgroi DC, Munson PJ, Esserman LJ,Liotta LA2005. Mapping molecular networks using proteomics: a visión for patient-tailored combination therapy. *J. Clin. Oncol*, 23 pp. 3614-3621.

Prasad N, Bridges AB, Lang CC, Clarkson PB, MacLeod C, Pringle TH, Struthers AD, MacDonald TM1. 997. Brain natriuretic peptide concentrations in patients with aortic stenosis. *Am Heart J*, 133,pp. 477–479.

Qi W, Mathisen P, Kjekshus J, Simonsen S, Bjørnerheim R, Endresen K, Hall C. Natriuretic peptides in patients with aortic stenosis. *Am Heart J*, 142, pp. 725–732.

Rajamannan N, Otto CM. 2004. Targeted Therapy to Prevent Progression of Calcific Aortic Stenosis. *Circulation*. 110; pp. 1180-1182 .

Righetti, P. G., Boschetti, E., Lomas, L. and Citterio, A. 2006. Protein equalizer technology: the quest for a "democratic proteome". *Proteomics*. Vol. 6, No. 14, pp. 3980–3992.

Roelofsen H, Dijkstra M, Weening D, de Vries MP, Hoek A, Vonk RJ. 2009. Comparison of isotope-labeled amino acid incorporation rates (CILAIR) provides a quantitative method to study tissue secretomes. *Mol Cell Proteomics*,8:316-24.

Rosseb AB, Pedersen TR, Boman K, Brudi P, Chambers JB, Egstrup K, Gerdts E, Gohlke-Brwolf C, Holme I, Kesniemi YA, Malbecq W, Nienaber CA, Ray S, Skjaerpe T,

Wachtell K, Willenheimer R, SEAS Investigators. 2008. Intensive lipid lowering with simvastatin and ezetimibe in aortic stenosis. N Engl *J Med,* 359, pp. 1343-56.

Roy S., Khanna S., Kuhn D.E., Rink C., Williams W.T., Zweier J.L. & Sen C.K (2006). Transcriptome analysis of the ischemia-reperfused remodeling myocardium: temporal changes in inflammation and extracellular matrix. *Physiol Genomics.* Vo. 25, No. 3, (May 2006), pp 364-74.

Schrader, M. & Schulz-Knappe, P. (2001) Peptidomics technologies for human body fluids. *Trends Biotechnol,* 19, S55–60.

Schulte, I., Tammen, H., Selle, H., Schulz-Knappe, P. Peptides in body fluids and tissues as markers of disease. *Expert Rev. Mol. Diagn.,* 5, 145 - 157.

Seam, N., Gonzales, D.A., Kern, S.J., Hortin, G.L., Hoehn, G.T., and Suffredini, A.F. (2007) Quality Control of Serum Albumin Depletion for Proteomic Analysis. *Clinical Chemistry.* Vol. 53, No. 11, pp. 1915–1920.

Sihlbom, C., Kanmert, I., von Bahr, H. and Davidsson, P.. 2008. Evaluation of the combination of bead technology with SELDI-TOF-MS and 2-D DIGE for detection of plasma proteins. *Journal of Proteome Research,* 7, 9, 4191– 4198.

Sitek B., Luttges J., Marcus K., Kloppel G.; Schmiegel W., Meyer H.E., Hahn S.A. & Stuhler K. (2005) Application of fluorescence difference gel electrophoresis saturation labelling for the analysis of microdissected precursor lesions of pancreatic ductal adenocarcinoma. *Proteomics.* Vol. 5, No. 10, (July 2005), pp. 2665-2679.

Slevin M, Elasbali AB, Miguel Turu M, Krupinski J, Badimon L, Gaffney J.2006. Identification of differential protein expression associated with development of unstable human carotid plaques. *Am J Pathol,* 168 (3), pp. 1004-1021

Stewart BF, Siscovick D, Lind BK, Gardin JM, Gottdiener JS, Smith VE, Kitzman DW, Otto CM. 1997. Clinical factors associated with calcific aortic valve disease. Cardiovascular Health Study. *J Am Coll Cardiol,* 29, pp. 630-4.

Stolle K., Weitkamp B., Rauterberg J., Lorkowski S. & Cullen P. (2004) Laser microdissection-based analysis of mRNA expression in human coronary arteries with intimal thickening. *J Histochem Cytochem.* Vol. 52, No. 11, (November 2004), pp. 1511-8.

Talwar S, et al. 2001. Plasma N-terminal pro BNP and cardiotrophin-1 are elevated in aortic stenosis. *Eur J Heart Fail,* 3, 15–19.

Tannu NS & Hemby SE. 2006. Two-dimensional fluorescence difference gel electrophoresis for comparative proteomics profiling. *Nat Protocols;* 1(4): 1732-1742.

Tian R., Zhang H., Ye M., Jiang X., Hu L., Li X., Bao X. and Zou H. (2007) Selective Extraction of Peptides from Human Plasma by Highly Ordered Mesoporous Silica Particles for Peptidome Analysis. Angew. *Chem. Int. Ed,* 2007, 46, 962 - 965.

Tirumalai R. S., Chan K. C., Prieto D. A., Issaq H. J., Conrads T.P. and Veenstra T.D. (2003) Characterization of the Low Molecular Weight Human Serum Proteome. *Mol Cell Proteomics,* 2, 1096 - 1103

Tsutamoto T, Wada A, Maeda K, Hisanaga T, Maeda Y, Fukai D, Ohnishi M, Sugimoto Y, Kinoshita M. 1997. Attenuation of compensation of endogenous cardiac natriuretic peptide system in chronic heart failure: prognostic role of plasma brain natriuretic peptide concentration in patients with chronic symptomatic left ventricular dysfunction. *Circulation,* 96, pp. 509–516.

Van der Pol E., Hoekstra A.G., Sturk A., Otto C., van Leeuwen T.G. & Nieuwland R. (2010) Optical and non-optical methods for detection and characterization of microparticles and exosomes. *J Thromb Haemost.* Vol. 8, No.12, (December 2010), pp. 2596-607.

Veenstra T.D., Conrads, T.P., Hood, B.L., Avellino, A.M., Ellenbogen, R.G. (2005) Biomarkers: Mining the Biofluid Proteome. *Molecular & Cellular Proteomics,* Vol. 4, No. 4, pp. 409-418.

Vivanco F, Mas S, Darde VM, De la Cuesta F, Alvarez-Llamas G, Barderas MG. 2007. Vascular proteomics. *Proteomics Clin. Appl, 1,* 1102–1122.

Vivanco F., De la Cuesta F., Barderas M.G., Zubiri I. & Alvarez-Llamas G. (2011) Principles, analysis and applications. In: Widley. Interscience Series On Mass Spectrometry. Edited by: Garcia A & Senis Y. Hardcover

Walter S. Speidl WS, Cimmino G, Ibañez B, Elmariah S, Hutter R, Garcia MJ, Fuster V, Goldman ME, Badimon JJ . 2010. Recombinant apolipoprotein A-I Milano rapidly reverses aortic valve stenosis and decreases leaflet inflammation in an experimental rabbit model. *Eur Heart J,* 31:2049-2057.

Wang, Y.Y., Cheng, P., & Chan, D.W. (2003) A simple affinity spin tube filter method for removing high-abundant common proteins or enriching low-abundant biomarkers for serum proteomic analysis. *Proteomics.* Vol. 3, No. 3, pp. 243–248.

Wu W.W., Wang G., Baek S.J. & Shen R.F. 2006. Comparative Study of Three Proteomic Quantitative Methods, DIGE, cICAT, and iTRAQ, Using 2D Gel- or LC-MALDI TOF/TOF. *Journal of Proteome Research,* 5, 651-658.

Yandle TG, et al. 1986. Radioimmunoassay and characterization of atrial natriuretic peptide in human plasma. *J Clin Endocrinol Meta.,* 63, 72–79.

Yandle TG, Richards AM, Gilbert A, Fisher S, Holmes S, Espiner EA. 1993. Assay of brain natriuretic peptide (BNP) in human plasma: evidence for high molecular weight BNP as a major plasma component in heart failure. *J Clin Endocrinol Metab,* 76, pp. 832–838.

Yetkin E, Walteriberger J. 2009. Molecular and cellular mechanism of aortic stenosis. *Int. J. Cardiology.* Doi:10.1016/j.ijcard.03.108.

Yocum A.K., Yu K., Oe T., Blair A. (2005) Effect of Immunoaffinity Depletion of Human Serum during Proteomic Investigations. *J Proteome Res.* Vol. 4, pp. 1722-1731.

Yu L, Guo Y, Zhang Z, Li Y, Li M, Li G, Xiong W, Zeng Y. SecretP: a new method for predicting mammalian secreted proteins. *Peptides,* 31(4):574-8.

Zhou H, Xu S, Ye M, Feng S, Pan C, Jiang X, Li X, Han G, Fu Y, Zou H. Zhou, H. J., Xu, S. Y., Ye, M. L., Feng, S., Pan, C., Jiang X. G., Li X., Han G. H., Fu Y., & Zou H. (2006) Zirconium phosphonate-modified porous silicon for highly specific capture of phosphopeptides and MALDI-TOF MS analysis. *J. Proteome Res,* 5, 2431–2437.

Zolotarjova N., Martosella J., Nicol G., Bailey J., Boyes B. E., and Barrett W. C. 2005. Differences among techniques for highabundant protein depletion. *Proteomics,* 5, 13, 3304–3313.

12

The Inflammatory Infiltrate in Calcific Aortic Stenosis is Characterized by Clonal Expansions of T Cells and is Associated with Elevated Proportions of Circulating Activated and Effector Memory CD8 T Cells

Robert Winchester and Susheel Kodali
Columbia University, College of Physicians and Surgeons
USA

1. Introduction

For some time, calcific aortic stenosis (CAS) had been considered as a "senile" or "degenerative" response to chronic hemodynamic stress and "wear and tear" on the valve (Pomerance 1972). The concept of inflammation in CAS was etched by Olssen and Otto and their colleagues who were among the first to clearly demonstrate a variable, but often quite appreciable T lymphocyte infiltration in this disease (Olsson, Dalsgaard, et al. 1994, Otto et al. 1994). Further work showed that most T cells infiltrating the valve are concentrated in regions of calcification or arrayed around newly appearing blood vessels that express VEGF, VEGF receptors, ICAM-1 and VCAM-1 (Mazzone et al. 2004, Soini et al. 2003, Wallby et al. 2002). The T cells within the valve tissue exhibit evidence of activation, including expression of CD25 and HLA-DR, while cells in the surrounding valvular mesenchymal tissues also strongly express HLA-DR, consistent with the release of inflammatory mediators such as interferon-γ from activated lymphocytes (Olsson, Dalsgaard, et al. 1994, Olsson, Rosenqvist, et al. 1994). The modified valve mesenchymal cells also express genes characteristic of osteoblasts suggesting that calcification results from an active, regulated osteogenic process (Mazzone et al. 2004, Rajamannan et al. 2003). Since CAS is more prevalent in anatomically variant bileaflet aortic valves and occurs at younger ages in this population, the finding of similar T lymphocyte infiltration in biscupid valves further emphasized the importance of this inflammation in the pathogenesis of CAS (Wallby et al. 2002). However questions regarding the immunologic nature of the T cell infiltrate in the valve, its significance and whether it is part of a broader systemic immune response remain unanswered.

Two principal immune scenarios could account for the conspicuous presence of T cells within CAS valve lesions. One possibility is that the infiltrating T cells consist of large numbers of unexpanded but clonally different lymphocytes that are recruited as a secondary consequence of attractive chemokines released by events such as valvular injury, atherosclerosis or non-antigen specific innate immune system activation of macrophages. This polyclonal T cell infiltration would be analogous to that found in stable atherosclerotic plaques (Li et al. 2005, Oksenberg et al. 1997, Stemme et al. 1991, Swanson et al. 1994). A second possibility is that the infiltrating T cells are made up by small numbers of highly expanded T cell clones. This would favor the interpretation that some features of an adaptive immune response occur within the valve characterized by selective expansion of certain clones possibly driven by a newly expressed antigen on the valve. This subsequently has the potential for enhanced T cell activation and mediator release associated with clonal expansion resulting in further valve injury.

These two primary scenarios can readily be distinguished by TCR repertoire analysis, which can delineate the clonal composition of the T cell infiltrate in the valve leaflet through structural features of the clonally specific β-chain T cell TCR. This would help determine whether the inflammatory infiltrate in the valve leaflet was primarily polyclonal, suggesting it was a secondary response to injury, or whether the infiltrate contained expanded T cell clones that would imply features of an adaptive immune response occurring within the valve leaflets (Wu et al. 2007).

1.1 T cell repertoire analysis background

T cells of either CD8 or CD4 lineage sets are distinguished by different clonally specific T cell receptors (TCRs) that define the T cell's clonotype and determine the clone's specific recognition of the peptide (p)-major histocompatibility complex (MHC). This recognition is the heart of the adaptive immune response. Ligation of a clonal TCR by the appropriate p-MHC complex initiates clonal proliferation of the T cells along with production of cytokines such as γ-interferon. The proliferating clonal progeny all share the same TCR clonotype.

The TCR consists of two chains, designated α and β. Each chain contains a variable and a constant region. In the case of the TCR β-chain, the variable region is composed of three recombined gene elements, the variable (V), diversity (D), and junctional (J) gene segments. The combination of these three segments form a hypervariable region, designated CDR3 that exhibits a clonotypically unique sequence of nucleotides. The amino acids encoded by these nucleotides are responsible for the specificity of the clone's TCR for a particular p-MHC complex.

The clonal proliferation that results from triggering the clone's TCR by this particular p-MHC increases the proportional representation of the responding T cell clones found in that site. The proportional representation of different clones in a T cell repertoire is determined by analysis of the nucleotide structure of the TCR β-chain using PCR analysis. This can be done by sequencing the PCR product and placing identical sequences into groups. The size of each group reflects the extent of clonal expansion and predominance as measured by the frequency distribution of the TCR β-chains from each clone, figure 1. For technical details of this methodology, see (Wu et al. 2007). Since the molecular events underlying the recombination of V, D, and J segments involve exonuclease nibbling from the ends of the joining segments, as well as the incorporation of additional non-germline nucleotides, the overall length of the β-chain is usually randomly altered by some dozens of nucleotides. The distribution of the β-chain lengths, plotted as a histogram, is a technically simpler characterization of the repertoire than detailed sequencing and provides a lower resolution sketch of the composition of an inflammatory repertoire or a given T cell population, figure 1. In this type of length-distribution analysis, sometimes called "spectratyping", a polyclonal repertoire without major clonal expansions exhibits a Gaussian-type of β-chain length distribution, while a repertoire containing a clonal expansion is characterized by a large peak at a particular β-chain length. The form of the plot can be either a histogram constructed in a spread-sheet program from the experimental results or a direct tracing of the distribution of the fluorescently-labeled PCR product from the machine performing the gel electrophoresis.

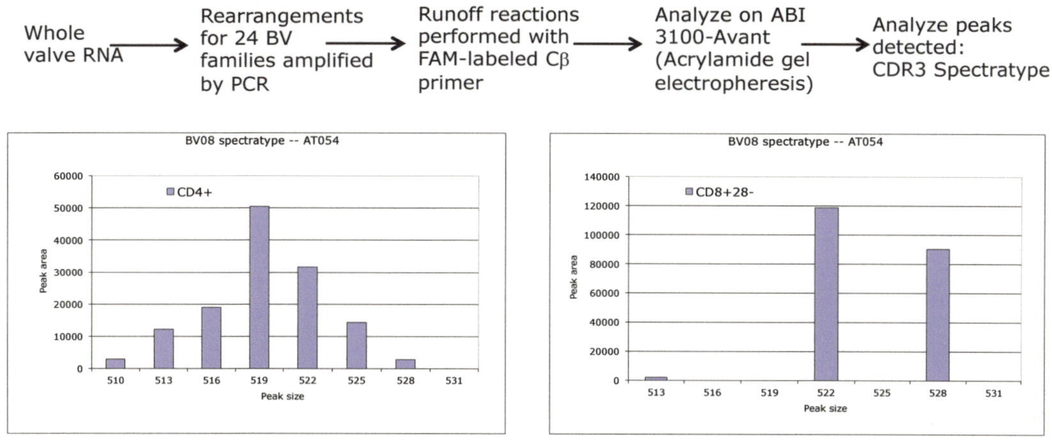

The spectratype peak distribution reflects the CDR3 length of the T cell receptor β chains:

-- may be *polyclonal* (normally distributed)
-- may be *oligoclonal* (several peaks, size is not normally distributed): antigen skew is suggested
-- may be *monoclonal* (single peak): strong antigen selection is suggested
-- no product amplified for that BV family

Fig. 1. An outline of the methods used to analyze the clonality of a T cell population.

The spectratype approach demonstrates the polyclonal characteristics of a CD4 T cell population in peripheral blood, left frame. This distribution of β-chain lengths would be similar to that given by the entrance of T cells into tissue that is a secondary consequence of chemokines released by non-specific inflammation. The right frame illustrates a highly oligoclonal pattern exhibited by the memory-effector T cell subset ($CD8^+CD28^-$) in blood. This antigen-driven pattern is composed of two major clones found at 522 and 528 nucleotides. Often the nucleotide size is converted to the length in amino acids of the hypervariable region of the CDR3 between two benchmarks in the V and J segments. The V segment gene elements are grouped into 24 BV families and typically a panel of 24 primers, each specific for a BV family, is used to assess repertoire complexity. Figure 1 shows the BV8 family distribution of β-chain lengths.

2. The inflammatory infiltrate in bicuspid and tricuspid valve calcific aortic stenosis is characterized by clonal expansions of T cells

These methods of repertoire analysis can be used to characterize the inflammatory infiltrate in the aortic valve. The TCR β-chain CDR3 length distribution in valves removed at surgery was found to be highly restricted, with skewed length spectra indicating the presence of a considerable number of oligoclonal expansions, (Wu et al. 2007) as illustrated below in Figure 2. Despite considerable heterogeneity, the majority of the infiltrating T cells in most valves and in most BV families consist of oligoclonal expansions, as shown by patterns containing one, two, or three peaks similar to those illustrated. The mean Hamming distance (mHD) is a statistical measure of the departure of the observed pattern of the valve repertoire from a reference polyclonal repertoire of control CD4 T cells from healthy individuals. The distance would be zero if the valve repertoire was identical to the reference, and 100 if it was completely different. The mHD across all expressed BV families was 60, range 45–80, illustrating the marked difference of the tricuspid aortic valve repertoire from the polyclonal reference repertoire ($p < 0.001$) and emphasizing the overall oligoclonal character of the T cell infiltrate in CAS valves (Winchester et al. 2011). Interestingly, some valves also had variable degree of polyclonal infiltration correlating with calcification severity. This same pattern of extensive oligoclonality and variable polyclonality was seen in bicuspid valves and their repertoire characteristics were indistinguishable from those of the tricuspid valves, Figure 2.

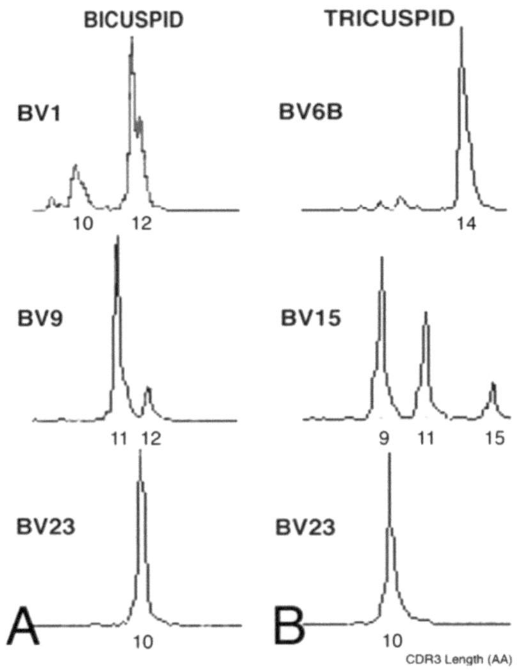

Fig. 2. Spectratype β-chain length distribution images illustrating the extensive oligoclonality in 3 BV families in a representative bicuspid (A) and tricuspid (B) CAS valve.

This counters the hypothesis that the repertoire of T cells infiltrating the valve leaflets is polyclonal and simply is a result of the presence of antecedent injury and inflammation. The presence of numerous clonal expansions in combination with a lesser, but variable degree of polyclonal infiltration argues for the interpretation that specific clonal expansions, likely induced by an adaptive immune response, are a component of CAS.

Since a few clones exhibited sequence homologies to clones previously identified in various inflammatory sites, such as multiple sclerosis lesions and HTLV-1 infection, (Wu et al. 2007), this suggests that a minority of CAS clones may be considered as bystander clones (McNally & Welsh 2002) related to the non antigen specific component of inflammation. However, the minor proportion of polyclonal, non-expanded T cells in many CAS samples compared to other inflammatory sites such as atherosclerotic plaques of inflamed synovia (Curran et al. 2004, Oksenberg et al. 1997, Stemme et al. 1991, Swanson et al. 1994), argues that inflammation-mediated T cell recruitment is not a general feature of CAS.

3. The inflammatory infiltrate in bicuspid and tricuspid valve calcific aortic stenosis is primarily associated with elevated proportions of circulating activated and effector memory CD8 T cells

The finding of clonal expansion in CAS valve leaflets raises the question of whether features of an ongoing systemic immune response would be present and be demonstrable in peripherally circulating T cells, implying that CAS had a systemic component. The alteration in T cell phenotype during an immune response, especially evident in the CD8 T cells, usually includes the transient expression of activation molecules, such as HLA-DR(Yu et al. 1980) and/or CD69, and the development of memory-effector cells particularly in sustained responses, defined by the loss of co-stimulatory CD28 molecules and acquisition of structures including natural killer receptors, e.g. CD57 (Brenchley et al. 2003, Hsu et al. 2006, Sallusto et al. 2004, Speiser et al. 1999). The presence of these features was studied by using flow cytometry to determine the expression of activation markers on the peripheral blood T cells and their subsets (Winchester et al. 2011). The combination of markers present can distinguish between naïve ($CD28^+$ and $CD57^-$) and memory effector ($CD28^-$ and $CD57^+$) T cells. Figure 3, next page, depicts four examples. Bicuspid valve sample B63 exhibits intense CD3 T cell activation as shown by the high proportion of T cells expressing HLA-DR, compared with a lower level in sample B48. The CD8 T cells of sample T54 exhibit extensive differentiation to $CD28^-$ memory effector status as shown by loss of CD28, versus a lesser degree of differentiation in sample T55.

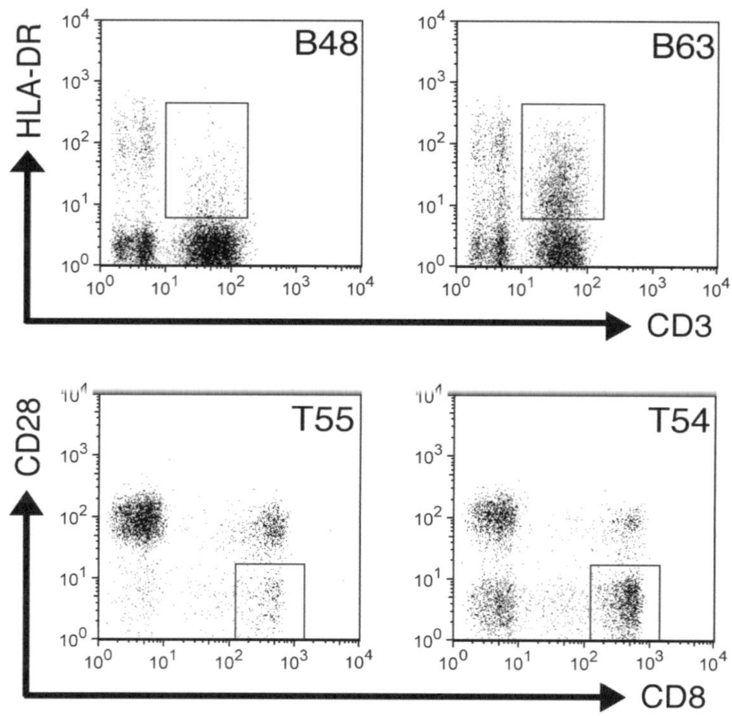

Fig. 3. Flow cytometry study of peripheral blood T lymphocytes from 4 CAS cases illustrates four different combinations of markers that identify activation (HLA-DR+) or varying degrees of differentiation to the $CD28^{null}$ memory-effector phenotype (CD28-).

The proportion of circulating CD3+ T cells expressing HLA-DR in CAS was considerably increased in the peripheral T cell compartment, range 4.7 to 32.9%, mean 16.1% and 16.3% in cases with tricuspid and bicuspid CAS valves, respectively, compared to the expected frequency of ≤ 5% in healthy controls (Winchester et al. 2011). The proportion of activated HLA-DR+ T cells correlated with a semiquantitative calcification score ranging from 1 through 8, correlation, $\rho = 0.530$, $p = 0.024$. Interestingly the percentage of the $CD8^+CD57^+$ T cell subset expressing HLA-DR ranged up to 49.9% and was greater than that found on the entire CD8 T cell subset in 11 of 14 CAS cases, indicating the CD8 T cells that have differentiated to a memory-effector phenotype continue to be strongly activated.

The proportion of circulating $CD8^+$ T cells that extinguished expression of CD28, one of the main markers of differentiation to the memory-effector phenotype, was substantially increased in tricuspid CAS, range 36.6 to 96%, mean 69.7% of CD8 T cells, and similarly in bicuspid CAS, range 20 to 85.5%, mean 65.8% (Winchester et al. 2011). Among tricuspid CAS cases the percentage of $CD8^+CD28^{null}$ T cells correlated with valve calcification severity ($\rho = 0.666$, $p = 0.003$). In the much younger bicuspid CAS patients, mean age 56± 18 years, the proportion of $CD8^+CD28^{null}$ T cells was more than double the level expected in normal age-matched individuals (Hsu et al. 2006). For all valve types, a greater proportion of $CD8^+CD28^{null}$ T cells was seen in cases where the valve calcification severity score was ≥ 4 ($p = 0.0006$), and the correlation with calcification score was $\rho = 0.590$, $p = 0.001$.

Because some of the findings of differentiation to memory effector phenotype are associated with physiologic aging and have been used to argue for immunologic senescence, immunosenescence, it was critical to study CAS occurring in bicuspid aortic valve cases, which occurs in individuals that are several decades younger. The results in those with bicuspid aortic valves were entirely similar to those in tricuspid aortic valve stenosis, indicating that this immune response was an intrinsic feature of CAS, and not likely a consequence of aging of the immune system.

The marked elevations in the level of activated CD8 T cells ($HLA\text{-}DR^+$ $CD69^+$) and extensive differentiation to memory effector phenotype ($CD28^-CD57^+$) are features indicative of an intense systemic immune response. These elevations generally parallel the infiltration of the valve by clonally expanded T cell populations. Furthermore, the extent of activation and expansion of the memory effector subsets in CAS cases was directly and strongly correlated with CAS severity (Winchester et al. 2011). Taken together with the elevated proportion of cells exhibiting differentiation to memory effector phenotype, these findings imply that a systemic immune response accompanies CAS.

In approximately half of the cases a lesser degree of activation and differentiation to the memory effector phenotype was found in the circulating CD4 T cell subset. The percentage of $CD4^+CD28^{null}$ T cells was moderately elevated, mean = 14.8%, range 2.6 to 50.5%, with a significant difference in mean frequency of the CD4+CD28- T cell subset between the atherosclerotic positive (19.36%) and negative (6.94%) subsets, p= 0.0074. (Winchester et al. 2011). Implicating this subset in the process of CAS, the number of $CD4^+CD28^{null}$ T cells was increased among cases with extensive valvular calcification, CAS score ≥4 ($p = 0.007$).

3.1 Immunostaining of CAS valves

Immunostaining of the valves was performed to define the phenotype and distribution of infiltrating T cells to aid in the interpretation of the repertoire analyses and relating the findings in the valve T cell infiltration to the phenotype found in blood (Winchester et al. 2011, Wu et al. 2007). The valve illustrated in figure 4 had a moderate level of polyclonality found by repertoire analysis, however upon staining, the large proportion of the infiltrating T cells exhibit the phenotype $CD8^{+}CD28^{-}$in the region of neovascularization. This is near a region of calcification at the lower left. There is considerable heterogeneity among different valves in terms of the number of infiltrating T cells and their immunophenotype found on immunostaining. Valves with multi or polyclonal T cell infiltration usually exhibited many regions of very abundant infiltration by CD8 and CD4 T cells. In contrast more oligoclonal samples had more sparse regions of T cell infiltration that predominantly stained for CD8. In all valves, the majority of CD8 T cells either lacked detectable expression of CD28 or staining was very dim, as shown in Figure 3. These $CD28^{null}$ or $CD28^{dim}CD8^{+}$ T cells were often found in proximity to sites of calcification or neovascularization, Figure 4. Reciprocally, in valves with greater proportions of polyclonal T cells, and with higher percentages of $CD4^{+}CD3^{+}$ T cells, more were $CD28^{brt}CD8^{-}$ (Winchester et al. 2011).

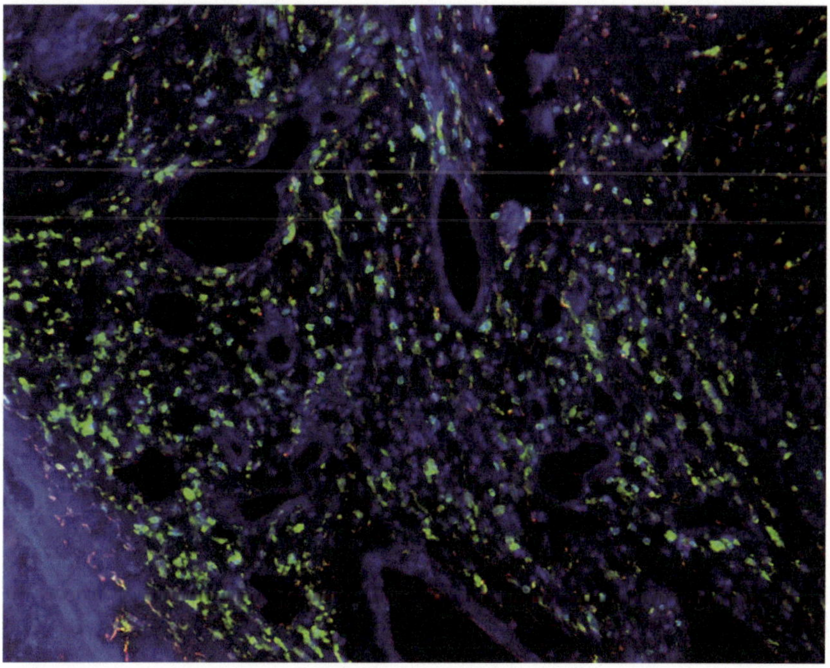

Fig. 4. An area of a tricuspid aortic valve exhibiting extensive neovascularization. It is stained for the expression of CD8 (green), CD28 (red-orange) and nuclei (Blue). The large proportion of the infiltrating T cells stain brightly for only the green fluorescence and have the phenotype $CD8^{+}CD28^{-}$.

4. Trafficking of the same T cell clones found expanded in the valve and T cell subsets in peripheral blood undergoing expansion

Trafficking of a subset of clones between the peripheral blood CD8 T cell subset and the infiltrate in a CAS valve is illustrated in figure 5 for three BV families. The darkened rectangles indicate that the same clone is found in the blood CD8 subset and in the valve.

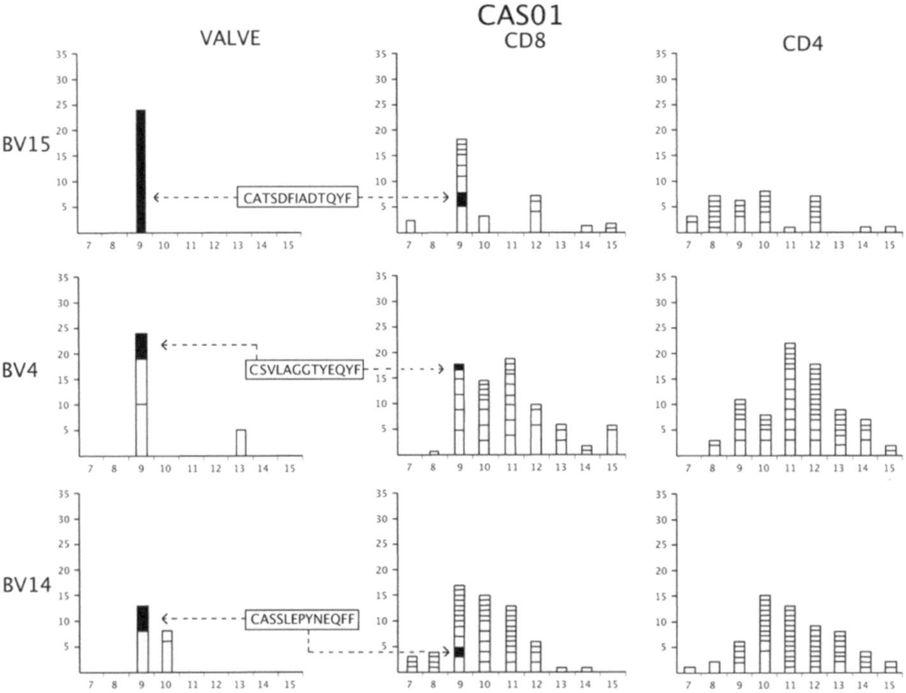

Fig. 5. An example of sharing of some clones expanded in the valve with the CD8 T cell subset. The repertoire analysis has been done by sequencing the TCR β-chain, and assembling the results into distribution histograms. The size of the rectangle denotes the clone size, with single sequence clones predominating in the CD4 subset.

In the initial study identifying clonal expansions in the valve, 24 of the valve-infiltrating T cell clones also had the same clone identified in blood. Importantly, 22 of these 24 shared clones were CD8 in lineage ($p=1.5x10^{-12}$) (Wu et al. 2007). As is seen in figure 5, in the valve, of the 9 expanded clones in the three examples, only three of these clones had clonal precursors identified in the blood, indicating evident clonal trafficking between the blood and the valve. Reciprocally a large number of clones are seen in the peripheral blood CD4 and CD8 subsets, of which only these 3 are found in the valve. This is an indication of the specificity of clonal entrance, and argues against passive streaming of clones from blood into the valve.

Further analysis and separation of the CD8 compartment of peripheral blood into the CD28+ naïve subset and the CD28- memory effector subset showed the large majority of T cell clones that were shared between the valve and the peripheral blood CD8 compartment were found in the memory effector $CD8^{+}CD28^{null}$ subset (Winchester et al. 2011), Table 1. Some clones were also shared with the CD8+CD28+ subset, and in each of these instances the clone was found expanded, indicating that it was proliferating and presumably in the process of differentiating to a memory effector phenotype. The clone with the clonotype sequence CASLALAFNEQFF, is an example of a clone in the process of this differentiation, and is found in both the CD8+CD28+ subset and the $CD8^{+}CD28^{null}$ subset (Winchester et al. 2011). These observations provide direct evidence supporting the association between the elevation in proportion of the $CD8^{+}CD28^{null}$ subset in blood and CAS severity. They show that the systemic immune response associated with CAS is an intrinsic part of the valve inflammation.

Additionally, one shared, but not expanded, clone in the CD4 blood subset was found with the clonotypic sequence CASSSKRLAGESGELFF, in a case that also had atherosclerotic disease. This instance of a minimally expanded clone that is shared between blood and the valve might reflect participation of the atherosclerotic process.

Case	TRBV-CDR3	Clonotypic CDR3 sequence	Valve clone size	Blood Subset	Blood clone size
T13	TRBV7-10	CASSQAPGKAFF	8	$CD28^+$ $CD8^+$	4
T13	TRBV7-12	CASSLDTRGDTQYF	4	$CD28^{null}$ $CD8^+$	38
T13	TRBV7-15	CASSSKRLAGESGELFF	1	$CD4^+$	1
T13	TRBV12-13	CASSRTSGVYNEQFF	11	$CD28^{null}$ $CD8^+$	22
T14	TRBV11-12	CASSLALAFNEQFF	18	$CD28^{null}$ and	3
				$CD28^+$ $CD8^+$	4
T14	TRBV11-17	CASSLNDRGVGLSSYEQYF	2	$CD28^+$ $CD8^+$	11

CDR3 length, number of amino acids in CDR3 loop according to IMGT nomenclature
Clone size refers to number of sequence of this clonotype recovered in a set of 40 sequences

Table 1. Shared T cell clonotypes recovered from aortic valve and peripheral blood

5. Discussion

Three central findings emerged from these studies on the immunological nature and significance of the T lymphocytes that infiltrate the valve leaflets in CAS: First, as shown by TCR β–chain sequencing and spectratype analysis, the T cell infiltrate in the CAS valves predominantly consists of expanded αβ TCR clones, with a varying component polyclonal T cell infiltration. This finding suggests that a major component of the T cell infiltrate in the leaflets in CAS appears to be due to antigen-induced proliferation of T cells. The extent of the clonal expansions correlated with the severity of CAS. Immunostaining revealed a large, but variable proportion of the infiltrating T cells were CD8 in lineage and exhibited the memory effector phenotype of extinguishing expression of CD28, supporting the interpretation of antigen induced differentiation. In addition to the clones some tissues exhibited a polyclonal infiltration of non-clonally expanded T cells indicative of non-antigen-specific inflammation and likely chemokine driven recruitment.

The second main finding was that the peripheral blood of CAS cases had greatly elevated levels of activated CD8 T cells ($HLA\text{-}DR^+$ and/or $CD69^+$) and extensive differentiation to memory effector phenotype ($CD28^-CD57^+$). These features in peripheral blood indicate an intense ongoing systemic immune response. The extent of activation and expansion of the peripheral blood memory effector subsets in CAS cases was directly and strongly correlated with CAS severity. The results in those with bicuspid CAS were entirely similar to those found in tricuspid CAS, indicating that this immune response was an intrinsic feature of CAS and not likely to be secondary to immunosenescence. It is possible that the significant elevations of CRP reported in CAS cases (Galante et al. 2001, Jeevanantham et al. 2007) is a constitutive component of the CD8 T cell activation and differentiation to a memory-effector phenotype, together reflecting the presence of a systemic adaptive immune response. A

lesser degree of activation and differentiation to the memory effector phenotype was found in the CD4 T cell subset in approximately half of the cases. This was highly correlated with the presence of atherosclerotic disease regardless of whether it appeared stable or not.
The third central finding was the demonstration that particular T cell clones found expanded within the valve were also expanded in peripheral blood, especially in the memory effector CD8 subset. This evidence of clonal trafficking between the blood and valve provides direct evidence linking events in blood to those in the valve and supports the association of the activation and expansion of the memory effector T cell subset in blood with the severity of CAS.
Several findings point to an important role of CD8 T cells and in particular the $CD8^{+}CD28^{null}$ T cells in CAS. They include identification of large numbers of T cells with this phenotype in the valve on immunostaining; activation and differentiation to memory-effector status among circulating lymphocytes, which strongly predominated in the CD8 T cell subset; as well as 8 instances of sharing of the same T cell clones expanded both in the valve and in the peripheral blood memory-effector $CD8^{+}CD28^{null}$ T cells (Winchester et al. 2011) Moreover, HLA-DR expression was particularly increased on the $CD8^{+}CD57^{+}$ T cell subset, indicating their continued activation. Together with the earlier findings where 23 of 24 clones identified both among the circulating lymphocytes and in the valve were CD8 lineage T cells (Wu et al. 2007) these data suggest the interpretation that the peptides driving this aspect of the immune response in CAS likely have a cytoplasmic origin, are presented in the context of class I MHC molecules and are recognized by CD8 T cells.
The selectivity of the process underlying the presence of the expanded T cells infiltrating the valve is supported by the absence of T cells from certain BV families in valve tissue (Winchester et al. 2011, Wu et al. 2007), the highly significant predominance of the CD8 subset among the clones shared with blood, the large proportion of clonal expansion in both blood CD4 and CD8 repertoires that were not identified in the valve and vice verse, the elevated proportion of expanded clones to unexpanded clones found in the valve, the structural homologies evident between CDR3 regions of unrelated clones as well as the frequent representation of the same CDR3 length in the valve (Wu et al. 2007). This selectivity is consistent with the operation of cognitive adaptive immune recognition events in the formation of the inflammatory infiltrate of the valve.

5.1 Atherosclerosis and CAS

CAS shares some risk factors with atherosclerosis and apoE knockout mice develop CAS (Ortlepp et al. 2003, Stewart et al. 1997, Tanaka et al. 2005). However, as emphasized by Otto et al.,(Otto & O'Brien 2001) CAS and atherosclerosis are not synonymous, given that only half of the patients with CAS have concomitant coronary artery disease, while the large majority of those with atherosclerosis do not develop CAS (Ortlepp et al. 2003). Additionally, bicuspid aortic valves are disproportionally affected with CAS further suggesting that factors distinct from atherosclerosis account for the development of CAS (Otto 2002). Moreover, the lack of clear efficacy of intensive lipid lowering therapy by statins in halting the progression of CAS (Cowell et al. 2005) suggests that processes other than those involved in atherosclerosis may be at play in CAS.
These facts notwithstanding, there is indirect evidence from our work that in CAS cases with evident atherosclerosis that the atherosclerotic process interacts with mechanisms responsible for CAS. Elevations in the $CD28^{null}$ CD4 T cell subset are well recognized in

unstable atherosclerotic disease (Liuzzo et al. 2000). In CAS peripheral blood, as discussed there was a significant difference in mean frequency of the CD4+CD28- T cell subset between the atherosclerotic positive (19.36%) and negative (6.94%) subsets, p= 0.0074. (Winchester et al. 2011). Implicating this subset in the process of CAS, the number of $CD4^{+}CD28^{null}$ T cells was increased among cases with extensive valvular calcification. Additionally, one instance of a shared, but not detectably expanded, clone between the CD4 blood subset was found (Table 1), in a case that also had atherosclerotic disease. It is possible this instance of a shared T cell clone reflects the contribution of the co-morbid atherosclerotic process (Oksenberg et al. 1997, Stemme et al. 1991). However, overt unstable atherosclerotic disease was not present in the CAS cases studied by us, suggesting that if the $CD4^{+}CD28^{null}$ T cell elevations in the subset of CAS cases with atherosclerotic is mechanistically linked to the atherosclerotic process, the role of this cellular subset in CAS differs from that proposed in unstable atherosclerosis. Moreover, as emphasized by Wu et al. (Wu et al. 2007), the overall oligoclonal nature and CD8 lineage of valve-infiltrating T cells and those expanded in blood that predominate in CAS contrast sharply with the findings reported in atherosclerosis (Oksenberg et al. 1997, Stemme et al. 1991). This underlines the fact that the predominant immune mechanism underlying the lymphocytic infiltration in CAS centered on CD8 T cells is distinct from that implicated in atherosclerosis.

5.2 Immunosenescence

In normal chronologic aging the prevalence of $CD28^{null}CD57^{+}$ T cells increases in the $CD8^{+}$ and, to a much lesser extent, in the $CD4^{+}$ compartment (Effros et al. 1994) along with large clonal expansions in this subset (Bandres et al. 2000, Posnett et al. 1994, Vallejo 2006). These expansions have been attributed in part to the sustained proliferation of $CD8^{+}$ T cells involved in maintaining viral latency to EBV and in responding to CMV. Effros and colleagues advanced the concept that $CD8^{+}CD28^{null}$ T cells are immunosenescent and that their expansion primarily down modulates both immune and non-immune functions and contributes to various age-related pathologies. Intriguingly in one sense, the present findings in tricuspid CAS are generally consistent with the association noted by Effros et al., especially given the advanced age of the tricuspid CAS cases, and in this respect tricuspid CAS can be added to conditions characterized by expansions of memory-effector T cells. (Effros et al. 2005, Goronzy & Weyand 2003, Hadrup et al. 2006, Hamann et al. 1999, Morley et al. 1995, Posnett et al. 1999, Posnett et al. 1994).

However, these data can be interpreted differently and studies presented in this chapter support the viewpoint that the mechanism differs from that proposed by Effros et al. in that CAS is not a secondary consequence of immunosenescence. The recent studies discussed in this chapter are consistent with the opposite possibility that a specific immune response involving the valve leaflets drives the activation and expansion of CD8 T cells and their maturation to $CD28^{null}$ phenotype. Accordingly we envision the expansion of the memory-effector subset to be a consequence of and a component of the immune response directed to the valve. This interpretation is supported by: a) The high expression of HLA-DR and CD69 on $CD8^{+}CD28^{null}$ T cells in CAS that distinguishes this condition from the $CD8^{+}CD28^{null}$ T cell populations in aging; b) The extent of the expansion of the $CD28^{null}CD8^{+}$subset that was directly and significantly correlated with the CAS severity score (p=0.003), but was independent of chronologic age; and c) Perhaps most consequentially, the complete resemblance of the findings in blood and in the valve between the much younger bicuspid valve CAS cases and the older tricuspid valve cases, emphasizing the importance of studying the much younger individuals who develop CAS in bicuspid aortic valves.

6. Conclusion

The results suggest that an ongoing systemic adaptive immune response is occurring in cases with bicuspid and tricuspid CAS, involving circulating CD8 T cell activation, clonal expansion and differentiation to a memory-effector phenotype, with trafficking of T cells in expanded clones between blood and the valve. The character of the immune response and the primary involvement of CD8 T cells suggests the T cell response is likely driven by a cellularly expressed antigen present in the valve leaflet, likely present in the cytoplasm of leaflet mesenchymal cells. The present studies raise several additional questions.

The first major question arises of what immune recognition event might be driving these immune events. Because CAS occurs in the setting of different clinical situations of bicuspid and tricuspid aortic valves and co morbidities including hypertension and atherosclerosis that have in common enhanced hemodynamic strain and diminished valvular compliance, one unifying hypothesis is that valve mesenchymal cells alter their transcriptional phenotype in response to enhanced strain, resulting in the cellular expression of stress-induced molecules. Peptides from these stress-induced molecules, to which the individual may not be fully tolerized, may be expressed in the context of class I MHC inducing an idiosyncratic autoimmune-like CD8 T cell immune response. This results in infiltration of the valve by expanding and activated T cell clones that recognize the stress neoantigen. Of course as in all autoimmune diseases the adaptive immune response to a self-antigen is not appreciably different from one to a pathogen, and the present studies leave open a range of possibilities as to the source and nature of the peptides driving this immune response. For several reasons, identification of the peptides recognized by the infiltrating T cell clones would be a central advance.

Since this hypothesis considers the expression of stress induced antigens in the valve as the driver of the systemic immune response identified in CAS cases, one approach to testing the hypothesis is to examine the effects of valve replacement surgery on the extent of the circulating CD8 T cell activation and differentiation to memory effector status. The hypothesis suggests that the level of activation and differentiation should return towards more normal levels. These studies are currently underway.

A second major question is what is the relevance of this immune response to CAS? It is possible these proliferating T cells release cytokines that alter the pattern of gene expression in the valve mesenchymal cells and recruit additional lymphocytes into the valve, suggesting that at a minimum one consequence of this inflammation is a further and potentially reversible decrease in valvular compliance. Support for this possibility comes in part from preliminary data in 8 cases where significant production of γ-interferon was found in the $CD8^{+}CD28^{null}$ T cell subset and from the earlier reports identifying HLA-DR expression on valve mesenchymal cells (Olsson, Rosenqvist, et al. 1994). This would be a positive feedback situation where the consequence of diminished valve compliance would presumably enhance the stress response of the mesenchymal cell leading to enhanced expression of stress antigens. It is also possible that the activated memory-effector CD8 T cells directly injure target valve cells and may additionally drive the development of heterotopic calcification, and neovascularization with precedent for development of analogous heterotopic calcification in the setting of the autoimmune $CD8^{+}CD28^{null}$ T cell response in diseases like psoriatic arthritis or ankylosing spondylitis.

Another major question is whether the extent of immune reactivity in blood could be a marker for the rate of progression of CAS, since both the extent of the changes in the blood and the infiltration in the valve vary considerably. However, the cross sectional nature of this study that demonstrated a correlation between intensity of CD8 T cell activation and differentiation to memory effector phenotype with calcification severity does not allow assessment of the predictive value of these measurements for the development of severe CAS. It is possible that low levels of CD8 T cell activation and differentiation to memory effector phenotype could be found to be a biomarker favoring slow progression of calcification and other features of the process. The use of tetramer technology with knowledge of the nature of the driving peptide would be the ideal way to specifically assess the intensity of this immune response and distinguish it from other CD8 T cell responses.

This line of immunologically oriented research work should add impetus to changing the view of CAS as an irreversible degenerative process, set the stage for identification of the target antigens driving this process, and give hope to the possibility of designing specific immunomodulatory therapy directed towards inhibiting the T cell clonal expansions or lymphocyte recruitment to diminish the relentless progression of this serious disease, for which currently valve replacement is the only treatment.

7. Acknowledgement

We are indebted to the many colleagues who have provided well-defined CAS cases and tissue samples for study, and who have contributed to data acquisition and analysis. We gratefully acknowledge the support of the USPHS, grant number R01HL084599.

8. References

Bandres, E., Merino, J., Vazquez, B., Inoges, S., Moreno, C., Subira, M. L. & Sanchez-Ibarrola, A. (2000) The increase of IFN-gamma production through aging correlates with the expanded CD8(+high)CD28(-)CD57(+) subpopulation. *Clin Immunol 96*(3): 230-235.

Brenchley, J. M., Karandikar, N. J., Betts, M. R., Ambrozak, D. R., Hill, B. J., Crotty, L. E., Casazza, J. P., Kuruppu, J., Migueles, S. A., Connors, M., Roederer, M., Douek, D. C. & Koup, R. A. (2003) Expression of CD57 defines replicative senescence and antigen-induced apoptotic death of CD8+ T cells. *Blood 101*(7): 2711-2720.

Cowell, S. J., Newby, D. E., Prescott, R. J., Bloomfield, P., Reid, J., Northridge, D. B. & Boon, N. A. (2005) A randomized trial of intensive lipid-lowering therapy in calcific aortic stenosis. *N Engl J Med 352*(23): 2389-2397.

Curran, S. A., FitzGerald, O. M., Costello, P. J., Selby, J. M., Kane, D. J., Bresnihan, B. & Winchester, R. (2004) Nucleotide sequencing of psoriatic arthritis tissue before and during methotrexate administration reveals a complex inflammatory T cell infiltrate with very few clones exhibiting features that suggest they drive the inflammatory process by recognizing autoantigens. *J Immunol 172*(3): 1935-1944.

Effros, R. B., Boucher, N., Porter, V., Zhu, X., Spaulding, C., Walford, R. L., Kronenberg, M., Cohen, D. & Schächter, F. (1994) Decline in CD28+ T cells in centenarians and in long-term T cell cultures: a possible cause for both in vivo and in vitro immunosenescence. *Exp Gerontol 29*(6): 601-609.

Effros, R. B., Dagarag, M., Spaulding, C. & Man, J. (2005) The role of CD8+ T-cell replicative senescence in human aging. *Immunol Rev 205*: 147-157.

Galante, A., Pietroiusti, A., Vellini, M., Piccolo, P., Possati, G., De Bonis, M., Grillo, R. L., Fontana, C. & Favalli, C. (2001) C-reactive protein is increased in patients with degenerative aortic valvular stenosis. *Journal of the American College of Cardiology 38*(4): 1078-1082.

Goronzy, J. J. & Weyand, C. M. (2003) Aging, autoimmunity and arthritis: T-cell senescence and contraction of T-cell repertoire diversity - catalysts of autoimmunity and chronic inflammation. *Arthritis Res Ther 5*(5): 225-234.

Hadrup, S. R., Strindhall, J., Kollgaard, T., Seremet, T., Johansson, B., Pawelec, G., thor Straten, P. & Wikby, A. (2006) Longitudinal studies of clonally expanded CD8 T cells reveal a repertoire shrinkage predicting mortality and an increased number of dysfunctional cytomegalovirus-specific T cells in the very elderly. *J Immunol 176*(4): 2645-2653.

Hamann, D., Kostense, S., Wolthers, K. C., Otto, S. A., Baars, P. A., Miedema, F. & van Lier, R. A. (1999) Evidence that human CD8+CD45RA+CD27- cells are induced by antigen and evolve through extensive rounds of division. *Int Immunol 11*(7): 1027-1033.

Hsu, H. C., Scott, D. K., Zhang, P., Zhou, J., Yang, P., Wu, Q., Schroeder, H. W., Jr., Gerald, L. B., Ravussin, E., Jazwinski, S. M. & Mountz, J. D. (2006) CD8 T-cell immune phenotype of successful aging. *Mech Ageing Dev 127*(3): 231-239.

Jeevanantham, V., Singh, N., Izuora, K., D'Souza, J. P. & Hsi, D. H. (2007) Correlation of high sensitivity C-reactive protein and calcific aortic valve disease. *Mayo Clinic proceedings. Mayo Clinic 82*(2): 171-174.

Li, Y., Schwabe, R. F., DeVries-Seimon, T., Yao, P. M., Gerbod-Giannone, M. C., Tall, A. R., Davis, R. J., Flavell, R., Brenner, D. A. & Tabas, I. (2005) Free cholesterol-loaded macrophages are an abundant source of tumor necrosis factor-alpha and interleukin-6: model of NF-kappaB- and map kinase-dependent inflammation in advanced atherosclerosis. *J Biol Chem 280*(23): 21763-21772.

Liuzzo, G., Goronzy, J. J., Yang, H., Kopecky, S. L., Holmes, D. R., Frye, R. L. & Weyand, C. M. (2000) Monoclonal T-cell proliferation and plaque instability in acute coronary syndromes. *Circulation 101*(25): 2883-2888.

Mazzone, A., Epistolato, M. C., De Caterina, R., Storti, S., Vittorini, S., Sbrana, S., Gianetti, J., Bevilacqua, S., Glauber, M., Biagini, A. & Tanganelli, P. (2004) Neoangiogenesis, T-lymphocyte infiltration, and heat shock protein-60 are biological hallmarks of an immunomediated inflammatory process in end-stage calcified aortic valve stenosis. *J Am Coll Cardiol 43*(9): 1670-1676.

McNally, J. M. & Welsh, R. M. (2002) Bystander T cell activation and attrition. *Curr Top Microbiol Immunol 263*: 29-41.

Morley, J. K., Batliwalla, F. M., Hingorani, R. & Gregersen, P. K. (1995) Oligoclonal CD8+ T cells are preferentially expanded in the CD57+ subset. *J Immunol 154*(11): 6182-6190.

Oksenberg, J. R., Stavri, G. T., Jeong, M. C., Garovoy, N., Salisbury, J. R. & Erusalimsky, J. D. (1997) Analysis of the T-cell receptor repertoire in human atherosclerosis. *Cardiovasc Res 36*(2): 256-267.

Olsson, M., Dalsgaard, C. J., Haegerstrand, A., Rosenqvist, M., Ryden, L. & Nilsson, J. (1994) Accumulation of T lymphocytes and expression of interleukin-2 receptors in nonrheumatic stenotic aortic valves. *J Am Coll Cardiol 23*(5): 1162-1170.

Olsson, M., Rosenqvist, M. & Nilsson, J. (1994) Expression of HLA-DR antigen and smooth muscle cell differentiation markers by valvular fibroblasts in degenerative aortic stenosis. *J Am Coll Cardiol 24*(7): 1664-1671.

Ortlepp, J. R., Schmitz, F., Bozoglu, T., Hanrath, P. & Hoffmann, R. (2003) Cardiovascular risk factors in patients with aortic stenosis predict prevalence of coronary artery disease but not of aortic stenosis: an angiographic pair matched case-control study. *Heart 89*(9): 1019-1022.

Otto, C. M. (2002) Calcification of bicuspid aortic valves. *Heart 88*(4): 321-322.

Otto, C. M., Kuusisto, J., Reichenbach, D. D., Gown, A. M. & O'Brien, K. D. (1994) Characterization of the early lesion of 'degenerative' valvular aortic stenosis. Histological and immunohistochemical studies. *Circulation 90*(2): 844-853.

Otto, C. M. & O'Brien, K. D. (2001) Why is there discordance between calcific aortic stenosis and coronary artery disease? *Heart 85*(6): 601-602.

Pomerance, A. (1972) Pathogenesis of aortic stenosis and its relation to age. *Br Heart J 34*(6): 569-574.

Posnett, D. N., Edinger, J. W., Manavalan, J. S., Irwin, C. & Marodon, G. (1999) Differentiation of human CD8 T cells: implications for in vivo persistence of CD8+ CD28- cytotoxic effector clones. *Int Immunol 11*(2): 229-241.

Posnett, D. N., Sinha, R., Kabak, S. & Russo, C. (1994) Clonal populations of T cells in normal elderly humans: the T cell equivalent to "benign monoclonal gammapathy". *J Exp Med 179*(2): 609-618.

Rajamannan, N. M., Subramaniam, M., Rickard, D., Stock, S. R., Donovan, J., Springett, M., Orszulak, T., Fullerton, D. A., Tajik, A. J., Bonow, R. O. & Spelsberg, T. (2003) Human aortic valve calcification is associated with an osteoblast phenotype. *Circulation 107*(17): 2181-2184.

Raulet, D. H. (2003) Roles of the NKG2D immunoreceptor and its ligands. *Nat Rev Immunol 3*(10): 781-790.

Sallusto, F., Geginat, J. & Lanzavecchia, A. (2004) Central memory and effector memory T cell subsets: function, generation, and maintenance. *Annu Rev Immunol 22*: 745-763.

Soini, Y., Salo, T. & Satta, J. (2003) Angiogenesis is involved in the pathogenesis of nonrheumatic aortic valve stenosis. *Hum Pathol 34*(8): 756-763.

Speiser, D. E., Valmori, D., Rimoldi, D., Pittet, M. J., Lienard, D., Cerundolo, V., MacDonald, H. R., Cerottini, J. C. & Romero, P. (1999) CD28-negative cytolytic effector T cells frequently express NK receptors and are present at variable proportions in circulating lymphocytes from healthy donors and melanoma patients. *Eur J Immunol 29*(6): 1990-1999.

Stemme, S., Rymo, L. & Hansson, G. K. (1991) Polyclonal origin of T lymphocytes in human atherosclerotic plaques. *Lab Invest 65*(6): 654-660.

Stewart, B. F., Siscovick, D., Lind, B. K., Gardin, J. M., Gottdiener, J. S., Smith, V. E., Kitzman, D. W. & Otto, C. M. (1997) Clinical factors associated with calcific aortic valve disease. Cardiovascular Health Study. *J Am Coll Cardiol 29*(3): 630-634.

Swanson, S. J., Rosenzweig, A., Seidman, J. G. & Libby, P. (1994) Diversity of T-cell antigen receptor V beta gene utilization in advanced human atheroma. *Arterioscler Thromb 14*(7): 1210-1214.

Tanaka, K., Sata, M., Fukuda, D., Suematsu, Y., Motomura, N., Takamoto, S., Hirata, Y. & Nagai, R. (2005) Age-associated aortic stenosis in apolipoprotein E-deficient mice. *J Am Coll Cardiol 46*(1): 134-141.

Vallejo, A. N. (2006) Age-dependent alterations of the T cell repertoire and functional diversity of T cells of the aged. *Immunol Res 36*(1-3): 221-228.

Wallby, L., Janerot-Sjoberg, B., Steffensen, T. & Broqvist, M. (2002) T lymphocyte infiltration in non-rheumatic aortic stenosis: a comparative descriptive study between tricuspid and bicuspid aortic valves. *Heart 88*(4): 348-351.

Winchester, R., Wiesendanger, M., O Brien, W., Zhang, H.-Z., Maurer, M. S., Gillam, L. D., Schwartz, A., Marboe, C. & Stewart, A. S. (2011) Circulating activated and effector memory T cells are associated with calcification and clonal expansions in bicuspid and tricuspid valves of calcific aortic stenosis. *Journal of Immunology (In Press).*

Wu, H. D., Maurer, M., Friedman, R. A., Marboe, C. C., Ruiz-Vazquez, E. M., Ramakrishnan, R., Schwartz, A., Tilson, M. D., Stuart, A. S. & Winchester, R. (2007) The Lymphocytic Infiltration In Calcific Aortic Stenosis Predominantly Consists of Clonally Expanded T Cells. *Journal of Immunology 178*: 5329-5339.

Yu, D. T., Winchester, R. J., Fu, S. M., Gibofsky, A., Ko, H. S. & Kunkel, H. G. (1980) Peripheral blood Ia-positive T cells. Increases in certain diseases and after immunization. *Journal of Experimental Medicine 151*: 91-100.

13

Natriuretic Peptides in Severe Aortic Stenosis - Role in Predicting Outcomes and Assessment for Early Aortic Valve Replacement

Aaron Lin and Ralph Stewart
Green Lane Cardiovascular Service, Auckland City Hospital, Auckland, New Zealand

1. Introduction

The natriuretic peptides are a group of endogenous, structurally related hormones with natriuretic, diuretic and peripheral vasodilatory actions. (Hunt, 1997; Yandle, 1986; Yandle, 1993) They serve an important regulatory role in response to acute increases in ventricular wall stress. A large number of cardiac conditions may cause an elevation of plasma levels of natriuretic peptides. Clinically, natriuretic peptides are of value in ruling out heart failure in patients presenting acutely to the emergency department with dyspnoea. (Maisel et al., 2002). Natriuretic peptides could also be useful in evaluating the severity and prognosis of patients with aortic stenosis (AS). Severe AS causes an increase in afterload and end-systolic left ventricular (LV) wall stress that, over time, leads to concentric myocardial hypertrophy. (Wachtell, 2008) This anatomical change of the LV is characterized at the molecular level by the re-expression of fetal isogenes, including increased gene expression of natriuretic peptides in the ventricular cardiomyocytes. (Sadoshima, 1992; Cameron, 1996)

This chapter reviews the existing data on natriuretic peptide measurement in AS, to summarize how these biomarkers can be utilized in clinical practice, and to explore their therapeutic implication concerning the optimal timing of aortic valve replacement in the setting of severe AS.

2. Management of severe Aortic Stenosis

2.1 Difficulty in determining the timing of valvular surgery

AS is a slowly progressive disease and current guidelines recommend that surgery is delayed until symptoms develop or LV function decreases. (Bonow et al., 2006) Initial symptoms experienced by patients with AS are often subtle and insidious and can be difficult to evaluate clinically. However, once significant symptoms develop, there is a dramatic change in patients' outlook with a reported average survival on medical therapy of less than 3 years. (Ross Jr, 1968; Frank, 1973) The risk of rapid clinical deterioration and poorer prognosis after symptom onset in some AS patients emphasizes the importance of early and accurate detection of AS related symptoms and timely referral for valvular surgery to avoid adverse cardiovascular outcomes in these patients.

Echocardiography is currently the gold standard for the non-invasive assessment of AS. The most widely used echocardiographic measures of AS severity in clinical practice are peak aortic velocity and aortic valve area determined by the continuity equation. (Otto, 1998) However, according to the current American College of Cardiology/American Heart Association guidelines, there is no single clinical, haemodynamic, or echocardiographic measure that has been adopted as a class I recommendation for valve replacement in the absence of symptoms in patients with isolated AS. (Bonow et al., 2006) This is because of the wide overlaps in haemodynamic and echocardiographic measures of severity between the symptomatic and asymptomatic patients, consistent with the known heterogeneous response to the pressure load of AS. (Otto, 2000)

There is also the problem of evaluating symptoms. Patients may not realize gradual onset of symptoms is due to disease progression. Also some patients may be unable to exercise because of non-cardiac comorbidities, or do not develop the classic symptoms of AS. This makes the determination of the optimal timing of aortic valve replacement (AVR) more challenging.

There is reluctance to perform surgery earlier than necessary because of a mortality rate for aortic valve surgery of approximately 3% to 5%, even in patients younger than 70 years, (Edwards et al., 2001) and prosthetic valve-related long-term morbidity. Conversely, patients who become symptomatic are at significant risk of developing adverse cardiac events while waiting for surgery, and peri-operative risk increases significantly with the severity of symptoms. (Rosenhek et al., 2002) These factors contribute to the controversy on the optimal timing of AVR in asymptomatic severe AS, because the risk of potential adverse cardiac complications from AS must be weighed against the risk of surgery in truly asymptomatic patients.

A non-invasive marker of early cardiac decompensation could be useful to risk stratify asymptomatic AS patients into those likely to derive benefit from surgery before the development of symptoms or irreversible LV impairment, from those who have a low risk of adverse events during follow-up.

2.2 Non-invasive biomarkers

Cardiac biomarkers are one solution to this dilemma. In recent years, biomarkers have become important tools for diagnosis, risk stratification and therapeutic decision making in cardiovascular diseases. To serve as markers of cardiac function, the biomarkers need to predict clinical and echocardiographic progression of disease. Echocardiographic assessment of AS requires trained and experienced sonographers with meticulous attention to the technical details of imaging and Doppler flow recording and accurate interpretation of findings. In contrast the introduction of fully automated assays with proven excellent test precision means that measurement of plasma levels of biomarkers is simple, reliable, not operator-dependent, relatively inexpensive, and reproducible.

Several biomarkers have been studied for this purpose. They include atrial natriuretic peptide (also known A-type natriuretic peptide, or ANP), brain natriuretic peptide (also known as B-type natriuretic peptide, or BNP), N-terminal BNP (the amino terminal part of BNP, or NT-BNP), N-terminal-proBNP (the amino terminal part of the BNP prohormone, or NT-proBNP), urodilatin, cardiotrophin-1, tumour necrosis factor-a (TNF-a) and TNF receptors 1 and 2. Of these the natriuretic peptides BNP and NT-proBNP predict adverse outcomes across a broad range of cardiac diseases in a great number of different clinical settings.

2.3 Natriuretic peptides

BNP was initially identified and described in 1988 after isolation from porcine brain. It was later recognised that BNP is predominately synthesized and secreted from the LV in response to increased ventricular wall stress. In the setting of volume and pressure overload, the increased wall stress initiates synthesis of the prehormone, pre-proBNP which is cleaved first to pro-BNP, then to the biologically active BNP and the inactive NT-proBNP fragments upon release into the circulation (Figure 1 and 2).

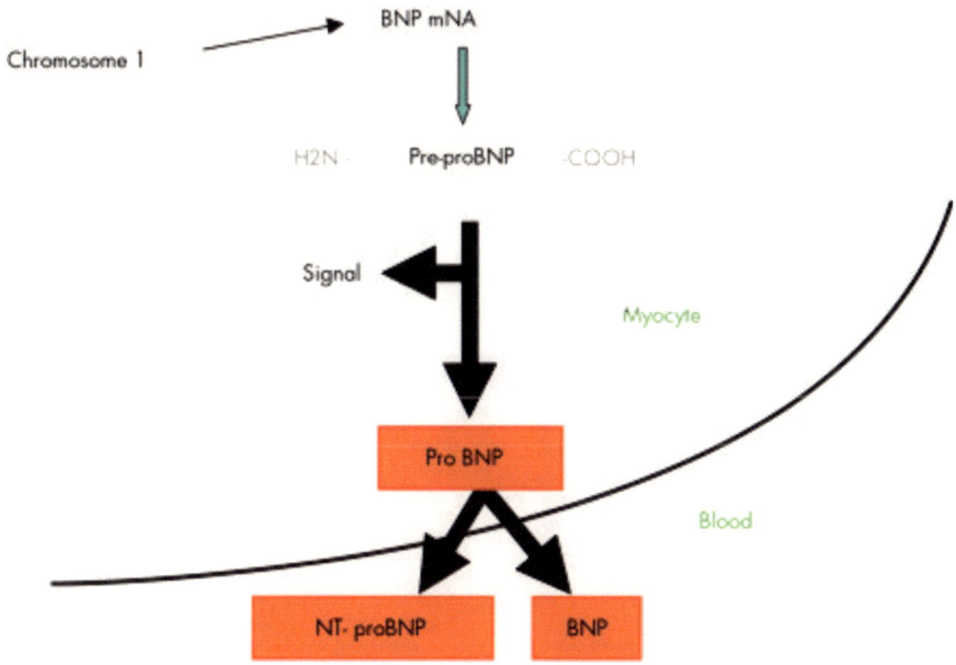

Fig. 1. Synthesis and secretion of B-type natriuretic peptide. (adapted from Bettencourt et al., 2005)

In contrast to BNP, ANP which is stored in granules within the atria and is released immediately after atrial stretch. (Yasue et al., 1994) Only small amounts of BNP are stored in granules. Rapid gene expression with de novo synthesis seems to be the underlying mechanism for the regulation of BNP secretion. (Yoshimura et al., 1993) However, the exact signalling pathways of natriuretic peptide secretion remain poorly defined. During the development of LV hypertrophy, gradual disappearance of natriuretic peptide clearance receptor mRNA had been found in the rat heart (Brown et al., 1993) and down-regulation of membrane-bound natriuretic peptide clearance receptor may, therefore, be a contributing factor to increased plasma natriuretic peptide levels.

As shown in Figure 3, in patients with normal LV systolic function and normal LA pressure, BNP and NT-proBNP levels correlate more significantly with LV mass index than ANP irrespective of aetiology. (Qi et al., 2001)

Because of differences in the excretion of BNP and NT-proBNP the absolute levels are not linearly correlated. BNP is cleared from plasma mostly by binding to the natriuretic peptide receptor type-C and through proteolysis by neutral endopeptidases. Direct renal filtration

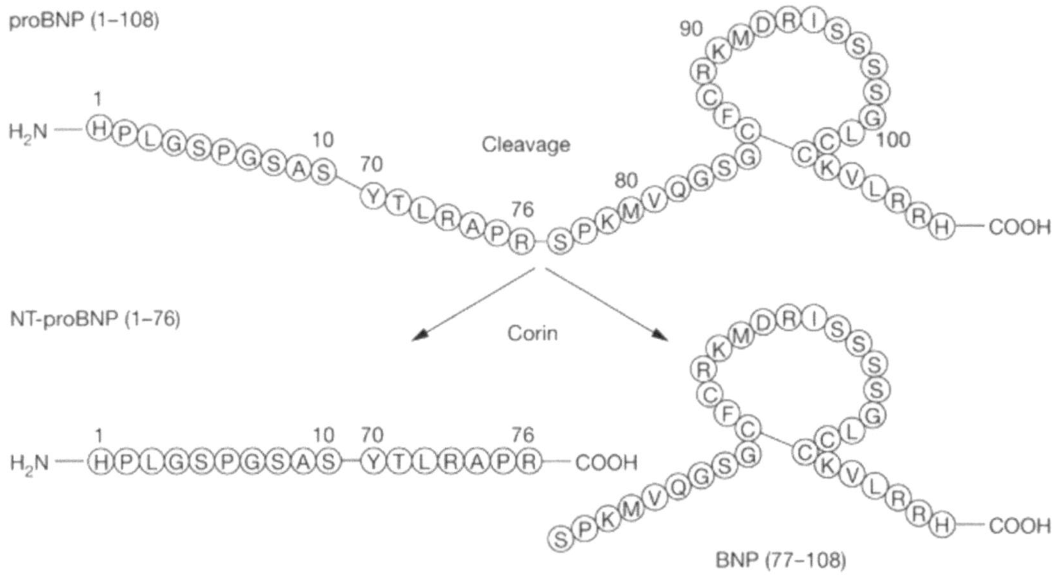

Fig. 2. Diagrammatic representation of the cleavage of the B-type natriuretic peptide prohormone. (adapted from Costello-Boerrigter et al., 2005)

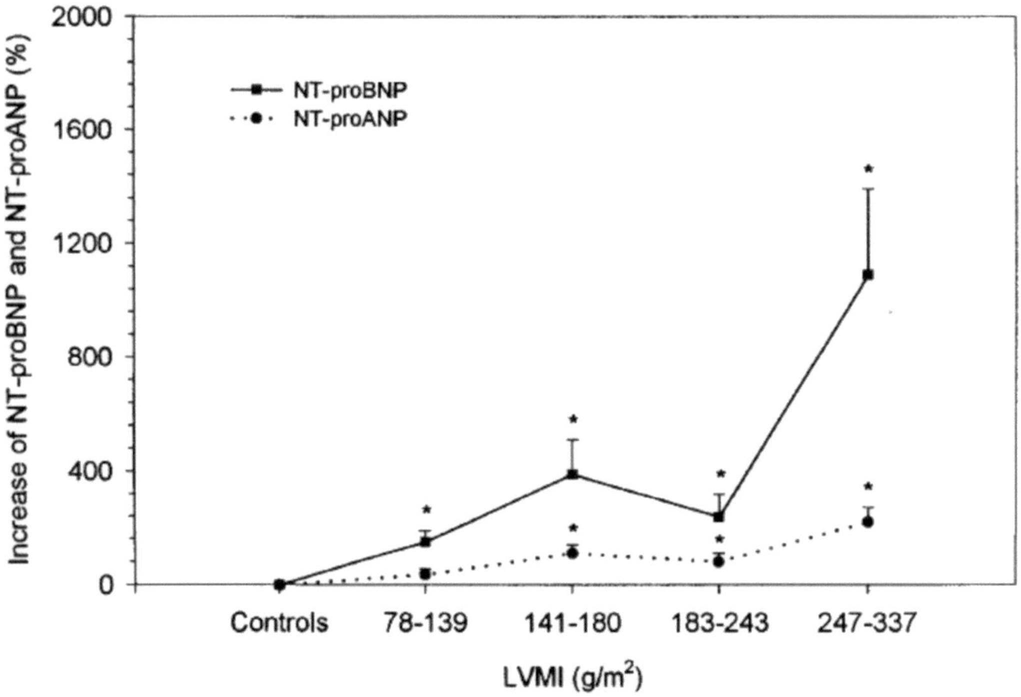

Fig. 3. Plot showing relation of NT-proBNP and NT-proANP to LVMI. *$P < .05$ vs control subjects. (adapted from Qi et al., 2001)

and passive excretion may also be responsible for some BNP clearance. In contrast, NT-proBNP has no specific clearance receptors and is mainly cleared by renal excretion. As a result, NT-proBNP has a longer half-life and circulates in higher concentrations in plasma. NT-proBNP is less influenced by short bursts of secretion, even though both molecules are released in equimolar proportions. (Qi, 2001; Boomsma, 2001)

ANP and NT-proANP are most closely associated with left atrial (LA) pressure as represented by pulmonary capillary wedge pressure (Qi et al., 2001) and the levels may result from increased LA pressure caused by LV systolic dysfunction and decompensation.

3. Natriuretic peptide levels in other cardiac and non-cardiac states

A number of cardiac and non-cardiac co-morbidities may influence natriuretic peptide levels. Cardiac examples include acute coronary syndromes, (de Lemos et al., 2001) mitral regurgitation, (Sutton et al., 2003) hypertrophic cardiomyopathy, (Hasegawa et al., 1993) advanced LV diastolic dysfunction, (Iwanaga et al., 2006) atrial fibrillation, (Iwanaga et al., 2006) and heart failure. Non-cardiac examples include severe respiratory disease, (Jensen et al., 1997) renal failure, (Jensen et al., 1997) fluid overload, and obesity. In patients with chronic kidney disease, decreased estimated glomerular filtration rate (GFR) is associated with increased plasma BNP and even greater elevation in NT-proBNP concentrations. Higher cut-off values for those with GFR <60mL/min/1.7m^2 have been suggested. (McCullough, 2003; Anwaruddin, 2006)

On average, obese patients tend to have lower plasma BNP and NT-proBNP levels than non-obese patients. (Das, 2005; Wang, 2005; Horwich, 2006) An inverse relationship between body mass index (BMI) and natriuretic peptides has been observed in patients both with and without heart failure. The underlying mechanism remains to be elucidated. Higher plasma BNP values within any body mass index category are associated with worse outcomes, (Horwich, 2006) although lower cut-offs are needed for diagnosing heart failure in obese patients.

It is unclear whether a single cut-point for the natriuretic peptides, as used for BNP in the diagnosis of heart failure (100 pg/mL), (Maisel et al., 2002) is appropriate for patients of all ages and both genders. Natriuretic peptide levels increase with aging in normal subjects and values are higher in women than in men with no cardiac disease after adjustment for age. (Wang, 2002; Gerber, 2003; Redfield, 2002) Some studies suggest BNP levels are related to oestrogen and/or testosterone levels, although results have been inconsistent. (Redfield, 2002; Costello-Boerrigter, 2006; Chang, 2007) These observations suggest the use of an age- and sex-specific threshold in different clinical settings could improve the diagnostic accuracy of natriuretic peptide levels and the clinical cut-off level should be elucidated in further studies. The specific assay used can also affect natriuretic peptide levels and contribute to different "normal" values.

4. Natriuretic peptides in aortic stenosis

Natriuretic peptide levels increase with the severity of aortic disease. (Gerber, 2003; Weber, 2005; Bergler-Klein, 2004; Weber, 2004) BNP and NT-proBNP levels correlate with peak-to-peak aortic valve and mean aortic gradient, and the correlation coefficients were stronger for BNP than for ANP. (Qi, 2001; Poulsen, 2007) Elevated BNP is also associated with lower AVA, (Gerber, 2003; Lim, 2004; Qi, 2001; Weber, 2003) although the correlation is lower than

with other echocardiographic parameters. The plasma level of BNP also increases with decrease in LV systolic function. These observations suggest serial measurements of BNP may be useful for monitoring patients with asymptomatic AS.
In the natural history of AS, a latent stage may exist during which LV hypertrophy compensates for the rise in afterload without producing a concomitant elevation of mean atrial pressure. As disease progresses, decompensation may occur with a reduction in the ratio between wall thickness and LV cavity size and a rise in atrial and pulmonary capillary wedge pressures.

4.1 Natriuretic peptides and functional status of AS patients

The transition from compensated to decompensated LV function may not be reliably detected by current echocardiographic measures such as ejection fraction, stroke volume, and transvalvular flow. In contrast, levels of natriuretic peptides correlate with the New York Heart Association (NYHA) symptom class and echocardiographic measures of LV dysfunction and therefore may be useful in indicating subtle LV pathology in asymptomatic patients. (Lim, 2004; Van Pelt, 2008; Weber, 2005; Gerber, 2005) Importantly, natriuretic peptide levels are on average higher in patients with NYHA class II symptoms than in patients with class I symptoms. This supports the notion that natriuretic peptide levels could be used to discriminate between early heart failure symptoms and normal effort tolerance (Figure 4). Interestingly, AVA is poorly correlated with the presence of symptoms. (Lim et al., 2004)

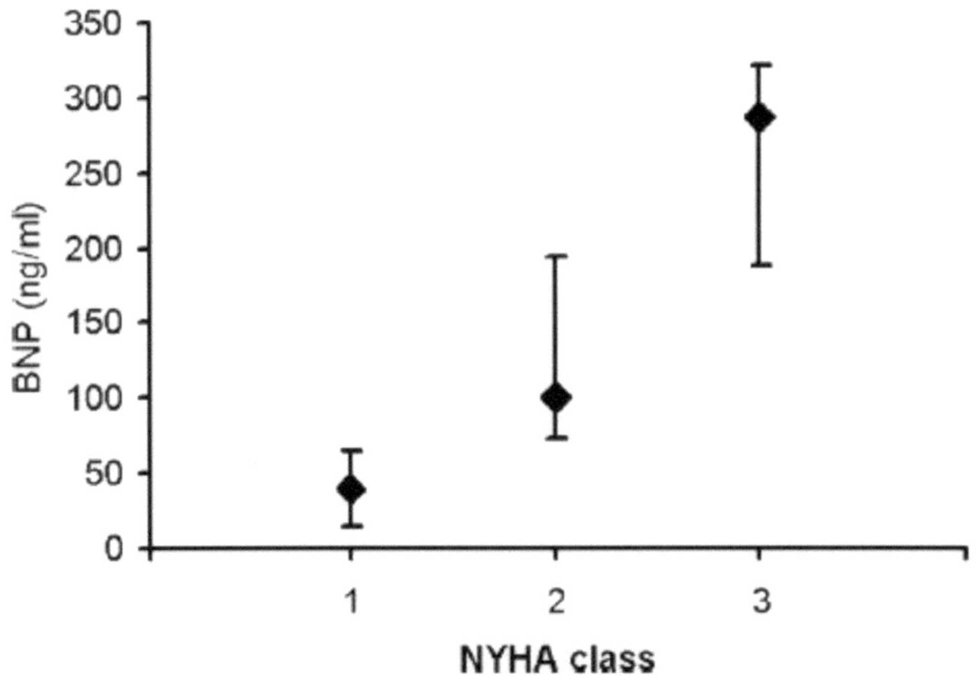

Fig. 4. Association between BNP levels (indicated as median and quartiles) and NYHA functional class (trend test, $p < 0.01$). (adapted from Lim et al., 2004)

In a study by Gerber et al and colleagues, 74 patients with severe AS were sub-grouped according to their AVA, symptom status, and LV EF. BNP and NT-proBNP levels were consistently higher in symptomatic patients referred for surgery whereas asymptomatic patients had lower natriuretic peptide levels (Figure 5). (Gerber et al., 2003)

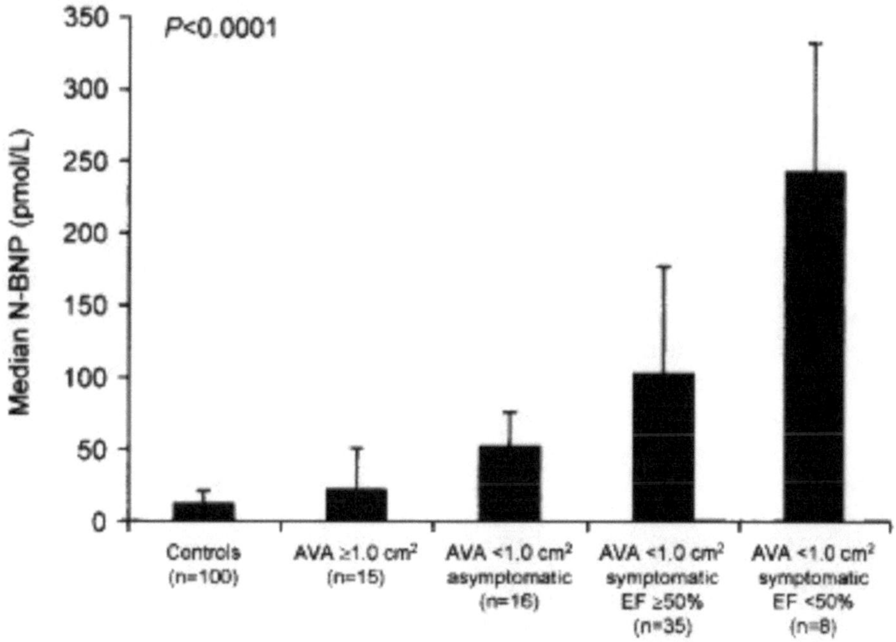

Fig. 5. Association between N-BNP levels and severity of aortic stenosis. The N-BNP levels (median [upper quartile]) in normal control subjects and in subgroups of patients with aortic stenosis by aortic valve area, symptoms, and LV systolic function are shown. AVA indicates aortic valve area; EF, ejection fraction. (adapted from Gerber et al., 2003)

Within each NYHA class, natriuretic peptide levels were not higher in patients with angina or syncope than in those without these symptoms, suggesting different pathophysiologies for these symptoms.

In a separate study, Gerber et al followed 29 asymptomatic patients with AS for an average of eighteen months. (Gerber et al., 2005) Patients with a plasma level of NT-proBNP that exceeded normal limits (>50 pmol/L) at baseline were more likely to develop symptoms earlier and significantly more often than those whose NT-proBNP levels were within normal limits. The average increase in NT-proBNP per year was also greater in patients who developed symptoms compared with those who remained asymptomatic. AVA, peak aortic velocity, and the ejection fraction were less reliable predictors of symptom onset. Similar findings were observed by Bergler-Klein et al in a group of 43 initially asymptomatic patients. (Bergler-Klein et al., 2004)

An abnormal blood pressure response to exercise is generally considered an indication for AVR in patients with asymptomatic AS. (Bonow et al., 2006) Exercise testing is recommended to assess AS patients with equivocal symptoms. However, there is sometimes reluctance to undertake an exercise test, or the patient may not be able to perform the test due to co-morbidities. A rise in plasma BNP may reflect early systolic dysfunction which results in a decrease in exercise capacity. Van Pelt et al demonstrated that AS patients with an increase in systolic BP of ≤20 mmHg during exercise had higher plasma levels of BNP than patients with an increase in systolic BP >20 mmHg. (Van Pelt et al., 2008) BNP was a superior predictor of abnormal blood pressure response than AVA, LV EF, diastolic function, and LV mass index. These observations support the use of BNP for monitoring asymptomatic patients or patients with equivocal symptoms, as well as patients who are unable to exercise. Newer echocardiographic methods such as tissue Doppler or speckle tracking methods which detect early deterioration of LV function also correlate with BNP levels. (Poulsen, 2007; Van Pelt, 2007)

4.2 Natriuretic peptides to predict outcome in asymptomatic severe AS

Echocardiography is the primary investigation for the assessment and monitoring of patients with AS, and the degree of aortic valve calcification, (Rosenhek et al., 2000) aortic valve area, parameters of LV function and LV hypertrophy each predict outcome in this group of patients, (Otto et al., 1997) although the severity of AS is the most important predictor. (Stewart et al., 2010) However, these echocardiographic parameters have only modest value in predicting individual risk. BNP levels have been shown to be independently prognostic of cardiovascular outcomes in patients with aortic stenosis who are treated without surgery (Figure 6). (Nessmith, 2005; Weber, 2006) BNP level is also an independent predictor for cardiovascular death in asymptomatic patients. (Lim et al., 2004) This may be explained if BNP is a more sensitive marker of early LV dysfunction than symptoms.

The risk of sudden cardiac death, (Pellikka, 2005; Rosenhek, 2000) as well as the risk of irreversible myocardial damage due to LV hypertrophy, (Lund et al., 2004) make risk stratification of patients with AS important. A comprehensive and objective approach that will facilitate decision making would, therefore, be of value.

A scoring system to predict adverse outcomes has been created by Monin et al for patients with asymptomatic severe aortic stenosis based on risk score including gender, BNP and peak aortic jet velocity at baseline. (Monin et al., 2009) These variables were chosen because each was independently associated with midterm adverse outcome. As no single value is an absolute criterion to define haemodynamic severity or to predict the development of symptoms, a continuous score integrating valve and ventricular related parameters may be more appropriate in selecting patients likely to benefit from early surgery. Independent predictors of outcome were female sex, peak aortic-jet velocity, and BNP at baseline. Accordingly, the score could be calculated as follows: Score = [peak velocity (m/s)×2]+(natural logarithm of BNP×1.5)+1.5 (if female sex). The use of aortic valve velocity and BNP emphasizes the haemodynamic effects at a valve level as well as the impact on the ventricle. Event-free survival after 20 months was 80% for patients within the first score quartile compared with only 7% for the fourth quartile. Areas under the receiver operating characteristic curves showed excellent performance of their risk score calculation. Future studies will also be needed to validate this strategy before implementing it as a risk calculator for bedside use.

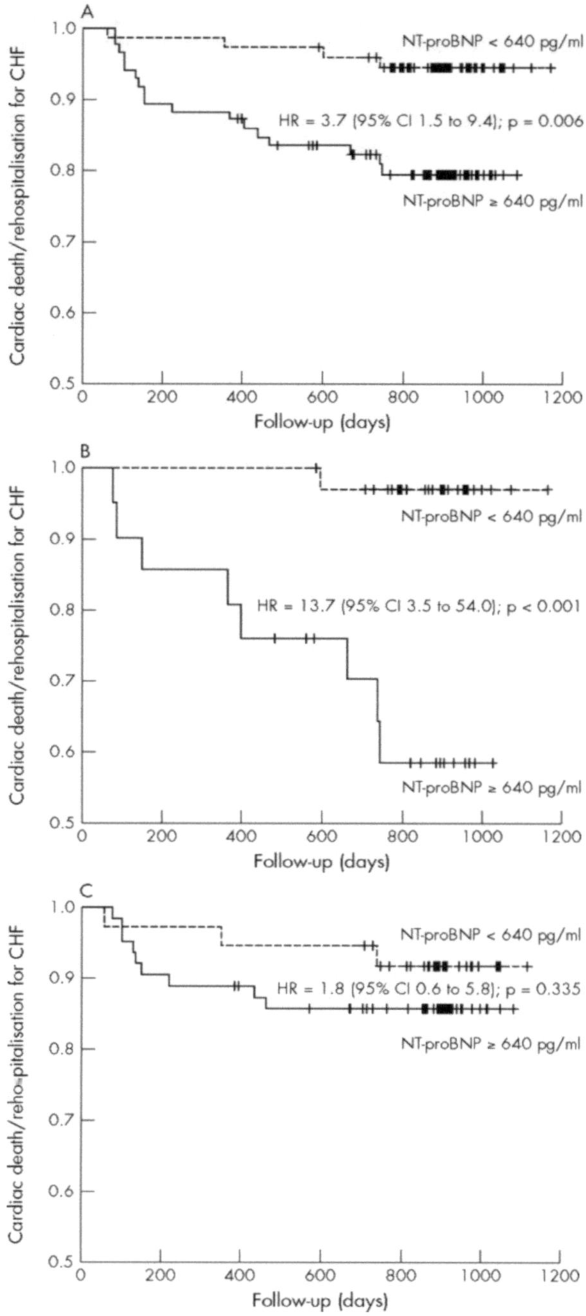

Fig. 6. Kaplan–Meier curves of event-free survival (freedom from cardiac death or rehospitalisation for decompensated heart failure (CHF)) of patients according to N-terminal pro-B-type natriuretic peptide (NT-proBNP) values above (solid line) and below (dotted line) a cut-off value of 640 pg/ml. (A) All patients. (B) Only conservatively treated patients. (C) Only surgically treated patients. CI, confidence interval; HR, hazard ratio. (adapted from Weber et al., 2006)

4.3 Natriuretic peptides and outcomes after aortic valve replacement

Preoperative NT-proBNP independently predicts perioperative and postoperative survival, necessity of intra-aortic balloon pump, postoperative symptomatic status, postoperative hospital stay, and postoperative LV function in patients undergoing heart surgery of various aetiologies. (Hutfless, 2004; Provenchere, 2006) Persistently elevated postoperative BNP levels are also associated with poorer outcomes and higher mortality after heart surgery. (Hutfless et al., 2004)

In symptomatic severe AS patients referred for AVR, preoperative natriuretic peptides were correlated with postoperative NYHA symptom class, LV function, and mortality. (Bergler-Klein, 2004; Predrazzini, 2008) Following AVR, BNP and NT-proBNP levels decrease over time, consistent with the expected haemodynamic improvement after valve replacement with relief of the LV afterload followed by reverse remodelling with gradual regression of LV hypertrophy. (Qi, 2002; Poulsen, 2007) The largest reduction is seen in patients with the largest postoperative valve area index. The postoperative decrease of NT-proBNP had also been demonstrated in some patients to be independently related to improvement of LV myocardial systolic longitudinal strain in echocardiography. (Van Pelt, 2007) However, BNP levels do not decrease in some patients. This may be due to persistent LV dysfunction or aortic prosthesis mismatch with a persistent residual LV outflow gradient from a small prosthetic valve orifice area. Patients who did not derive a symptomatic improvement from AVR were in lower NYHA class at baseline and had a tendency towards lower levels of NT-proBNP at study entry. (Weber et al., 2005)

5. BNP in low-flow, low-gradient aortic stenosis

The prognostic value of BNP in the particularly challenging subset of patients who have low-flow and low-gradient AS has also been studied. It is critical from the perspective of therapeutic decisions to make the distinction between severe AS and pseudo-severe AS who have a high operative mortality (Monin, 2003; Connolly, 2000) and a poor prognosis. It remains unclear which patients would derive benefit from AVR and which could be treated medically. In severe AS, the LV systolic dysfunction is related to the duration and severity of AS. In pseudo-severe AS, LV dysfunction from other causes results in low forward flow and reduced valve opening which overestimates the severity of AS. Dobutamine stress echocardiography (DSE) is potentially useful in distinguishing the two conditions (Blais, 2006; De Filippi, 1995) by assessing the response of valve area and gradient to a dobutamine-induced flow increase. Nonetheless, this differentiation remains difficult and it is uncertain whether DSE can reliably predict the outcome with surgery. (Monin, 2003; Quere, 2006)

Bergler-Klein and colleagues reported on 69 low-flow, low-gradient patients who underwent inotropic challenge and related the outcome to their BNP levels (Figure 7). (Bergler-Klein et al., 2007) The study included 29 patients with severe AS and 40 patients with pseudo-severe AS. BNP levels were higher in patients with true AS when compared with pseudo-AS, a finding consistent with the concept that BNP is elevated in AS due to the effect on wall tension and ventricular stretch associated with the increased after-load in addition to the failing LV. Nonetheless, a significant overlap of BNP values was observed between groups.

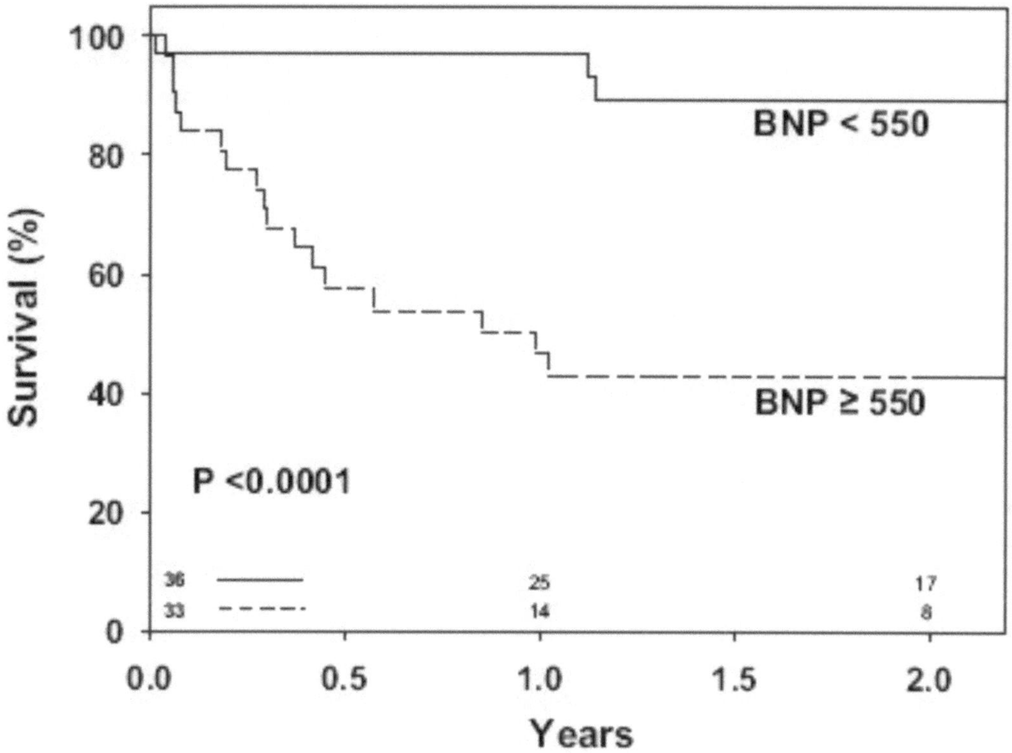

Fig. 7. Kaplan-Meier survival curve for the entire study population according to baseline BNP<550 or ≥550 pg/mL. A BNP of >550 pg/mL was found to be associated with a poor outcome for both groups, with only 47% of such patients surviving for 1 year compared with 97% survival in patients with lower BNP values. (adapted from Bergler-Klein et al., 2007))

BNP level >550 pg/mL remained the strongest independent predictor of survival when factors such as New York Heart Association functional class, LV EF, contractile reserve, the status of true or pseudo-AS, medical versus surgical therapy, and other clinical variables such as coronary artery disease or diabetes were considered. Therefore, BNP could potentially be used to improve risk stratification and management of this group of patients. However, BNP is non-specific with plasma levels increasing with heart failure due to many causes. More data will be required before BNP can be formally used for therapeutic recommendations.

6. Conclusion

Together with clinical and echocardiographic parameters, measurement of BNP may improve risk stratification and management of patients with AS. BNP and NT-proBNP are important prognostic markers and predictors of symptom-free survival in patients with severe AS. A patient with severe AS and a high plasma level of BNP is likely to carry a high risk of adverse events, and aortic valve replacement should be considered. Measurement of BNP may complement clinical and echocardiographic evaluation, allow more reliable follow-up, and improve the optimal timing of AVR surgery by early identification of the transition from compensated to decompensated LV function. Serially rising levels could also be helpful in identifying patients with LV dysfunction, but current evidence for such use is limited. Clinical judgment will be needed to interpret the significance of a BNP measurement in patients with AS.

7. Acknowledgements

We thank Charlene Nell, Team Support Administrator, Green Lane Cardiovascular Research Unit, for excellent secretarial assistance.

8. References

Anwaruddin, S.; Lloyd-Jones, D.; Baggish, A.; Chen, A.; Krauser, D.; Tung, R.; Chae, C. & Januzzi, J. Jr. (2006). Renal function, congestive heart failure, and amino-terminal pro-brain natriuretic peptide measurement: results from the ProBNP Investigation of Dyspnea in the Emergency Department (PRIDE) study. *Journal of the American College of Cardiology,* Vol.47, No.1, (January 2006), pp. 91–97, ISSN: 0735-1097.

Bergler-Klein, J.; Klaar, U.; Heger, M.; Rosenhek, R.; Mundigler, G.; Gabriel, H.; Binder, T.; Pacher, R.; Maurer, G. & Baumgartner, H. (2004). Natriuretic peptides predict symptom-free survival and postoperative outcome in severe aortic stenosis. *Circulation,* Vol.109, No.19, (May 2004), pp. 2302–2308, ISSN: 0009-7322.

Bergler-Klein, J.; Mundigler, G.; Pibarot, P.; Burwash, I.; Dumesnil, J.; Blais, C.; Fuchs, C.; Mohty, D.; Beanlands, R.; Hachicha, Z.; Walter-Publig, N.; Rader, F. & Baumgartner, H. (2007). B-type natriuretic peptide in low-flow, low-gradient aortic stenosis: relationship to hemodynamics and clinical outcome: results from the Multicenter Truly or Pseudo-Severe Aortic Stenosis (TOPAS) study. *Circulation,* Vol.115, No.22, (June 2007), pp. 2848–2855, ISSN: 0009-7322.

Bettencourt, P. (2005). Clinical usefulness of B-type natriuretic peptide measurement: present and future perspectives. *Heart,* Vol.91, No.11, (November 2005), pp. 1489-1494, ISSN: 1468-201X.

Blais, C.; Burwash, I.; Mundigler, G.; Dumesnil, J.; Loho, N.; Rader, F.; Baumgartner, H.; Beanlands, R.; Chayer, B.; Kadem, L.; Garcia, D.; Durand, L. & Pibarot, P. (2006). Projected valve area at normal flow rate improves the assessment of stenosis severity in patients with low-flow, low-gradient aortic stenosis: the multicenter TOPAS (Truly Or Pseudo-Severe Aortic Stenosis) study. *Circulation,* Vol.113, No.5, (February 2006), pp. 711–721, ISSN: 0009-7322.

Bonow, R.; Carabello, B.; Chatterjee, K.; de Leon, A. Jr; Faxon, D.; Freed, M.; Gaasch, W.; Lytle, B.; Nishimura, R.; O'Gara, P.; O'Rourke, R.; Otto, C.; Shah, P.; Shanewise, J.; Smith, S., Jr; Jacobs, A.; Adams, C.; Anderson, J.; Antman, E.; Fuster, V.; Halperin, J.; Hiratzka, L.; Hunt, S.; Lytle, B.; Nishimura, R.; Page, R. & Riegel, B. (2006). ACC/AHA 2006 guidelines for the management of patients with valvular heart disease: a report of the American College of Cardiology/American Heart Association Task Force on Practice Guidelines (writing Committee to Revise the 1998 guidelines for the management of patients with valvular heart disease) developed in collaboration with the Society of Cardiovascular Anesthesiologists endorsed by the Society for Cardiovascular Angiography and Interventions and the Society of Thoracic. *Journal of the American College of Cardiology,* Vol.48, No.3, (August 2006), pp. e1–e148, ISSN: 0735-1097.

Boomsma, F. & van den Meiracker, A. (2001). Plasma A- and B-type natriuretic peptides: physiology, methodology and clinical use. *Cardiovascular Research,* Vol.51, No.3, (August 2001), pp. 442-449, ISSN: 1755-3245.

Brown, L.; Nunez, D. & Wilkins, M. (1993). Differential regulation of natriuretic peptide receptor messenger RNAs during the development of cardiac hypertrophy in the rat. *Journal of Clinical Investigation,* Vol.92, No.6, (December 1993), pp. 2702-2712, ISSN: 0021-9738.

Cameron, V.; Aitken, G.; Ellmers, L.; Kennedy, M. & Espiner, E. (1996). The sites of gene expression of atrial, brain, and C-type natriuretic peptides in mouse fetal development: temporal changes in embryos and placenta. *Endocrinology,* Vol.137, No.3, (March 1996), pp. 817-824, ISSN: 0013-7227.

Chang, A.; Abdullah, S.; Jain, T.; Stanek, H.; Das, S.; McGuire, D.; Auchus, R. & de Lemos, J. (2007). Associations among androgens, estrogens, and natriuretic peptides in young women: observations from the Dallas Heart Study. *Journal of the American College of Cardiology,* Vol.49, No.1, (January 2007), pp. 109-16, ISSN: 0735-1097.

Connolly, H.; Oh, J.; Schaff, H.; Roger, V.; Osborn, S.; Hodge, D. & Tajik, A. (2000). Severe aortic stenosis with low transvalvular gradient and severe left ventricular dysfunction: result of aortic valve replacement in 52 patients. *Circulation,* Vol.101, No.16, (April 2000), pp. 1940–1946, ISSN: 0009-7322.

Costello-Boerrigter, L. & Burnett, J., Jr. (2005). The prognostic value of N-terminal proB-type natriuretic peptide. *Nature Clinical Practice. Cardiovascular Medicine,* Vol.2, No.4, (April 2005), pp. 194-201, ISSN: 1759-5002.

Costello-Boerrigter, L.; Boerrigter, G.; Redfield, M.; Rodeheffer, R.; Urban, L.; Mahoney, D.; Jacobsen, S.; Heublein, D. & Burnett, J., Jr. (2006). Amino terminal pro-B-type natriuretic peptide and B-type natriuretic peptide in the general community: determinants and detection of left ventricular dysfunction. *Journal of the American College of Cardiology,* Vol.47, No.2, (January 2006), pp. 345–53, ISSN: 0735-1097.

Das, S.; Drazner, M.; Dries, D.; Vega, G.; Stanek, H.; Abdullah, S.; Canham, R.; Chung, A.; Leonard, D.; Wians, F., Jr. & de Lemos, J. (2005). Impact of body mass and body composition on circulating levels of natriuretic peptides: results from the Dallas Heart Study. *Circulation,* Vol.112, No.14, (October 2005), pp. 2163-2168, ISSN: 0009-7322.

De Filippi, C.; Willett, D.; Brickner, E.; Appleton, C.; Yancy, C.; Eichhorn, E. & Grayburn, P. (2005). Usefulness of dobutamine echocardiography in distinguishing severe from nonsevere valvular aortic stenosis in patients with depressed left ventricular function and low transvalvular gradients. *American Journal of Cardiology,* Vol.75, No.2, (January 1995), pp. 191–194, ISSN: 0002-9149.

de Lemos, J.; Morrow, D.; Bentley, J.; Omland, T.; Sabatine, M.; McCabe, C.; Hall, C.; Cannon, C. & Braunwald, E. (2001). The prognostic value of B-type natriuretic peptide in patients with acute coronary syndromes. *New England Medical Journal.* Vol.345, No.14, (October 2001), pp. 1014-1021, ISSN: 0028-4793.

Edwards. F.; Peterson, E.; Coombs, L.; DeLong, E.; Jamieson, W.; Shroyer, A. & Grover, F. (2001). Prediction of operative mortality after valve replacement surgery. *Journal of the American College of Cardiology,* Vol.37, No.3, (March 2001), pp. 885–892, ISSN: 0735-1097.

Frank, S.; Johnson, A. & Ross, J., Jr. (1973) Natural history of valvular aortic stenosis. *British Heart Journal,* Vol.35, No.1, (January 1973), pp. 41–46, ISSN: 1468-201X.

Gerber, I.; Stewart, R.; Legget, M.; West, T.; French, R.; Sutton, T.; Yandle, T.; French, J.; Richards, A. & White, H. (2003) Increased plasma natriuretic peptide levels reflect symptom onset in aortic stenosis. *Circulation,* Vol.107, No.14, (April 2003), pp. 1884–1890, ISSN: 0009-7322.

Gerber, I.; Legget, M.; West, T.; Richards, A. & Stewart, R. (2005). Usefulness of serial measurement of N-terminal pro-brain natriuretic peptide plasma levels in asymptomatic patients with aortic stenosis to predict symptomatic deterioration. *American Journal of Cardiology,* Vol.95, No.7, (April 2005), pp. 898–901, ISSN: 0002-9149.

Hasegawa, K.; Fujiwara, H.; Doyama, K.; Miyamae, M.; Fujiwara, T.; Suga, S.; Mukoyama, M.; Nakao, K.; Imura, H. & Sasayama, S. (1993). Ventricular expression of brain natriuretic peptide in hypertrophic cardiomyopathy. *Circulation,* Vol.88, No.2, (August 1993), pp. 372-380, ISSN: 0009-7322.

Horwich, T.; Hamilton, M. & Fonarow, G. B-type natriuretic Peptide levels in obese patients with advanced heart failure. (2006). *Journal of the American College of Cardiology,* Vol.47, No1, (January 2006), pp. 85-90, ISSN: 0735-1097.

Hunt. P.; Richards, A.; Nicholls, M.; Yandle, T.; Doughty, R. & Espiner, E. (1997). Immunoreactive amino-terminal pro-brain natriuretic peptide (NT-PROBNP): a new marker of cardiac impairment. *Clinical Endocrinology (Oxf).* Vol.47, No.3, (September 1997), pp. 287-296, ISSN: 1365-2265.

Hutfless, R.; Kazanegra, R.; Madani, M.; Bhalla, M.; Tulua-Tata, A.; Chen, A.; Clopton, P.; James, C.; Chiu, A. & Maisel, A. (2004). Utility of B-type natriuretic peptide in predicting postoperative complications and outcomes in patients undergoing heart surgery. *Journal of the American College of Cardiology,* Vol.43, No.10, (May 2004), pp. 1873–1879, ISSN: 0735-1097.

Iwanaga, Y.; Nishi, I.; Furuichi, S.; Noguchi, T.; Sase, K.; Kihara, Y.; Goto, Y. & Nonogi, H. (2006). B-type natriuretic peptide strongly reflects diastolic wall stress in patients with chronic heart failure: comparison between systolic and diastolic heart failure. *Journal of the American College of Cardiology,* Vol.47, No.4, (February 2006), pp. 742–748, ISSN: 0735-1097.

Jensen, K.; Carstens, J.; Ivarsen, P. & Pedersen, E. (1997). A new, fast and reliable radioimmunoassay of brain natriuretic peptide in human plasma: reference values in healthy subjects and in patients with different diseases. *Scandinavian Journal of Clinical and Laboratory Investigation,* Vol.57, No.6, (October 1997), pp. 529-540, ISSN: 0036-5513.

Lim, P.; Monin, J.; Monchi, M.; Garot, J.; Pasquet, A.; Hittinger, L.; Vanoverschelde, J.; Carayon, A. & Gueret, P. (2004). Predictors of outcome in severe aortic stenosis and normal left ventricular function: role of B-type naturetic peptide. *European Heart Journal,* Vol.25, No.22, (November 2004), pp. 2048 –2053, ISSN: 1522-9645.

Lund, O.; Erlandsen, M.; Dorup, I.; Emmertsen, K.; Flo, C. & Jensen, F. (2004). Predictable changes in left ventricular mass and function during ten years after valve replacement for aortic stenosis. *Journal of Heart Valve Disease,* Vol.13, No.3, (May 2004), pp. 357–368, ISSN: 0966-8519.

Maisel, A.; Krishnaswamy, P.; Nowak, R.; McCord, J.; Hollander, J.; Duc, P.; Omland, T.; Storrow, A.; Abraham, W.; Wu, A.; Clopton, P.; Steg, P.; Westheim, A.; Knudsen, C.; Perez, A.; Kazanegra, R.; Herrmann, H. & McCullough, P. for Breathing Not Properly Multinational Study Investigators. (2002). Rapid measurement of B-type natriuretic peptide in the emergency diagnosis of heart failure. *New England Medical Journal,* Vol.347, No.3, (July 2002), pp. 161-167, ISSN: 0028-4793.

McCullough, P.; Duc, P.; Omland, T.; McCord, J.; Nowak, R.; Hollander, J.; Herrmann, H.; Steg, P.; Westheim, A.; Knudsen, C.; Storrow, A.; Abraham, W.; Lamba, S.; Wu, A.; Perez, A.; Clopton, P.; Krishnaswamy, P.; Kazanegra, R. & Maisel, A. for Breathing Not Properly Multinational Study Investigators. (2003). B-type natriuretic peptide and renal function in the diagnosis of heart failure: an analysis from the Breathing Not Properly Multinational Study. *American Journal of Kidney Disease,* Vol.41, No.3, (March 2003), pp. 571–579, ISSN: 0272-6386.

Monin, J.; Quere, J.; Monchi, M.; Petit, H.; Baleynaud, S.; Chauvel, C.; Pop, C.; Ohlmann, P.; Lelguen, C.; Dehant, P.; Tribouilloy, C. & Gueret, P. (2003). Low gradient aortic stenosis: operative risk stratification and predictors for long-term outcome: a multicenter study using dobutamine stress hemodynamics. *Circulation,* Vol.108, No.3, (July 2003), pp. 319–324, ISSN: 0009-7322.

Monin, J.; Lancellotii, P.; Monchi, M.; Lim, P.; Weiss, E.; Piérard, L. & Gueret P. (2009). Risk score for predicting outcome in patients with asymptomatic aortic stenosis. *Circulation,* Vol.120, No.1, (July 2009), pp. 69–75, ISSN: 0009-7322.

Nessmith, M.; Fukuta, H.; Brucks, S. & Little, W. (2005). Usefulness of an elevated B-type natriuretic peptide in predicting survival in patients with aortic stenosis treated without surgery. *American Journal of Cardiology,* Vol.96, No.10, (November 2005), pp. 1445–1448, ISSN: 0002-9149.

Otto, C.; Burwash, I.; Legget, M.; Munt, B.; Fujioka, M.; Healy, N.; Kraft, C.; Miyake-Hull, C. & Schwaegler, R. (1997). Prospective study of asymptomatic valvular aortic stenosis. Clinical, echocardiographic, and exercise predictors of outcome. *Circulation,* Vol.95, No.9, (May 1997), pp. 2262–2270, ISSN: 0009-7322.

Otto, C. (1998). Aortic stenosis: clinical evaluation and optimal timing of surgery. *Cardiology Clinics,* Vol.16, No.3, (August 1998), pp. 353–373, ISSN: 0733-8651.

Otto, C. (2000). Aortic stenosis: listen to the patient, look at the valve. *New England Journal of Medicine,* Vol.343, No.3, (August 2000), pp. 652–654, ISSN: 0028-4793.

Pedrazzini, G.; Masson, S.; Latini, R.; Klersy, C.; Rossi, M.; Pasotti, E.; Faletra, F.; Siclari, F.; Minervini, F.; Moccetti, T. & Auricchio, A. (2008). Comparison of brain natriuretic peptide plasma levels versus logistic EuroSCORE in predicting in-hospital and late postoperative mortality in patients undergoing aortic valve replacement for symptomatic aortic stenosis. *American Journal of Cardiology,* Vol.102, No.6, (September 2008), pp. 749–754, ISSN: 0002-9149.

Pellikka, P.; Sarano, M.; Nishimura, R.; Malouf, J.; Bailey, K.; Scott, C.; Barnes. M. & Tajik, A. (2005). Outcome of 622 adults with asymptomatic, hemodynamically significant aortic stenosis during prolonged follow-up. *Circulation,* Vol.111, No.24, (June 2005), pp. 3290–3295, ISSN: 0009-7322.

Poulsen, S.; Sogaard, P.; Nielsen-Kudsk, J. & Egeblad, H. (2007). Recovery of left ventricular systolic longitudinal strain after valve replacement in aortic stenosis and relation to natriuretic peptides. *Journal of the American Society of Echocardiography,* Vol.20, No.7, (July 2007), pp. 877–884, ISSN: 0894-7317.

Provenchere, S.; Berroeta, C.; Reynaud, C.; Baron, G.; Poirier, I.; Desmonts, J.; Iung, B.; Dehoux, M.; Philip, I. & Bénessiano, J. (2006). Plasma brain natriuretic peptide and cardiac troponin I concentrations after adult cardiac surgery: association with postoperative cardiac dysfunction and 1-year mortality. *Critical Care Medicine,* Vol.34, No.4, (April 2006), pp. 995–1000, ISSN: 0090-3493.

Qi, W.; Mathisen, P.; Kjekshus, J.; Simonsen, S.; Bjornerheim, R.; Endresen, K. & Hall, C. Natriuretic peptides in patients with aortic stenosis. *American Heart Journal,* Vol. 142, No.4, (October 2001), pp. 725–32, ISSN: 0002-8703.

Qi, W.; Mathisen, P.; Kjekshus, J.; Simonsen, S.; Endresen, K.; Bjornerheim, R. & Hall, C. The effect of aortic valve replacement on n-terminal natriuretic propeptides in patients with aortic stenosis. *Clinical Cardiology,* Vol.25, No.4 (April 2002), pp. 174–78, ISSN: 1932-8737.

Quere JP, Monin JL, Levy F, Petit H, Baleynaud S, Chauvel C, Pop C, Ohlmann P, Lelguen C, Dehant P, Gueret P, Tribouilloy C. Influence of preoperative left ventricular contractile reserve on postoperative ejection fraction in low-gradient aortic stenosis. *Circulation,* Vol.113, No.14, (April 2006), pp. 1738–1744, ISSN: 0009-7322.

Redfield, M.M.; Rodeheffer, R.J; Jacobsen, S.J.; Mahoney, D. W.; Bailey, K. R. & Burnett, J. C. Plasma brain natriuretic peptide concentration: impact of age and gender. *Journal of the American College of Cardiology,* Vol.40, No.5, (September 2002), pp. 976–82, ISSN: 0735-1097.

Rosenhek, R.; Binder, T.; Porenta, G.; Lang, I.; Christ, G.; Schemper, M.; Maurer, G. & Baumgartner, H. Predictors of outcome in severe, asymptomatic aortic stenosis. *New England Journal of Medicine,* Vol.343, No.9, (August 2000), pp. 611–617, ISSN: 0028-4793.

Rosenhek, R.; Maurer, G. & Baumgartner H. Should early elective surgery be performed in patients with severe but asymptomatic aortic stenosis? *European Heart Journal,* Vol.23, No.18, (September 2002), pp. 1417–1421, ISSN: 1522-9645.

Ross, J. Jr. & Braunwald, E. Aortic stenosis. *Circulation,* Vol.38, Suppl 1, (July 1968), pp. 61–67, ISSN: 0009-7322.

Sadoshima, J.; Jahn, L. & Takahashi, T. Molecular characterization of the stretch-induced adaptation of cultured cardiac cells: an in vitro model of load-induced cardiac hypertrophy. *Journal of Biological Chemistry,* Vol.267, No.15, (May 1992), pp. 10551-60, ISSN: 0021-9258.

Stewart, R.A.; Kerr, A.J.; Whalley, G.A.; Legget, M.E.; Zeng, I.; Williams, M.J.; Lainchbury, J.; Hamer, A.; Doughty, R.; Richards, M.A. & White, H.D. The New Zealand Heart Valve Study Investigators. Left ventricular systolic and diastolic function assessed by tissue Doppler imaging and outcome in asymptomatic aortic stenosis. *European Heart Journal,* Vol.31, No.18, (September 2010), pp. 2216-22, ISSN: 1522-9645.

Sutton ,T.M.; Stewart, R.A.H.; Gerber, I.L.; West, T. M.; Richards, A. M.; Yandle, T. G. & Kerr, A. J. Plasma natriuretic peptide levels increase with symptoms and severity of mitral regurgitation. *Journal of the American College of Cardiology,* Vol.41, No.12, (June 2003), pp. 2280-2287, ISSN: 0735-1097.

Van Pelt, N.C.; Stewart, R.A.; Legget, M.E.; Whalley, G. A.; Wong, S. P.; Zeng, I.; Oldfield, M. & Kerr, A. J. Longitudinal left ventricular contractile dysfunction after exercise in aortic stenosis. *Heart,* Vol.93, No.6, (June 2007), pp. 732–738, ISSN: 1468-201X

Van Pelt, N.C.; Kerr, A.J.; Legget, M.E.; Pasupati, S.; Wahlley, G.; Wong S.; Zeng, I. & Stewart RAH. Increased B-type natriuretic peptide is associated with an abnormal blood pressure response to exercise in asymptomatic aortic stenosis. *International Journal of Cardiology.* Vol.127, No.3 , (July 2008), pp. 313–320, ISSN: 0167-5273.

Wachtell, K. Left ventricular systolic performance in asymptomatic aortic stenosis. *European Heart Journal Supplements,* Vol.10, Suppl E, (July 2008), pp. E16 -E22, ISSN: 1522-9645.

Wang, T.J.; Larson, M.G.; Levy, D.; Leip, E. P.; Benjamin, E. J.; Wilson, P. W.; Sutherland, P.; Omland, T. & Vasan, R. S. Impact of age and sex on plasma natriuretic peptide levels in healthy adults. *American Journal of Cardiology,* Vol.90, No.3, (August 2002), pp. 254–258, ISSN: 0002-9149.

Wang, T.J.; Larson, M.G.; Levy, D.; Benjamin, E.J.; Leip, E.P.; Wilson, P.W.; Vasan, .R.S. Impact of obesity on plasma natriuretic peptide levels. *Circulation,* Vol.109, No.5, (February 2004), pp. 594-600, ISSN: 0009-7322.

Weber, M.; Arnold, R. & Rau M. N-terminal pro brain type natriuretic peptide is a highly sensitive biochemical marker for surgical therapy in patients with aortic stenosis. *Circulation,* Vol.108, (2003), pp. IV-513, ISSN: 0009-7322.

Weber, M.; Arnold, R.; Rau, M.; Brandt, R.; Berkovitsch, A.; Mitrovic, V. & Hamm, C. Relation of N-terminal pro-B-type natriuretic peptide to severity of valvular aortic stenosis. *American Journal of Cardiology,* Vol.94, No.6, (September 2004), pp. 740–745, ISSN: 0002-9149.

Weber, M.; Arnold, R., Rau, M.; Elsaesser, A.; Brandt, R.; Mitrovic, V. & Hamm, C. Relation of N-terminal pro B-type natriuretic peptide to progression of aortic valve disease. *European Heart Journal,* Vol.26, No.10, (May 2005), pp. 1023–1030, ISSN: 1522-9645.

Weber, M.; Hausen, M.; Arnold, R.; Nef, H.; Moellman, H.; Berkowitsch, A.; Elsaesser, A.; Brandt, R.; Mitrovic, V. & Hamm, C. Prognostic value of N-terminal pro-B-type natriuretic peptide for conservatively and surgically treated patients with aortic valve stenosis. *Heart,* Vol.92, No.11, (November 2006), pp. 1639–1644, ISSN: 1468-201X.

Yandle, T.G.; Espiner, E.A.; Nicholls, M.G. & Duff, H. Radioimmunoassay and characterization of atrial natriuretic peptide in human plasma. *Journal of Clinical Endocrinology Metabolism,* Vol.63, No.1, (July 1986), pp. 72-79, ISSN: 1945-7197.

Yandle, T.G.; Richards, A.M.; Gilbert, A.; Fisher, S.; Holmes, S. & Espiner, E. A. Assay of brain natriuretic peptide (BNP) in human plasma: evidence for high molecular weight BNP as a major plasma component in heart failure. *Journal of Clinical Endocrinology Metabolism,* Vol.76, No.4, (April 1993), pp. 832-838, ISSN: 1945-7197.

Yasue, H.; Yoshimura, M.; Sumida, H.; Kikuta, K.; Kugiyama, K.; Jougasaki, M.; Ogawa, H.; Okumura, K.; Mukoyama, M. & Nakao, K. Localization and mechanism of secretion of B-type natriuretic peptide in comparison with those of A-type natriuretic peptide in normal subjects and patients with heart failure. *Circulation,* Vol.90, No.1, (July 1994), pp. 195–203, ISSN: 0009-7322.

Yoshimura, M.; Yasue, H.; Okumura, K.; Ogawa, H.; Jougasaki, M.; Mukoyama, M.; Nakao, K. & Imura, H. Different secretion patterns of atrial natriuretic peptide and brain natriuretic peptide in patients with congestive heart failure. *Circulation*, Vol.87, No.2, (February 1993), pp. 464–9, ISSN: 0009-7322.

14

Cellular and Neuronal Aspects in Aortic Stenosis

J. Ker[1] and WFP Van Heerden[2]
[1]*Physician, University of Pretoria, Pretoria,*
[2]*Pathologist, University of Pretoria, Pretoria,*
South Africa

1. Introduction

For quite some time the physiological approach to cardiac valve function held the belief that these are purely passive structures merely moving in response to changes in transvalvular pressure generated by atrial and ventricular contractions [1, 2, 3]. Today, this "passive hypothesis" is being challenged as numerous studies have shown that mammalian cardiac valves are capable of independent contraction during various stages of the cardiac cycle [1, 4, 5]. In order to understand this concept and the pathophysiological implications for valvular disorders, one would need to understand the cellular components and appreciate the neural network innervating the diverse cellular milieu of the cardiac valve as we understand it today.

The diverse cellular population of the aortic valve, together with its neuronal network will be discussed in order to clarify the cellular and neuronal aspects of the complex and still incompletely understood process of aortic stenosis.

2. Macro structure of the aortic valve

As a unit, the aortic valve is composed of four parts: the aortic annulus, the aortic valvular cusps, the sinuses of Valsalva and the sinotubular junction [3]. The three semi-lunar cusps are attached at their base to a crown-shaped annulus [3]. The interaction between the cusps and the root is extremely important to ensure adequate coronary blood flow. Proper closure of the cusps in diastole helps to preserve the shape of the aortic root and this ensures the creation of vortices of blood flow in the sinuses of Valsalva which is a major determinant of coronary blood flow [3].

The aortic cusps are composed of three layers: the fibrosa, the spongiosa and the ventricularis [3]. The fibrosa lines the aortic side and is rich in collagen fibers, whereas the ventricularis lines the ventricular side and is rich in elastin fibers [3, 6]. The spongiosa lies between these two layers and is composed primarily of proteoglycans [3, 6].

3. Cellular components of the aortic cusps

Both sides of the aortic valve cusps, the fibrosa and ventricularis, are lined by endothelial cells [1, 2, 3]. These valvular endothelial cells are able to respond to stress placed on the cusps, particularly shear stress and can produce several vasoactive mediators, such as nitric oxide, endothelins and prostaglandins [1, 7, 8], thus translating mechanical stimuli into biological responses, referred to as mechanotransduction [3]. The actual release of these various vasoactive mediators can be effected by neurotransmitters such as acetylcholine and substance P, released by nerve endings innervating the valvular cusps [7, 8]. These substances released by the endothelium can in turn stimulate the local nerve terminals and elicit various reflex responses [1, 9]. The role of this "endothelium-cusp-nerve interaction" in health and disease is an interesting and yet insufficiently explained arena in the healthy and diseased aortic valve.

Below the layer of endothelial cells lining the outer and inner layer of the aortic cusps (the fibrosa and ventricularis), the extracellular matrix is found, composed of elastin, collagen and proteoglycans [10]. In addition to the elastin, collagen and proteoglycans in this extracellular matrix, a population of valve interstitial cells can be found [2, 3]. These consist of fibroblasts, smooth muscle cells and myofibroblasts [2, 3, 11]. The proportion of these different cells comprising the interstitial cell component will depend on the condition and state of health of the valve [2]. These cells possess important secretory and proliferative properties to repair and maintain the extracellular matrix [2, 3]. They also have contractile properties and express the same structural genes as cardiac muscle, such as cardiac troponin T, I and C, cardiac myosin light chain and beta myosin heavy chain [2, 12]. Immunohistological studies have shown that almost 60% of aortic valve interstitial cells can express alpha-smooth muscle actin [2, 13].

The most recently identified cell type in the aortic valve is a population of resident stem cells which lie within the cusps [3, 14]. These cells are hematopoietic in origin with later mobilization towards the valve cusps [15].

The human aortic valve is an avascular structure, but is innervated by a network of afferent and efferent nerves [3].

4. The aortic neural network

The neural innervation of the aortic valve arise from two sources, the ventricular endocardial plexus [1] and the aortic adventitial wall [16]. These nerves are found in the entire leaflet, except at the coapting edge [1]. Compared to the two coronary leaflets, the noncoronary leaflet displays an attenuated density of innervation and the density of innervation declines in all the leaflets with advancing age [1]. This decline in valvular neural innervation with age seems to be limited to the aortic valve [1]. It seems that each cardiac valve is independently innervated with no nerve fibers extending between valves [2]. The thin aortic nerves display a circumferential pattern within each leaflet [2, 17]. Morphologically and neurochemically these valvular nerve endings appear similar to the nerve endings found in the epicardium and endocardium of the human heart [1, 18]. Aortic nerve terminals has been found to express immunoreactivity for tyrosine hydroxylase, neuropeptide Y, acetylcholinesterase, substance P and vasoactive intestinal peptide (VIP) [1, 2, 19]. These various neurotransmitters also have neuromodulatory effects, regulating the activity of several populations of neurons in the valve [2].

Thus, it is clear that there exists a rich cellular milieu inside the cusps of the aortic valve, with a rich supply of nerve endings, each one releasing neurotransmitters with diverse

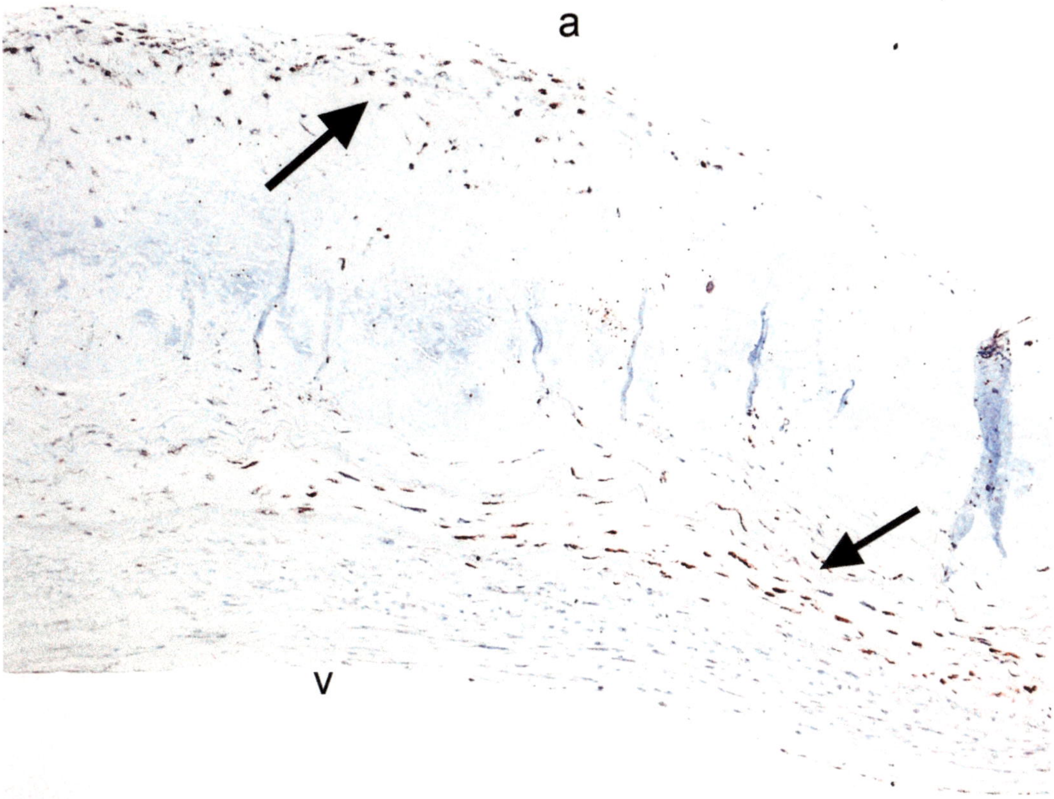

Fig. 1. S-100 staining of a stenotic valve shows the presence of positive spindle shaped cells suggestive of Schwann cells (arrows). (original magnification X 100).

physiological effects, effecting a complex array of contractile, secretory and homeostatic actions [2]. (Fig. 1). The aortic valve can thus be seen as a structure that is regulated by a local neural network very similar to the gastrointestinal tract, bronchial tree and blood vessels [2].

5. Diverse cellular changes in aortic stenosis

A cell not seen in the normal aortic valve is the osteoblast. However, during the inflammatory process leading to ultimate aortic stenosis, aortic valve myofibroblasts may differentiate into osteoblasts and thus contribute towards valve calcification [20]. (Fig 2).
Normal aortic valves are avascular and the oxygen demand of the cellular milieu is supplied by diffusion [21]. However, in the stenotic aortic valve a vascularization process is part of the pathogenesis of aortic stenosis [22]. (Fig 3).
The presence of myofibroblasts is associated with expression of alpha smooth muscle actin and osteoblastic markers such as osteocalcin and bone sialoprotein [23]. This contributes to fibrosis of the leaflets and the formation of calcified nodules [23]. Distinction between smooth muscle cells and myofibroblasts is difficult as both cell types express alpha-smooth muscle actin. It is possible to distinguish between these two groups of cells with h-caldesmon

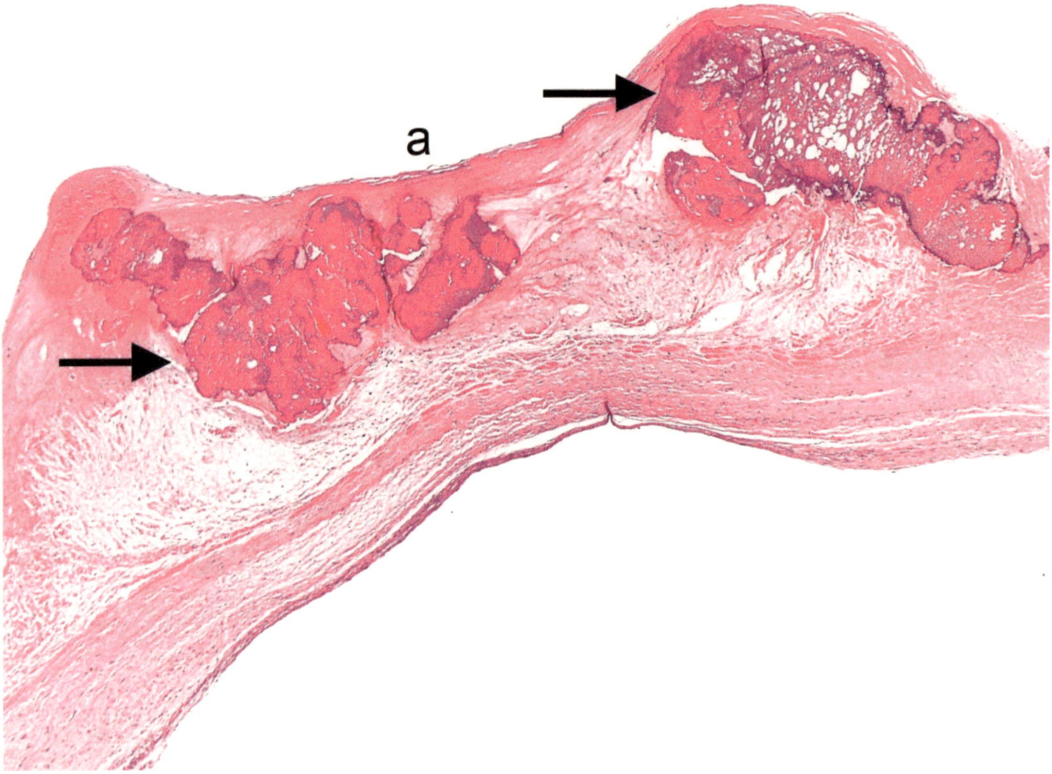

Fig. 2. Low power photomicrograph of a stenotic aortic valve shows the presence of calcifications (arrows) on the aortic side (a) of the valve (original magnification X40).

immunohistochemical evaluation. H-caldesmon is specific for smooth muscle cells and do not react with myofibroblasts [24]. (Figs 4 & 5).

6. Possible future therapeutic implications of cellular and neuronal aspects of aortic stenosis

From the preceding discussion it is clear that there are numerous possibilities for the development of new therapeutic agents in order to arrest the progression of the complex process of aortic stenosis. In the early stages the increase in smooth muscle cells and myofibroblasts may be inhibited by yet to be discovered inhibitors of differentiation.

The process of angiogenesis in the valve leaflet may be blocked, as well as the differentiation of valvular myofibroblasts into osteoblasts with subsequent calcification.

It is also possible that the still incompletely understood effects of neuronal stimulation of the valvular interstitial cells may play a causal role in the initial process of aortic stenosis and that these neurons may lend themselves susceptible to future inhibition by therapeutic agents.

Lastly, the possible therapeutic role of native stem cells inside the valvular cusps are endless and only the future will tell.

In conclusion, it can be said that the possible future therapy of the process of aortic stenosis may become a purely medical one, with surgery limited to cases discovered in the end stage of this complex process.

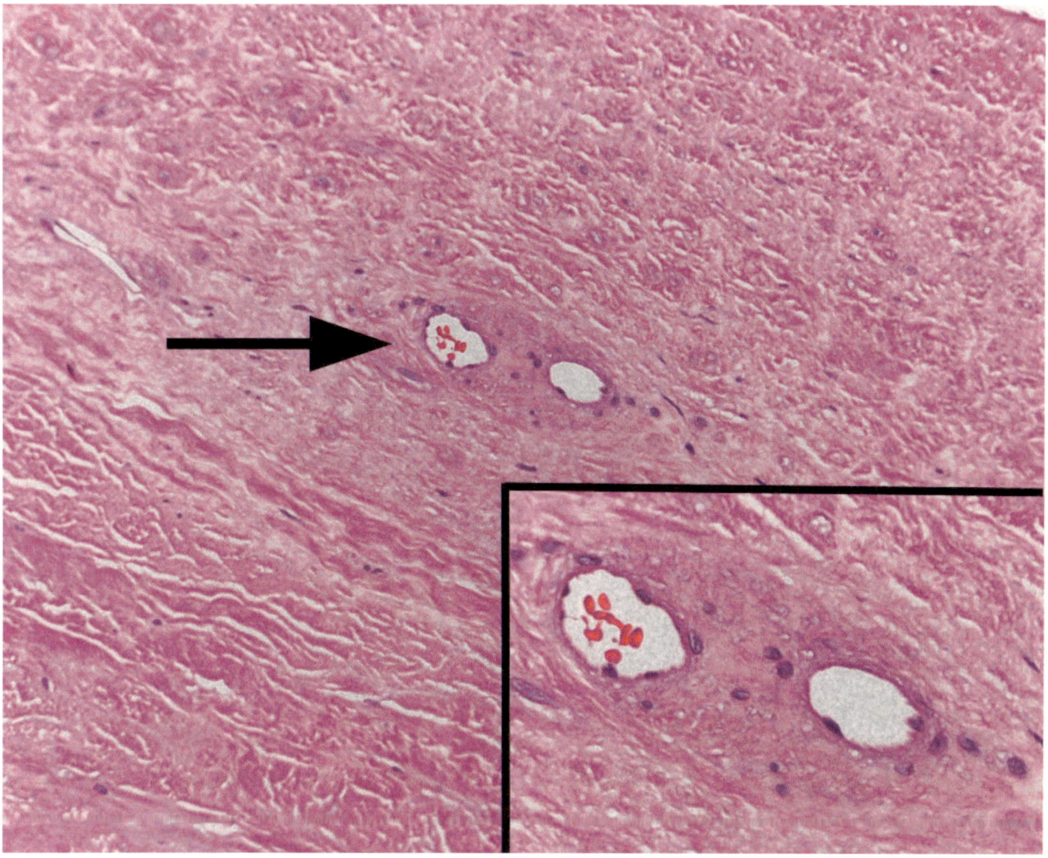

Fig. 3. Small blood vessels (arrow) in a stenotic aortic valve. (original magnification X 100). Inset: Higher magnification of the blood vessels. (original magnification X 200).

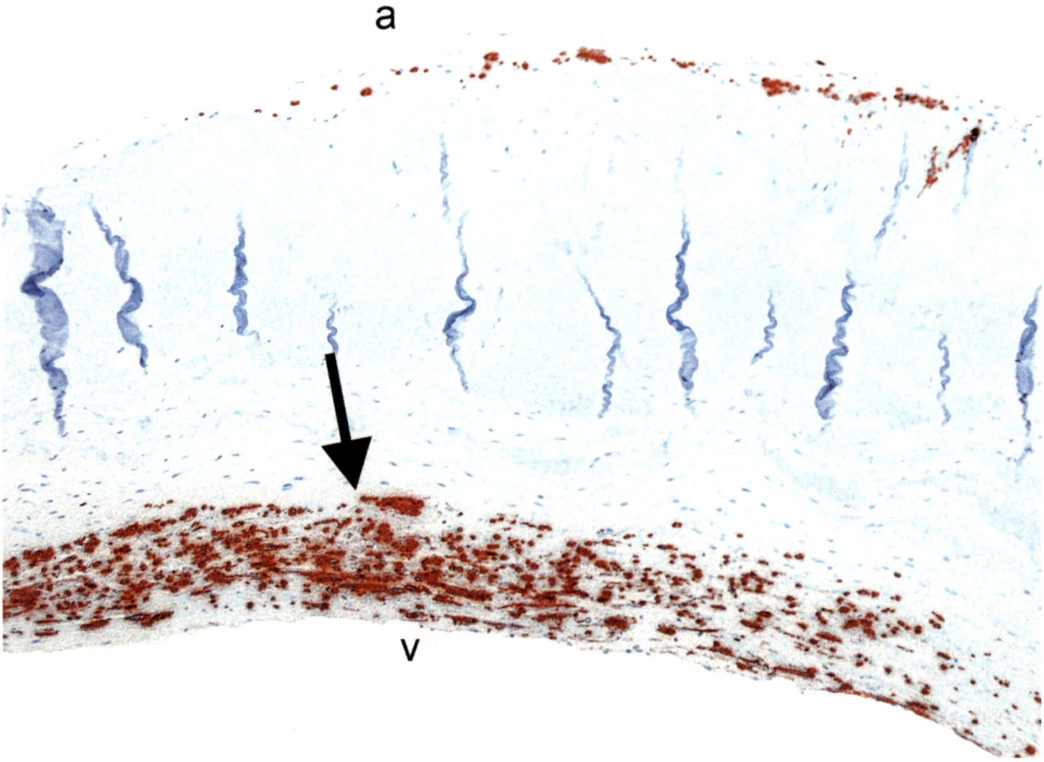

Fig. 4. Immunohistochemical staining of a decalcified stenotic aortic valve with smooth muscle actin (SMA) shows the presence of numerous positive cells (smooth muscle cells and myofibroblasts) (arrow) on the ventricular side (v) of the valve. Fewer positive cells are present on the aortic side (a). (original magnification X 100).

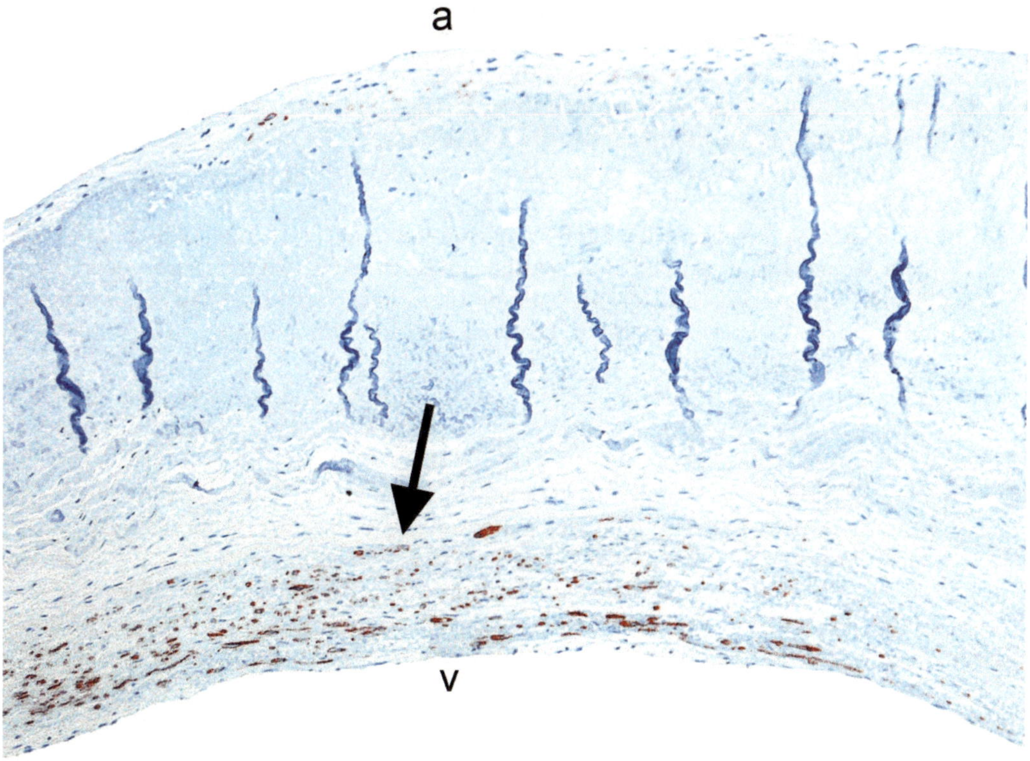

Fig. 5. H-caldesmon immunohistochemical stain (specific for smooth muscle cells) of the same area as in Fig. 4 demonstrates the portion of SMA positive cells that are smooth muscle cells (arrow). The SMA positive cells that did not stain with h-caldesmon are myofibroblastic in nature. (original magnification X 100).

7. References

[1] Marron K, Yacoub MH, Polak JM, Sheppard MN, Fagan D, Whitehead BF, de Leval MR, Anderson RH, Wharton J. Innervation of human atrioventricular and arterial valves. Circulation 1996; 94:368-375.

[2] El-Hamamsy I, Yacoub MH, Chester AH. Neuronal regulation of aortic valve cusps. Current Vascular Pharmacology 2009; 7:40-46.

[3] El-Hamamsy I, Chester AH, Yacoub MH. Cellular regulation of the structure and function of aortic valves. Journal of Advanced Research 2010; 1:5-12.

[4] Braunwald E, Rockoff SD, Newland-Oldham H Jr, Ross J Jr. Effective closure of the mitral valve without atrial systole. Circulation 1966; 33: 404-409.

[5] Sonnenblick EH, Napolitano LM, Daggett WM, Cooper T. An intrinsic neuromuscular basis for mitral valve motion in the dog. Circ Res. 1972; 31:417-430.

[6] Stella JA, Sacks MS. On the biaxial mechanical properties of the layers of the aortic valve leaflet. J Biomech Eng 2007; 129(5):757-766.

[7] Ku DD, Nelson JM, Caulfield JB, Winn MJ. Release of endothelium relaxing factors from canine cardiac valves. J Cardiovasc Pharmacol. 1990; 16:212-218.

[8] Siney L, Lewis MJ. Nitric oxide release from porcine mitral valves. Cardiovasc Res. 1993; 27: 1657-1661.
[9] Hainsworth R. Reflexes from the heart. Physiol Rev. 1991; 71:617-658.
[10] Yacoub MH, Cohn LH. Novel approaches to cardiac valve repair: from structure to function: part I. Circulation 2004; 109(8):942-950.
[11] Taylor PM, Batten P, Brand NJ, Thomas PS, Yacoub MH. The cardiac valve interstitial cell. Int J Biochem Cell Biol. 2003; 35(2):113-118.
[12] Roy A, Brand NJ, Yacoub MH. Molecular characterization of interstitial cells isolated from human heart valves. J Heart Valve Dis 2000; 9:459-464; discussion 64-65.
[13] Taylor PM, Allen SP, Yacoub MH. Phenotypic and functional characterization of interstitial cells from human heart valves, pericardium and skin. J Heart Valve Dis 2000; 9:150-158.
[14] Chen JH, Yip CYY, Sone ED, Simmons CA. Identification and characterization of aortic valve mesenchymal progenitor cells with robust osteogenic calcification potential. Am J Pathol 2009; 174:1109-1119.
[15] Visconti RP, Ebihara Y, LaRue AC, Fleming PA, McQuinn TC, Masuya M. An in vivo analysis of hematopoietic stem cell potential: hematopoietic origin of cardiac valve interstitial cells. Circ Res 2006; 98(5): 690-696.
[16] Kawano H, Shirai T, Kawano Y, Okada R. Morphological study of vagal innervation in human semilunar valves using a histochemical method. Jpn Circ J 1996; 60: 62-66.
[17] De Biasi S, Vitellaro-Zuccarello L. Intrinsic innervation of porcine semilunar heart valves. Anat Embryol (Berl) 1982; 165: 71-79.
[18] Marron K, Wharton J, Sheppard MN, Fagan D, Royston D, Kuhn DM, de Leval MR, Whitehead B, Anderson RH, Polak JM. Distribution, morphology and neurochemistry of endocardial and epicardial nerve terminal arborizations in the human heart. Circulation 1995; 92: 2343-2351.
[19] Steele PA, Gibbins IL, Morris JL. Projections of intrinsic cardiac neurons to different targets in the guinea-pig heart. J Auton Nerv Syst 1996; 56: 191-200.
[20] Yu PJ, Skolnick A, Ferrari G, Heretis K, Mignatti P, Pintucci G, Rosenzweig B, Diaz-Cartelle J, Kronzon I, Perk G, Pass HI, Galloway AC, Grossi EA, Grau JB. Correlation between plasma osteopontin levels and aortic valve calcification: potential insights into the pathogenesis of aortic valve calcification and stenosis. Journal of Thoracic and Cardiovascular Surgery 2009; 138(1): 196-199.
[21] Hammon JW (Jr), O`Sullivan MJ, Oury J, Fosburg RG. Allograft cardiac valves. A view through the scanning electron microscope. Journal of Thoracic and Cardiovascular Surgery 1974; 68: 352-360.
[22] Chalajour F, Treede H, Ebrahimnejad A, Lauke H, Reichenspurner H, Ergun S. Angiogenic activation of valvular endothelial cells in aortic valve stenosis. Experimental Cell Research 2004; 298: 455-464.
[23] Benton JA, Kern HB, Leinwand LA, Mariner PD, Anseth KS. Statins block calcific nodule formation of valvular interstitial cells by inhibiting alpha-smooth muscle actin expression. Arterioscler Thromb Vasc Biol. 2009; 29: 1950-1957.
[24] Ceballos KM, Nielsen GP, Selig MK, O'Connell JX. Is anti-h-caldesmon useful for distinguishing smooth muscle and myofibroblastic tumors? An immunohistochemical study. Am J Clin Pathol 2000; 114: 746-753.

Part 5

Associated Disorders with Aortic Stenosis

15

Severe Calcific Aortic Valve Stenosis and Bleeding: Heyde's Syndrome

Giampaolo Zoffoli et al.*
Department of Cardiac Surgery, Venezia-Mestre, Italy

1. Introduction

In 1958 Dr. Edward C. Heyde, an internist living and working in Vancouver, WA, first reported in a letter to the New England Journal of Medicine, 10 cases of calcific aortic stenosis and grastrointestinal bleeding. The association between severe calcific aortic stenosis and iron deficency anemia due gastrointestinal bleeding, from colonic angiodysplasia was described as Heyde syndrome. A letter appearing shortly after confirmed an odd ratio of almost 3.0 between the two diseases. (1)

In the same year Goldman noted that within the population of severe aortic stenosis there was a three fold higher prevalence of gastrointestinal bleeding, and few years later Cattell published a more drastic position, due to the the fact that patient with aortic stenosis could bleed from a lesion in the ascending colon which has not been demonstrated by the pathologist, and recommended blind right haemicolectomy as a treatment for recurrent anaemia.

Dystrophic calcification of heart valves was first described by dr. Monckeberg in 1904.

With the advent of the extracorporeal circulation discovered by Gibbon in 1954, applied to cardiac surgery operations, a new frontiere for valve disease was achieved, and valve therapy radically changed in those years, in favour of valve replacement.

Unfortunately for many years the association between these two condition has been underestimated and it has not been verified with a methodological approach intil the '80s, when Greenstein and King reported in two different publications this association between aortic stenosis and bleeding. (2,3).

In a first attempt to treat this syndrome, an empirical approach was used with blood transfusion; but in those years it has been noticed that, after aortic valve replacement, there was a complete cessation of the bleeding, and the restoring of the normal gastrointestinal mucosa.

By 1987, 30 cases of upper and lower gastrointestinal angiodysplasia had been cured by AVR. Angiodysplasia might remain visible at endoscopy even after AVR, but only 1 of the 30 cases ever developed recurrent gastrointestinal bleeding.

Patients with Heyde syndrome who are treated by intestinal resection generally continue to bleed from other sites, while AVR usually cures the clotting disorder and anaemia. A

*Domenico Mangino, Andrea Venturini, Angiolino Asta, Alberto Terrini, Chiara Zanchettin, Francesco Battaglia and Elvio Polesel
Department of Cardiac Surgery, Venezia-Mestre, Italy

retrospective study of 91 patients with aortic stenosis and chronic unexplained gastrointestinal bleeding revealed that bleeding ceased in 93% of patients treated by valve replacement, compared with 5% of those managed surgically, with or without bowel resection.
We have to remember that prosthetic valves may encroach on valvular orifices causing mild stenosis (patient-prosthesis mismatch).
It is important to consider the possible presence of Heyde syndrome if metallic AVR is being considered, as there is a need for lifelong anticoagulation subsequently.
Despite the small interest within the scientific community, this syndrome has been a matter of debate but no explanation for this link has been found.
Aortic stenosis is now the most acquired valvular lesion in the elderly. The prevalence of critical aortic stenosis is 1-2% at 75 years, rising to 6% at 85 years.
Angiodysplasia is present in 3% of population that undergo to colonoscopies, and may occur anywhere in the gastrointestinal tract, but is most common in the ascending colon, especially in the cecum (37%).
Several studies have tried to define prevalence and etiopathology of this syndrome, but results remained unclear so far, because aortic stenosis may be easily detected in later symptomatic stages, while colon angiodysplasia will not always result in anemia, or routine investigations may not reveal that they are the cause of a patient's anemia, and it is likely that many mild cases remain undiagnosed.
Some early studies on Heyde syndrome showed a correlation of a typical murmur of aortic stenosis with idiopathic gastrointestinal bleeding, while later studies have used echocardiographic and endoscopic diagnoses. Colonoscopy is the most common investigation used to visualise the colon, but colonoscopic diagnoses are usually used in retrospective studies. Many studies have not distinguished bleeding from non-bleeding angiodysplasia.
According to Yoshida and co-workers, in a recent study, severe aortic stenosis is found in up to 15–25% of patients with repeated bleeding.(22) Mehta *et al.* investigated 29 patients with gastrointestinal angiodysplasia detected on endoscopy with echocardiography, but found no cases of aortic stenosis.(23) Similarly, Oneglia *et al.* investigated 59 patients and found that only one had aortic stenosis.(24)
In a prospective, case-matched study of 40 patients who were found to have angiodysplasia, Bhutani and colleagues found no increased prevalence of aortic stenosis. (25)
Pate and colleagues studied 3.8 million discharge summaries retrospectively, and found a significant association ($P<0.0001$) between aortic stenosis and gastrointestinal bleeding presumed to be due to angiodysplasia. Age was statistically significant as a confounding factor, as patients who had been diagnosed with both conditions were older than patients with only one or neither ($P<0.0001$). In another retrospective case-note study of 3,623 patients with either aortic or mitral stenosis, gastrointestinal bleeding was found to be significantly more common in the aortic stenosis group ($P<0.001$).
In a study of patients diagnosed with angiodysplasia of the gastrointestinal tract over a 10-year period, echocardiography significantly correlated with aortic stenosis but not with mitral stenosis. Significant aortic stenosis was 2.6 times more common than in controls, and severe aortic stenosis was 4.1 times more common than in the general population. The study included patients diagnosed by angiography as well as endoscopy in contrast to the study of Bhutani *et al.*.
Only several years later the letter from dr. Heyde, this haemorragic syndrome, basicly an acquired coagulopathy, was associated with acquired type 2A von Willebrand syndrome, which is characterised by the loss of the largest multimers of von Willebrand factor. (4,5,6)

Proteolysis of von Willebrand factor as it passes through the stenotic valve is one of the proposed causes of the bleeding. High shear forces can induce structural changes in the shape of the von Willebrand factor molecule, leading to exposure of the bond between amino acids Tyr842 and Met843, which is sensitive to the action of a specific von Willebrand protease. (8,9,10)

This results in proteolysis of the highest-molecular-weight multimers of von Willebrand factor, which are the most effective in platelet-mediated hemostasis under conditions of high shear stress. (11)

Yoshida and colleagues showed electrophoretic deficits of large multimers of vWF in patients with aortic stenosis which resolved postoperatively, but no differences in pre- and postoperative vWF were found in patients with severe mitral regurgitation. (22)

In mild to moderate cases of von Willebrand disease, a therapy based on Desmopressin (DDAVP), that releases Factor VIII storage pools, is used with a moderate success.

The concept of proteolysis of the highest-molecular-weight multimers of von Willebrand factor, under conditions of high shear stress, is further supported by the recent demonstration that this biologic abnormalities can be corrected by valve replacement. (12,13,14)

So many authors have hypothesised that acquired von Willebrand syndrome could be a common feature in patients with aortic stenosis. Moreover Vincentelli et al. argue that severe forms of Heyde's syndrome might be sufficient reason for aortic valve replacement, even if the stenosis is otherwise clinically unimportant and is not likely to cause complications.(16)

In 1971, Boss and Rosenbaum described distension of vessels in the intestinal mucosa in post-mortem cases of aortic stenosis and attributed the blood loss to this (26). Low-grade chronic hypoxia may stimulate reflex sympathetic vasodilation and smooth muscle relaxation, progressing to true ectasia of vessel walls.

Another theory is that colonic mucosal hypoxia might be caused by cholesterol emboli from the aortic valve or by the altered pulse waveform in aortic stenosis. Angiodysplasia have been described in hypertrophic cardiomyopathy, in which is also found alteration of the pulse waveform.

Several studies comparing cases of aortic and mitral valve stenosis have shown a higher prevalence of gastrointestinal bleeding in the former. Other valvular lesions might cause chronic hypoxia in the intestinal mucosa, but do not induce altered pulse waveforms. Some found no association of aortic stenosis with angiodysplasia but found a high frequency of colonic polyps and tumours whereas others have suggested that Heyde syndrome is the end result of senile degeneration of both aortic valvular and gastrointestinal mucosal tissue.

In an elderly patient with established aortic stenosis, development of iron deficiency anaemia should raise the possibility of Heyde syndrome. Initial investigations should explore other possibilities such as underlying gastrointestinal malignancy, coeliac disease or nutritional deficiency. The presence of angiodysplasia on sigmoidoscopy or colonoscopy (figure 1) or a failure of the investigations to find any clear site of gastrointestinal bleeding, should raise the possibility of Heyde syndrome. For patients in whom initial investigations show no abnormality, angiodysplasia may be diagnosed by capsule endoscopy.

Patients presenting with gastrointestinal bleeding should be examined carefully for aortic stenosis and there should be a low threshold for arranging echocardiogram in patients with normal colonoscopies or proven arteriovenous malformations.

In vWS-2A, routine screening tests for vWS are usually normal. The gold standard is gel electrophoresis of vWF. vWS-2A is characterised by absence of large vWF multimers seen on SDS-agarose electrophoresis. The sensitivity of various tests for vWS-2A has been ranked as

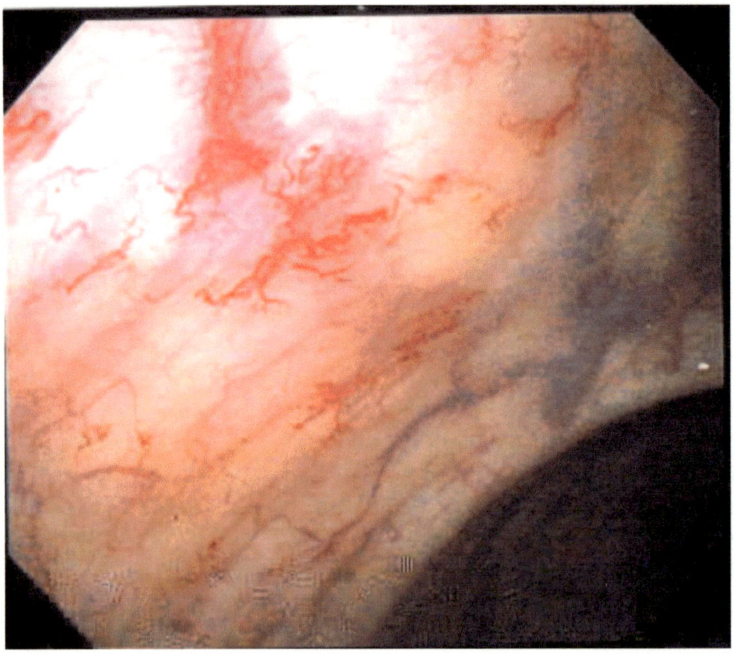

Fig. 1. Colonscopy showing the presence of angiodysplasia.

follows: gel electrophoresis (most sensitive), PFA-100 closure time, skin bleeding time, vWF ristocetin cofactor activity and vWF antigen level (least sensitive).
So many authors nowadays affirm that Heyde syndrome refers to a triad of aortic stenosis, acquired coagulopathy (von Willebrand syndrome type IIA) and anemia due to bleeding from intestinal angiodysplasia or from an idiopathic site. (21)
The purpose of the present study is to evaluate the prevalence and the determinants of haemostatic abnormalities in patients withaortic stenosis and their clinical consequences.

2. Materials and methods

Between January 2005 and January 2009, 588 patients underwent aortic-valve replacement (AVR) for degenerative calcific aortic stenosis in our Institution.
312 patients (53%) underwent AVR alone, in 91 patients (15.6%) was associated a mitral valve procedure, and in 32.2% (188 patients) a concomitant coronary artery by-pass graft procedure was performed. 18 patients (3%) presented an history of haemorrhage, which causes seemed to be unexplained. We took into consideration this population that presented the association of gastrointestinal bleeding and severe aortic stenosis, in which we would hypothesised that an acquired von Willebrand syndrome could be present as a determinant of haemostatic abnormalities. Four (22%) of these 18 patients had an intestinal resection previous to cardiac surgery, with persisting gastrointestinal bleeding at six months after resection.

3. Screening bleeding diathesis

Only bleeding during the six months preceding evaluation was taken into account. Bleeding symptoms were evaluated by the use of a standardised screening questionnaire. The same evaluation was repeated six months postoperatively in the group positive for bleeding.

4. Echocardiographic evaluation

Using an HP Sonos 5500 echocardiographic system, an investigator assessed the haemodynamic performance of the aortic valve by transthoracic echocardiography at base line and at seven days and six months postoperatively. The mean and peak transvalvular pressure gradients were calculated with the modified Bernoulli equation, and the effective orifice area (EOA) was calculated by the continuity equation. At seven days and six months postoperatively, a mismatch between the patient and prosthesis was defined as an indexed EOA of less than 0.85 cm^2 per square meter of body-surface area. The echocardiographic data are presented in Table 1.

Variable	Severe Aortic Stenosis
Max Gradient(mmHg)	73.3 +/- 12.7
Effective orifice area (cm^2)	0.67 +/- 0.1
Indexed effective orifice area (cm^2/m^2 of body surface area)	0.39 +/- 0.16
Ejection fraction (EF) %	55 +/- 7

Table 1. Mean (+/- SD) Echocardiographic data

5. Blood collection and laboratory assays

In patients with severe aortic stenosis associated to an history of haemorrhage, blood samples were collected the day before surgery, seven days, and six months after surgery. Plasma von Willebrand factor antigen was measured by immunoturbidimetry. Functional analysis of von Willebrand factor was performed by measuring its collagen-binding activity with an enzyme-linked immunosorbent assay,[15] with the use of equine type 1 collagen (Horm, Nycomed). The ratio between collagen binding and von Willebrand factor antigen was calculated (the normal value is greater than 0.7).

Event	N° of patients
Epistaxis	12
Gingivorrhagia	14
Gastrointestinal Haemorrhage	16
Ecchymosis	6

Table 2. Hemorrhagic disorders

6. Results

Mean age were 75.5 years, 50% of patients were male; all patients were operated of AVR alone, mean effective orifice area was 0.67 cm^2, with an average maximum gradient of 73.3 mmHg +/- 12.7mmHg, and a mean ejection fraction (EF) of 55% +/-7.

6.1 Prevalence of pre-operatory bleeding

18 patients of 588 (3%) had episodes of bleeding in the six months before surgery. Epistaxis occurred in 12 patients, gingivorrhagia in 14, gastrointestinal haemorrhage in 14, and 6 patients had episodes of spontaneous ecchymosis. 12 of 18 patients had an history of major bleeding (epistaxis, gastrointestinal) that needed transfusion.

6.2 Base-line biologic data

At base line, before operation, levels of von Willebrand factor antigen were normal in all patients (more than 0.5 IU per milliliter).

6.3 Surgical treatment

All patients received a biologic prosthesis porcine valve (Medtronic Hancock II) or a pericardial bioprosthesis (Edwards Magna). No mechanical prosthesis were implanted. Anticoagulant therapy for three months were given at 9 patients (50%), in the other 9 patients 100 mg per day of Acetylsalicylate Acid was started first, without anticoagulant.

7. Immediate postoperative results

The median blood loss 24 hours after valvular replacement was 550 ml (range, 250 to 2120). The postoperative blood loss in patients with preoperative history of bleeding was almost the same than in those without previous episodes. No patients underwent re-operation for bleeding after surgery. No patients died at 30 days follow up.
The levels of von Willebrand factor antigen were normal pre-operatively, at six days and at six months after surgery, in all patients examined.

7.1 Six months follow-up

All patients were analysed at six months follow-up. No valve stenosis or other valve malfunction that required reoperation were detected.
In no one patient was observed epistaxis or gastrointestinal haemorrhage or any other kind of bleeding episodes at six months follow-up. No valve mismatch between patients and prosthesis was observed. The platelet counts were normal, (except for the patient that had pre-operative trombocitemia). No correlation between type of prosthesis (pericardial or porcine) and changes in haemostatic values was found, and there was no effects correlated to the anticoagulant therapy which nine patients (50%) underwent for three months.

8. Discussion

The objective of this study was to evaluate the frequency and determinants of acquired von Willebrand syndrome in consecutive patients undergoing valve replacement for severe aortic stenosis presenting a concomitant history of bleeding. Investigation showed that bleeding (mostly from the gastrointestinal mucosa, or epistaxis) was present in about 3% percent of the patients with severe aortic stenosis, although some authors reported a strongly higher prevalence (up to 20%). (16)
Veyradier and colleagues have shown that vascular malformations, such as angiodysplasia, are at high risk of bleeding in patients with aortic stenosis, since effective haemostasis in these high-shear-stress lesions requires the presence of high-molecular-weight multimers of von Willebrand factor. (6) However we observed that von Willebrand factor abnormalities weren't present in our series, and there was no correlation with the pressure gradient and the stenosis-induced shear stress, indicating that von Willebrand factor abnormalities are not related to the severity of aortic stenosis. This disaccording with other authors that linked haemostatic defect to direct proteolysis of the largest multimers of von Willebrand factor. (16) We demonstrated that the relation between severe aortic stenosis and bleeding is present in a considerable quote of patients (3%).

In our series we used only biologic valve prosthesis, and no correlation between type of prosthesis (pericardial or porcine) and changes in haemostatic values was found. There was no effects correlated to the anticoagulant therapy which nine patients (50%) underwent for three months. As long as a mismatch between patient and prosthesis is avoided, whether mechanical prostheses can be safely implanted in patients who have a history of severe bleeding remains debatable. Additional studies are required to confirm that preoperative hemorrhagic syndrome does not have to be considered in deciding between a biologic and a mechanical valve substitute in patients with aortic stenosis.
In our series all patients had a surgical grade of stenosis, with high trans-valvular gradients, and the most important finding was that no one of them had higher surgical bleeding after valve replacement. We didn't notice a straight correlation between pre-operative and post-operative bleeding, but probably all patients with severe aortic stenosis without valve replacement are also at high risk for bleeding during noncardiac surgery. Those patients who have an history of bleeding, mostly from the gastrointestinal mucosa, or an history of epistaxis, have to sustain many admissions to the Hospital, with many exams or surgical operations to control bleeding and its complications. However, the therapeutic possibilities for the control of bleeding are limited. (17) At the present time, it is well accepted that patients with severe aortic stenosis who become symptomatic require aortic-valve replacement. (18) However, only cardiac symptoms are considered in the evaluation of the indications for valve replacement. (19) As suggested by some authors, the best correction for bleeding in those patients is probably achieved by valve replacement. (13) Further prospective studies are needed to determine whether haemostatic disturbances should be taken into account in the indications for valve replacement. Warkentin and colleagues recently reported long-lasting correction (lasting more than 10 years) of clinical and biologic hemostatic abnormalities in two patients who had undergone surgical treatment of severe aortic stenosis with acquired von Willebrand syndrome and bleeding.(20) In our patients no more episodes of bleeding were reported after surgery, even in the group with anticoagulants. In consideration of the very low mortality and morbidity of the procedure, and considering that at a six month follow-up all patients were still free from bleeding episodes, we consider that the best correction for bleeding in those patients is probably achieved by valve replacement.

9. References

[1] Heyde EC. Gastrointestinal bleeding in aortic stenosis. N Engl J Med 1958;259:196-196

[2] Greenstein RJ, McElhinney AI, Reuben D, Greenstein AJ. Colonic vascular ectasias and aortic stenosis: coincidence or casual relationship? Am J Surg 1986;151:347-351.

[3] King RM, Pluth JR, Giuliani ER. The association of unexplained gastrointestinal bleeding with calcific aortic stenosis. Ann Thorac Surg 1987;44:514-516.

[4] Warkentin TE, Moore JC, Morgan DG. Aortic stenosis and bleeding gastrointestinal angiodysplasia: is acquired von Willebrand's disease the link? Lancet 1992;340:35-37.

[5] Gill JC, Wilson AD, Endres-Brooks J, Montgomery RR. Loss of the largest von Willebrand factor multimers from the plasma of patients with congenital cardiac defects. Blood 1986;67:758-761.

[6] Veyradier A, Balian A, Wolf M, et al. Abnormal von Willebrand factor in bleeding angiodysplasias of the digestive tract. Gastroenterology 2001;120:346-353.

[7] Federici AB, Rand JH, Bucciarelli P, et al. Acquired von Willebrand syndrome: data from an international registry. Thromb Haemost 2000;84:345-349. [Erratum, Thromb Haemost 2000;84:739.]

[8] Tsai HM, Sussman II, Nagel RL. Shear stress enhances the proteolysis of von Willebrand factor in normal plasma. Blood 1994;83:2171-2179.
[9] Dent JA, Berkowitz SD, Ware J, Kasper CK, Ruggeri ZM. Identification of a cleavage site directing the immunochemical detection of molecular abnormalities in type IIA von Willebrand factor. Proc Natl Acad Sci U S A 1990;87:6306-6310.
[10] Siediecki CA, Lestini BJ, Kottke-Marchant KK, Eppell SJ, Wilson DL, Marchant RE. Shear-dependent changes in the three-dimensional structure of human von Willebrand factor. Blood 1996;88:2939-2950.
[11] Sugimoto M, Matsui H, Mizuno T, et al. Mural thrombus generation in type 2A and 2B von Willebrand disease under flow conditions. Blood 2003;101:915-920.
[12] Cappell MS, Lebwohl O. Cessation of recurrent bleeding from gastrointestinal angiodysplasias after aortic valve replacement. Ann Intern Med 1986;105:54-57.
[13] Anderson RP, McGrath K, Street A. Reversal of aortic stenosis, bleeding gastrointestinal angiodysplasia, and von Willebrand syndrome by aortic valve replacement. Lancet 1996;347:689-690.
[14] Pareti FI, Lattuada A, Bressi C, et al. Proteolysis of von Willebrand factor and shear stress-induced platelet aggregation in patients with aortic valve stenosis. Circulation 2000;102:1290-1295.
[15] Favaloro EJ, Henniker A, Facey D, Hertzberg M. Discrimination of von Willembrandt's disease (vWD) subtypes: direct comparison of von Willembrandt factor: collagen binding assay (VWF:CBA) with monoclonal antibody (MAB) based von Willembrandt fator-capture system. Thromb Haemost 2000;84:541-7.
[16] Vincentelli A, Susen S, Le Tourneau T, Six I, Fabre Olivier, Juthier F, Bauters A, Decoene C, Goudemand J, Prat A, Jude B, Aquired von Willembrand Syndrome in aortic stenosis. N Eng J Med, July 24, 2003.
[17] Veyradier A,Jenkins CS,Fressinaud E, Meyer D.: Acquired von Willebrand syndrome:frompathophysiology to management. Thromb Haemost 2000;84:175-82.
[18] Carabello BA .Aortic stenosis.N Engl J Med 2002;346:677-82.
[19] Bonow RO,Carabello B,de Leon AC,et al.ACC/AHA guidelines for the management of patients with valvular heart disease: executive summary:a report of the American College of Cardiology/American Heart Association Task Force on Practice Guidelines (Committee on Management of Patients with Valvular Heart Disease).J Heart Valve Dis 1998;7:672-707.
[20] Warkentin TE,Moore JC,Morgan DG. Gastrointestinal angiodysplasia and aortic stenosis.N Engl J Med 2002;347:858-9.
[21] Massyn M.W., Khan S.A., Heyde syndrome: a common diagnosis in older patients with severe aortic stenosis. Age and ageing 2009;38: 267-270.
[22] Yoshida K, Tobe S., Kawata M, et al.: Acquired and reversible von Willebrand disease with high shear stress aortic valve stenosis. Ann Thorac Surg 2006;81:490-4.
[23] Mehta PM, Heinsimer JA, Bryg RJ, et al. Reassessment of the association between gastrointestinal arteriovenous malformations and aortic stenosis. Am J Med 1989;86:275
[24] Oneglia C, Sabatini T, Rusconi C, et al. Prevalence of aortic valve stenosis in patients affected by gastrointestinal angiodysplasia. Eur J Med 1993;2:75-8.
[25] Bhutani MS, Gupta SC, Markert RJ, et al. A prospective controlled evaluation of endoscopic detection of angiodysplasia and its association with aortic valve disease. Gastrointest Endosc 1995;42:398-402.
[26] Boss EG, Rosenbaum JM, Bleeding from the right colon associated with aortic stenosis. Am J Dig Dis 1971;16:269-75.

16

Hybrid Procedure in Neonatal Critical Aortic Stenosis and Borderline Left Heart: Buying Time for Left Heart Growth

Ward Y. Vanagt[1,2], Stephen C. Brown[1,3] and Marc Gewillig[1]
[1]Paediatric Cardiology, University hospitals Leuven
[2]Cardiovascular Research Institute, Maastricht University,
[3]University of the Free State,
Belgium
The Netherlands
South Africa

1. Introduction

Infants with "borderline" left ventricles due to congenital aortic valve stenosis may be critically ill soon after birth since the left ventricle may be unable to sustain the complete systemic circulation.

In these hearts, the stroke volume of the left ventricle is markedly decreased because of diminutive left ventricular internal dimensions. As the arterial duct closes in the first hours after birth, the left ventricle becomes responsible for generating the full systemic output. If the left heart is of borderline dimensions, this may lead to shock and even death.

However, postnatal loading and growth conditions of the left ventricle differ significantly from foetal life and in so doing influence the postnatal course. Left ventricular growth potential remains and is likely to be stimulated by these physiological changes. Some may occur rapidly following birth whilst others may take weeks to months.

Infants with borderline left ventricles present the physician with a unique dilemma: is this child able to tolerate a biventricular circulation or should one rather embark on a univentricular strategy? In recent years, experience with the hybrid procedure for hypoplastic left heart syndrome showed that indications may be extended to patients with critical aortic stenosis and borderline left heart. A hybrid procedure typically consists of surgical bilateral banding of the branch pulmonary arteries in combination with placement of a stent in the ductus arteriosus after balloon angioplasty of the stenosed aortic valve (Fig 1). As a result, a parallel circulation is created and the right heart can support the left heart to maintain adequate systemic output. This "buys time" to observe the growth potential of the left heart and allows the physician more room to make an informed decision regarding univentricular or biventricular long-term strategy.

In this chapter we describe the background, possibilities, technical aspects and results of this strategy in neonates with critical aortic stenosis and borderline left heart.

2. Background of borderline left ventricle

It is not entirely clear exactly what is referred to when using the term "borderline left heart". Some refer to quantitative and others to qualitative characteristics. The fact remains that it is

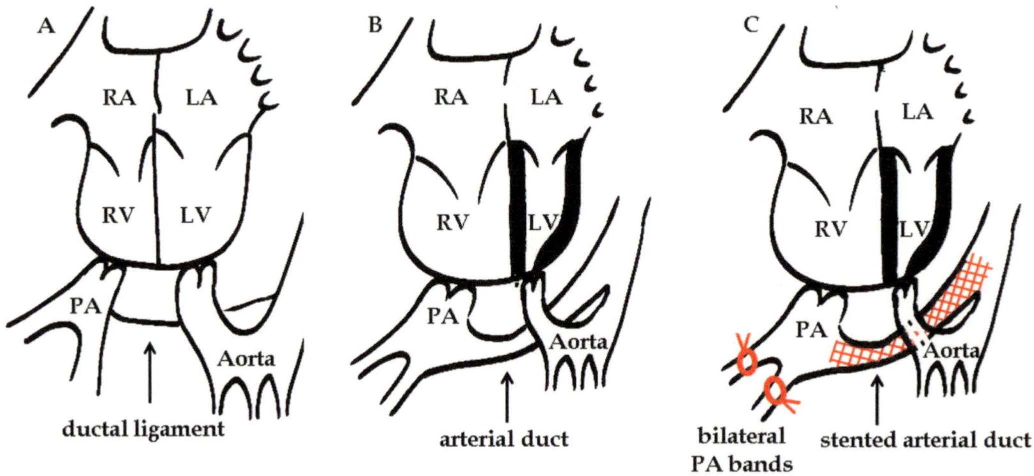

Fig. 1. Schematic drawing of a normal neonatal heart with constriction of the arterial duct (A), a borderline left heart with aortic stenosis, left ventricular hypertrophy, open arterial duct (B) and a borderline left heart after the hybrid procedure with bilateral banding of the pulmonary arteries (PA), stent in the arterial duct (C). RA: right atrium, RV: right ventricle, LA: left atrium, LV: left ventricle.

difficult to define and that a more comprehensive approach is required when facing a left ventricle that is smaller than normal.

In essence, a normal left ventricle should be able to provide satisfactory forward flow by means of generating and maintaining sufficient stroke volume and aortic pressure as well as being compliant enough to keep left atrial and pulmonary venous pressures low. A borderline left ventricle may thus be recognised by being smaller than normal (quantitative) combined with functional (qualitative) inabilities to provide either forward flow and/or leading to excessive pulmonary venous congestion.

In a comprehensive review Corno identified risk factors such as quantitative measurements of left ventricular enddiastolic dimensions, aortic and mitral valve orifices indexed for body surface area (Corno, 2005). Associated abnormalities such as younger age, endocardial fibroelastosis, non-compaction of the left ventricle, aortic coarctation, mitral valve abnormalities and pulmonary hypertension are also important risk factors to be considered (Hickey et al., 2007). In the end, both objective measurements and clinical judgment need to be taken into account when deciding what is considered a borderline left ventricle. This is important, especially since the decision whether to proceed to univentricular or biventricular repair, will be influenced by how borderline left heart is defined.

3. Pathophysiological and clinical correlates

3.1 Deleterious factors in borderline left ventricle with aortic stenosis

Prenatally, the foetal left ventricle receives 40% of the combined cardiac output: 10% of the cardiac output enters the left atrium via the pulmonary veins whilst 30% of the combined cardiac output is received due to right-to-left shunting over the foramen ovale. Good ventricular filling is a prerequisite for adequate cardiac growth. In the normal heart, the neonatal transition from a foetal parallel circulation to a circulation in series requires the left ventricle to generate sufficient aortic pressure and output. Simultaneously, left atrial pressure has to remain low and pulmonary artery pressure has to decrease to normal levels within weeks. In infants with aortic stenosis and borderline left ventricle, symptoms occur during or after the transition from the parallel foetal circulation to the circulation in series when the arterial duct closes.

3.1.1 Foetus

In infants with severe left ventricular outflow tract obstruction such as critical aortic stenosis, left ventricular pressure overload results in significant left ventricular hypertrophy while pressure overload and subendocardial ischemia induce endocardial fibroelastosis. Myocardial hypertrophy and endocardial fibroelastosis result in decreased ventricular volumes and myocardial compliance. The limited blood flow results in reduction of growth of the left ventricular cavity. The foramen ovale may also be restrictive, thereby further limiting left ventricular filling and subsequently growth by up to 75%. Similarly, reduced mitral inflow as a result of mitral valve abnormalities will further compromise foetal left ventricular growth.
Antenatally, the circulation of foetuses with borderline left hearts does not lead to problems. Adequate systemic perfusion is maintained despite the small size of the left ventricle due to increased right-to-left shunting over the ductus arteriosus. Therefore, overall foetal development and somatic growth are usually not jeopardized by a borderline left heart.

3.1.2 After birth

In the delivery room, the newborn with borderline left heart (Fig 2) will be hemodynamically stable as long as the arterial duct remains open. Patients with a severely restrictive, hypoplastic left ventricle and absence of atrial left-to-right shunting, may present with symptoms appearing immediately after birth. However, the latter subset of patients is not the topic of this chapter.

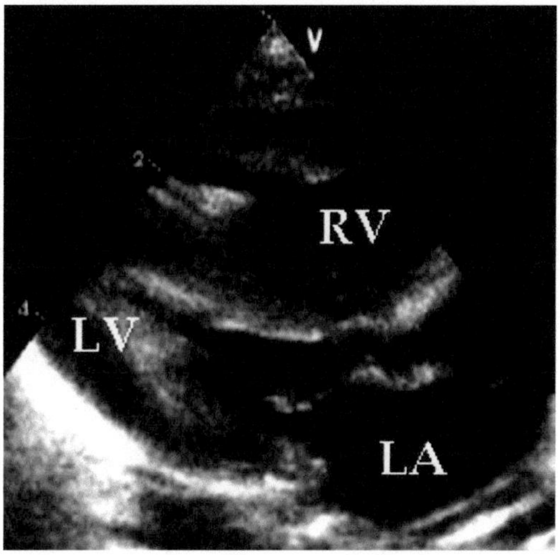

Fig. 2. Echocardiographic parasternal long axis view of borderline left heart in a neonate with aortic stenosis, left ventricular hypertrophy, and endocardial fibroelastosis.

3.1.3 Circulatory failure in the first postnatal days

Acute failure occurs when closure of the arterial duct results in low systemic output due to insufficient left heart size and function. As indicated in the definition of borderline left heart, failure may be due to an inability to generate proper flow and pressure (forward failure) with or without left atrial hypertension and pulmonary venous congestion (retrograde failure). The extent of systemic under perfusion is variable and includes cold extremities, pallor and decreased peripheral pulses. When systemic output is further compromised, hypoperfusion of internal organs results in progressive metabolic acidosis. In the most severe cases, closure of the arterial duct rapidly results in severe arterial hypotension, shock and death. Associated lesions, such as coarctation of the aorta, may even further compromise circulation.

3.1.4 Chronic circulatory failure

Cardiac failure can occur in weeks to months after birth due to pulmonary hypertension. After birth, pulmonary venous return to the left atrium is greater than before resulting in increased left ventricular preload. If the left ventricular cavity is too small or if left ventricular filling is restricted (especially in the presence of mitral valve stenosis or impaired left ventricular compliance), left-to-right shunting over the interatrial septum increases. When interatrial communication as well as left ventricular filling are restrictive, it will lead to left atrial congestion, retrograde pulmonary venous and arterial hypertension and/or pulmonary oedema.

Severe pulmonary hypertension can manifest several months after birth with low output cardiac failure. In these patients with severe pulmonary hypertension, compression of the small left ventricle may occur due to septal deviation as a result of the markedly enlarged hypertensive right ventricle (Smallhorn, 2009), thereby further compromising left ventricular function and growth.

3.2 Favourable factors promoting postnatal left ventricular growth

Following birth, several circulatory factors change significantly compared to foetal conditions. These changes in preload, afterload and growth factors promote growth of the left ventricle.

3.2.1 Increased preload

After birth, pulmonary flow will significantly increase with augmented pulmonary venous return to the left heart. Preload to the left ventricle will therefore always increase after birth, giving rise to the phenomenon of "unfolding" of the left ventricle (Fig. 3). This is often observed where, within minutes after birth, the left ventricle enlarges in infants where foetal ultrasound demonstrated asymmetric four chamber views with small left ventricles. The overall increased flow also results in catch-up growth. Such catch-up growth, however, may take weeks or months to occur.

3.2.2 Reduced afterload

The neonate with critical aortic stenosis will typically be offered percutaneous balloon angioplasty of the aortic valve, thereby decreasing the pressure overload of the left ventricle. This will eventually result in reduction of hypertrophy, increased left ventricular volumes and better compliance with improved filling. These changes may take weeks or even

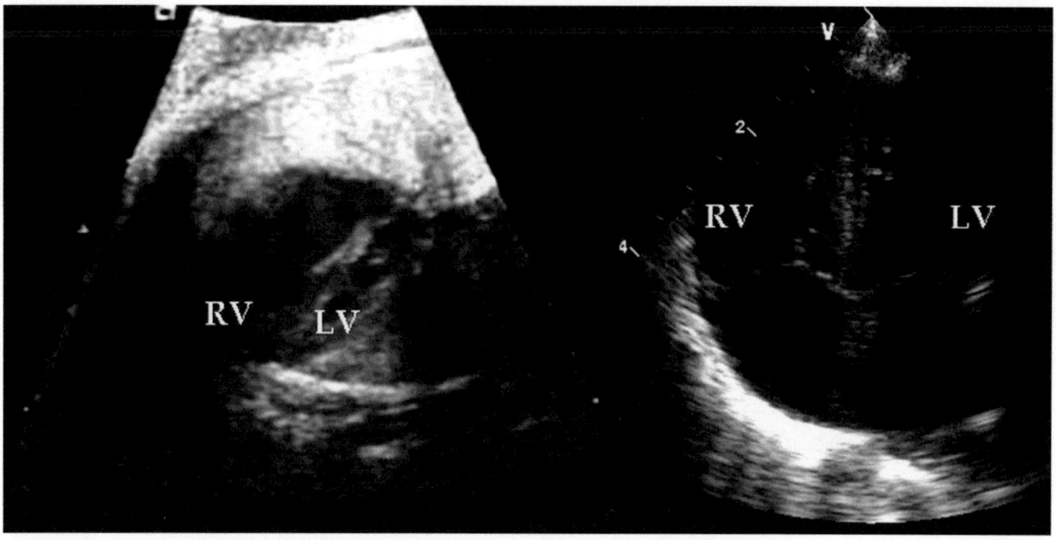

Fig. 3. Four chamber echocardiographic views demonstrating small left ventricle (due to restrictive atrial flow) in foetus (left) and unfolding of the left ventricle 4 hours after birth (right).

months before a significant clinical effect can be observed. In a series of 53 neonates undergoing aortic valve balloon angioplasty, significant growth of aortic valve annulus, aortic sinus, and left ventricular dimensions z-score have been demonstrated (Han et al., 2007).

3.2.3 Growth factors

Insulin and insulin-like growth factor I levels are increased in foetuses of mothers with pre-existing or gestational diabetes. Circulating insulin-like growth factor I in the foetus is a very potent cardiac growth factor, inducing cardiac hypertrophy and hyperplasia (Hayati et al., 2004). Furthermore, insulin-like growth factor I is known to mediate many of the anabolic effects of growth hormone on the heart (Hayati et al., 2004). After birth, insulin levels will drop to normal ranges, removing the pathological stimulus for cardiac hypertrophy. Similarly, increased maternal cortisol levels during late pregnancy induce foetal cardiac hypertrophy (Reini et al., 2008). Again, the effect of postnatal remodelling and the regression of hypertrophy can only be observed after some weeks to months.

4. Treatment options in patients with borderline left ventricle

4.1 Decision making in the neonatal phase

A treatment strategy has to be chosen in the neonatal phase, and previously implied an early choice for either a biventricular or univentricular strategy. On the extreme ends of the spectrum of decreased left heart size and aortic stenosis, the decision concerning the definitive strategy can readily be made in the neonatal phase (Fig. 4). On the one end, hypoplastic left heart syndrome will be palliated by a univentricular strategy. On the other end of the spectrum with a near-normal sized left ventricle, a biventricular repair is the rule. However, in true borderline cases, this early decision proves to be difficult due to lack of guidelines with clear -cut predictability.

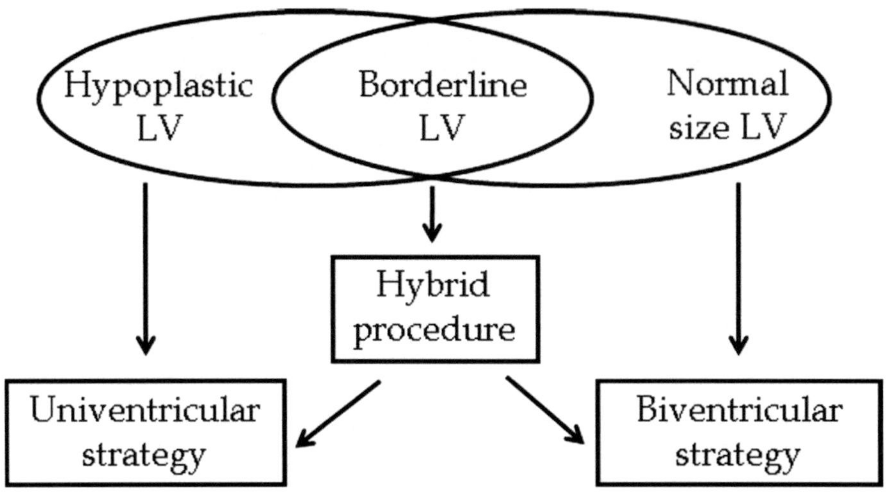

Fig. 4. Options in decision-making in the neonatal phase.

Several scoring systems such as the Rhodes score (Rhodes et al., 1991), Colan score (Colan et al., 2006) and the Univentricular Repair Survival Advantage Tool (Hickey et al., 2007) exist to predict the optimal type of repair. These scoring systems use several left ventricular parameters in an equation, the result of which above or below a given cut-off value generates the predicted most favourable treatment strategy. The Rhodes score involves the variables of body surface area, indexed aortic root size, left ventricle to heart long axis ratio and indexed mitral valve area (Rhodes et al., 1991). In the Colan score, the equation is based on body surface area, aortic annulus z-score, left ventricle to heart long axis ratio and degree of endocardial fibroelastosis (Colan et al., 2006). The Univentricular Repair Survival Advantage Tool is based on morphologic, functional and pathologic information; the exact equation is not published but the score can be calculated at the freely accessible Congenital Heart Surgeons' Society website www.chss.org (Hickey et al., 2007).

A recent small series, however, demonstrated that the results of the aforementioned scoring systems never provided unanimous recommendations regarding the optimal type of repair for the individual patient with borderline left heart (Davis et al., 2011). This important observation emphasizes the true "borderline" characteristics of this disease entity. Another issue to consider is the fact that body surface area, aortic and mitral valve diameters may change very little in the first 2 - 3 weeks, whilst left ventricular enddiastolic dimensions and compliance may change markedly; these are not taken into account in scoring systems. The main issue still remains - what is best: living with a restrictive biventricular circulation or a good univentricular circulation?

4.2 Univentricular strategy

The univentricular strategy typically implies three consecutive surgical procedures: reconstruction of the aortic arch and main pulmonary artery (Damus-Kaye-Stansel & Norwood I) with atrial septectomy and creation of a shunt to the pulmonary artery in the neonatal phase, followed approximately four to six months later by creation of a partial cavo-pulmonary connection (Glenn shunt) and finally completion of the total cavopulmonary connection at the age of two to four years (Fontan circuit). When a univentricular strategy is followed from the neonatal phase, conversion to biventricular physiology may no longer be an option or may be extremely difficult.

Risk factors for increased mortality after univentricular repair consist of tricuspid valve regurgitation, presence of a large ventricular septal defect and smaller indexed dominant ventricular length (Hickey et al., 2007). Despite major improvement in survival rates of the Norwood stage I procedure, infants undergoing this procedure still face a mortality risk of 10-30%, depending on risk factors and the experience level of the team (Bacha, 2006, Stasik et al., 2006). In a recent study, survival rate of the Norwood stage I procedure exceeded 90% in an experienced unit after the initial learning curve (Rychik et al., 2010).

4.3 Biventricular strategy

The biventricular approach consists of treatment of left ventricular outflow obstruction, typically by balloon angioplasty of the aortic valve in a neonate. Surgical aortic valvotomy or the Ross-Konno procedure are alternative options usually performed at a later stage. In case of concomitant coarctation of the aorta, coarctectomy should be performed.

When a biventricular strategy is chosen early but eventually fails, usually due to low cardiac output or pulmonary hypertension, this can lead to death of the patient; otherwise conversion to a univentricular circulation is associated with markedly increased risk (Davis et al., 2011, Pizarro et al., 2009). Decreased survival rates after biventricular repair are found in patients with small left ventricular outflow tract size, small aortic arch size, presence of endocardial fibroelastosis or left ventricular dysfunction (Hickey et al., 2007). Inappropriate pursuit of biventricular repair occurs more often and entails poorer survival rates as compared to inappropriate univentricular repair (Hickey et al., 2007).

4.4 Strategies in the presence of indecision

The immediate decision can be delayed by prolonged infusion of prostaglandins. This will give the clinician one to two weeks to decide by allowing time for the left ventricle to unfold and left ventricular volumes to exhibit a "creep" phenomenon. Serial echocardiography to assess left ventricular dimensions and forward flow is imperative.

In patients with borderline left heart, a hybrid procedure may be considered since it "buys time" while the options for an eventual biventricular or univentricular strategy are kept open. Meanwhile, growth of the left heart is allowed and can be closely monitored. The postponement of immediate decision making offers a chance to fully explore the growth potential of the left heart and avoids the risks of early pursuit of an inappropriate strategy.

A more difficult group comprises infants where biventricular repair is considered and significant pulmonary hypertension develops after ductal closure. In these, usually with systemic or suprasystemic right heart pressures, options are limited: one can create a "reversed" central shunt between pulmonary artery and aorta and re-band the pulmonary arteries or consider a Damus-Kaye type procedure with a large central shunt, but run the risk of shunt blockage because of the underlying pulmonary hypertension. However, these late "change of mind" -procedures are associated with considerable morbidity and mortality.

5. Advantages of the hybrid procedure in borderline left ventricles

The hybrid approach was initially developed as an alternative to the Norwood I procedure for hypoplastic left heart syndrome. Factors driving the concept of the hybrid route were the relatively high mortality rates of surgical stage I (5-30%) and a relatively bloodless intervention avoiding cardiopulmonary bypass.

In the setting of a borderline left ventricle this approach has distinct advantages:

- the hybrid procedure allows the physician to buy time for decision making in neonates with borderline left heart, as previously mentioned.
- in patients with increased operative risk for the first stage in a univentricular strategy (birth weight < 2.5 kg, prematurity < 34 weeks gestational age, genetic malformations, additional cardiac anomalies), the hybrid procedure offers an alternative, lower risk approach (Bacha, 2006).
- initial cardiopulmonary bypass surgery is avoided. In case a univentricular strategy is eventually selected, the hybrid approach allows for postponement of the Norwood I procedure to a later moment when it can be combined with the creation of the Glenn shunt. However, only two instead of three cardiopulmonary bypass procedures are thus necessary to reach the Fontan circulation, since the hybrid procedure is performed off-pump (Akintuerk et al., 2002, Venugopal et al., 2010). In addition, when the child is older and larger cardiopulmonary bypass surgery and circulatory arrest are better tolerated (Bacha, 2006, Corsini et al., 2011).

6. Technical considerations

The goal is to create a balanced pulmonary and systemic circulation in parallel, with sufficient oxygenation of blood in addition to adequate systemic perfusion simultaneously maintaining low pulmonary vascular resistances. Application of the hybrid procedure in the setting of a borderline left heart aims to buy time allowing the left heart to grow without being exclusively responsible for systemic output.

In order to achieve this, left ventricular outflow tract obstruction is treated, the arterial duct is stented to provide adequate systemic perfusion, whilst the branch pulmonary arteries are banded to protect the pulmonary vasculature from excessive flow and pressure (Fig. 1). If the interatrial communication is significantly restrictive, atrial left-to-right shunting may be improved by percutaneous intervention.

Ideally, the procedure is performed in a "hybrid" theatre, where both cardiopulmonary bypass and catheterization equipment is present (Bacha, 2006). In many centres, the surgical procedure and catheterisation procedure are performed separately, albeit with only a short time interval between the events.

6.1 Prostaglandin infusion

Prostaglandin E_1/Alprostadil is administered for temporary maintenance of arterial duct patency. Prostaglandin E_1 causes vasodilatation by its effect on vascular and ductus arteriosus smooth muscle (Roth, 2008). Given the short half-life of 5-10 minutes of this drug, it is administered by continuous intravenous infusion. The onset of action is usually within 30 minutes after administration is started and the maximum effect is observed after 1.5-3 hours (Roth, 2008). More than 70% is metabolized in the lungs, and 90% is excreted as metabolites in the urine within 24 hours (Roth, 2008). Concomitant use of antihypertensive drugs can increase the risk of hypotension. The major adverse effect seen in 10% of newborns is apnoea requiring endotracheal intubation and artificial ventilation, with children < 2 kg being at increased risk (Roth, 2008). Other side effects such as flushing, bradycardia, tachycardia, hypotension, gastro-intestinal disturbances, oedema, seizures, electrolyte abnormalities, hypoglycemia, disturbed platelet aggregation and infection are seen less frequently.

6.2 Balloon dilation of the aortic valve

Standard techniques of balloon valvulopolpasty in infants have been previously described (Kasten-Sportes et al., 1989). In order to reduce the risk of aortic regurgitation, balloon size should not be too large and an overall ratio of not more than 0.9 is recommended. In one large study on balloon dilation of the aortic valve in neonates, aortic regurgitation occurred in 15% (McElhinney et al., 2005). Rapid right ventricular pacing to improve balloon stability may be used, but is hardly ever required in these infants. Many interventionalists prefer a retrograde approach, but the procedure can be performed anterograde as well. Alternatively, a carotid artery approach provides easy, rapid access but concerns exist regarding stenosis of the carotids on long-term follow-up.

6.3 Stenting of the arterial duct

Meticulous attention should be paid to the technique of ductal stenting. Stents can be introduced directly into the pulmonary artery after bilateral branch banding during the initial procedure or, alternatively, percutaneously a few days after surgery.
Prostaglandin infusion may be stopped 4 - 12 hours prior to ductal stenting, but in our experience, this is usually not needed in these cases. Stent selection is based upon ductal anatomy. In general, the diameter should be at least the size of the thoracic aorta and it is important that the whole length of the arterial duct should be covered by the stent. Positioning of the stent at the aortic junction of the ductus is of utmost importance: it should not protrude into the lumen of the aorta, since this will preclude percutaneous management in the future. At the pulmonary end, the stent should extend beyond the ductus-pulmonary artery junction. Pre-mounted self expandable stents are preferred since it averts the need for long sheaths and the ductus in these cases is usually wide and curved e.g. OptiMed® sinus stent range (Optimed Medizinische Instrumente GmbH, Ettlingen, Germany) and Andramed® U-Flex (Andramed, Reutlingen, Germany) both 5 F systems. Self expandable stents are available in open- as well as closed-cell designs. Closed-cell stents can easily be repositioned before full expansion but have less grip. Open-cell designs on the other hand, have the advantage that it anchors itself to the wall of the ductus and can therefore not be repositioned. In the presence of a stenotic ductus, a balloon expandable stent could be selected e.g. Palmaz® Blue™ stents (Cordis Corporation, a Johnson & Johnson company; Warren, NJ) - these are mostly closed-cell designs. Generally ductal stents would be in the range of 5 -7 mm in diameter with lengths varying between 10 and 20 mm.
Delivery of the ductal stent can be performed in the hybrid suite. After direct puncture of the right ventricular outflow tract or main pulmonary artery, a short sheath is placed by the surgeon 2-3 mm inside the vessel and secured by means of a purse-string suture (Bacha, 2006). Heparin should be administered at this stage. A guidewire (0.014" or 0.018") is passed through the ductus into the descending aorta. Angiography is performed to assess ductal anatomy and position of the pulmonary artery bands. The balloon-deployable or self-

expandable stent is then advanced over the guide wire and positioned to cover the entire ductal length. A second stent can be used if necessary. Control angiography is performed after stent placement to confirm correct positioning (Fig 5).
Percutaneous stents can be delivered either antegradely or retrogradely. Premounted stents are delivered using 5 F or 6F short sheaths. Overall, we prefer the antegrade placement of stents 1 - 3 days after pulmonary artery banding during which a balloon septostomy can be performed if necessary. Technique is similar, but sometimes a long delivery sheath to navigate the curves of the right ventricle may be required although it is rarely necessary.

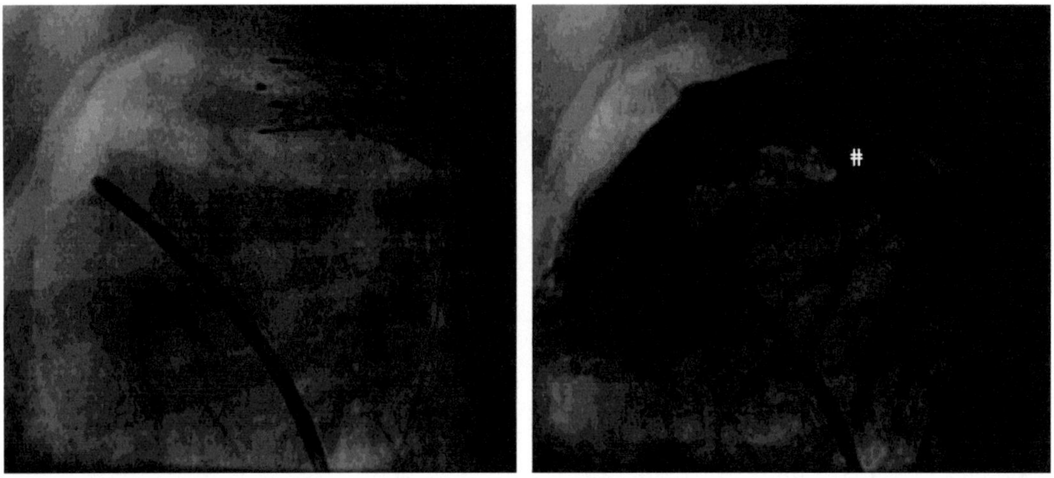

Fig. 5. Angiographic views of stent in the arterial duct. Pre and post contrast views showing patent stent in ductus (*) and pulmonary artery branch band (#) during contrast injection.

During the procedure, careful attention should be paid to the aortic arch and any associated abnormalities amenable to catheter intervention, for example coarctation of the aorta, should be addressed.
In a study of 58 patients undergoing the hybrid procedure, mortality related to percutaneous ductal stenting was 1.7% (Akinturk et al., 2007). Complications of ductal stenting include vascular injury, constriction of the ductus due to passage of the guide wire, insufficient coverage of the ductus necessitating re-intervention, ductal stent migration and thrombosis of the stent (Holzer et al., 2010).

6.4 Bilateral banding of the pulmonary arteries

Banding of the branch pulmonary arteries is performed to decrease pulmonary overflow and improve the balance of the systemic and pulmonary flows. Furthermore, banding provides protection of the pulmonary vasculature in order to be able to pursue a univentricular circulation or cardiac transplantation later in life (Pizarro et al., 2009). In a mathematical model of the circulation after the hybrid procedure in hypoplastic left heart syndrome, computational results indicate that the balance between systemic and pulmonary blood flow is sensitive to the degree of pulmonary artery banding rather than to the size of the ductal stent (Corsini et al., 2011).
By means of median sternotomy, bilateral banding of the branch pulmonary arteries is performed. The chest retractor has to be placed in such a way as to be removable during

fluoroscopy in the hybrid theatre. At our institution, Gore-Tex rings with diameters as suggested by Galantowicz are used: 3.0mm for infants < 2.5kg and 3.5mm for infants over 2.5kg (Galantowicz et al., 2008). The ring is cut through, placed around the artery and closed again using a 7/0 polypropylene stitch. The Gore-Tex rings are then fixed to the branch pulmonary arteries with a 7/0 polypropylene stitch. Rings should be placed close to the bifurcation of the pulmonary artery. This configuration creates breakable bands and is thus amenable to future percutaneous interventions. We have demonstrated that percutaneous saturations could be markedly improved after careful balloon angioplasty of such bands (Brown et al., 2010). The advantage of this concept is that, in a borderline left ventricle demonstrating growth, nonsurgical re-establishment of flows is possible (Brown et al., 2010).

Mortality for pulmonary arterial banding is as low as 1.7% as demonstrated by the Giessen experience which included 58 patients undergoing the hybrid procedure (Akinturk et al., 2007). Complications consist of band migration and pulmonary artery distortion which may require further intervention. Especially distal migration of bands to the hilus is an important cause of morbidity and need for surgical re-intervention.

6.5 Creating or enlarging the interatrial communication

If the interatrial septum is markedly restrictive, it should be addressed. In the vast majority of patients balloon septostomy will be adequate. Complication rates are low if the interatrial septum has normal anatomy, but much higher in the presence of abnormal anatomy (Holzer et al., 2008).

However, in the infant with a borderline left ventricle, mild restriction in order to force flow through the mitral valve is preferable and septostomy is rarely required. In our experience, infants with borderline left ventricles requiring septostomy often have less favourable long-term outcome and rarely proceed to biventricular repair.

7. Intermediate follow-up of hybrid procedures

Most of the data regarding the outcome of hybrid procedures have been obtained in infants with hypoplastic left heart syndrome. Hospital survival after the hybrid stage I procedure in infants with hypoplastic left heart has ranged from 70-90% (Bacha, 2006). In a series of 14 high-risk patients of whom 11 had hypoplastic left heart syndrome, in-hospital survival of the hybrid strategy was 11/14 (79%), death being caused by ductal stent embolization in one infant, progressive cardiac dysfunction in another, sepsis after cardiac arrest, extracorporeal membrane oxygenation and cardiac transplantation in one patient (Bacha et al., 2006). Reports have demonstrated that there is an initial learning curve and, in an expert center, in-hospital survival of hybrid stage I palliation in 40 infants with hypoplastic left heart syndrome was as high as 98% (Galantowicz et al., 2008). Between stage I and II palliation, 2 deaths occurred due to infection, 3 deaths were related to the stage II procedure and 1 death took place in-between stage II and III palliation (Galantowicz et al., 2008). This results in an overall survival of 83%, with interstage mortality and reintervention rate being similar as reported with consecutive Norwood procedures (Galantowicz et al., 2008). Other units have reported similar results (Honjo et al., 2009).

If growth of the left ventricle occurs and biventricular repair is considered, by using a hybrid procedure, it can be accomplished by either percutaneous or surgical means.

Percutaneous biventricular repair would consist of balloon angioplasty to remove the breakable bands and closure of the ductus arteriosus with a device (Brown et al., 2009). Redo aortic valve angioplasty may also be required at the time of intervention. Surgical alternatives would include removal of the bands plus ductal clipping with or without removal of stent or variants of the Ross-Konno procedure. In order to facilitate biventricular repair, aggressive left heart rehabilitation by resection of endocardial fibroelastosis and mitral valve cleavage have also been employed (Emani et al., 2009).
On the other hand, those who qualify for univentricular repair should proceed to stage II options as mentioned.

8. Left heart growth and decision making after the hybrid procedure

8.1 Growth of left heart

Current experience suggests that left heart structures are capable of growing under certain physiologic conditions and in several series of hypoplastic left heart syndrome, results show that some patients proceeded to biventricular repair. In an interesting chick model, it was demonstrated that restriction of flow gave rise to left ventricular hypoplasia and that restoration of flow resulted in physiological growth associated with myocyte hyperplasia (deAlmeida et al., 2007). Recently it was shown that when there is very low flow in the left heart leading to left heart hypoplasia during mid and late gestation, the left ventricle still retained the potential to grow to adequate size for support of a biventricular circulation (Vogel et al., 2010). There is only scant data available concerning growth of left heart structures after the hybrid procedure in infants with borderline left heart and consist mostly of isolated case reports. Ballard described a small series of patients with borderline left heart: all seven patients underwent a hybrid procedure, after which aortic discriminant score (12.12x(body surface area) + 0.59x(aortic annulus z-score) + 5.73x(left ventricle long axis/heart long axis) -7.02) increased in all patients. Four of the seven patients had aortic valve stenosis and were considered inappropriate for biventricular repair in the neonatal phase. After the hybrid procedure, growth of left heart structures allowed for biventricular repair in three out of four patients (Ballard et al., 2010).
In a large study of infants with valvular aortic stenosis undergoing balloon angioplasty during the neonatal phase, the vast majority of patients with a z-score < -1 for aortic annulus size and left ventricular size prior to balloon valvuloplasty, demonstrated normalization of the z-score value within 1-2 years (McElhinney et al., 2005). In another series, aortic valve annulus, aortic sinus, and left ventricular dimension z-scores increased significantly over time, while mitral valve z-score remained below normal during follow-up (Han et al., 2007).

8.2 Decision making during follow-up after the hybrid procedure

The anatomic and physiologic variability makes it impractical to regard a single therapeutic approach optimal for all infants with borderline left hearts. Contemporary experience suggests a rethinking of current strategies and evaluation of new therapeutic options. To the best of our knowledge, there is presently no scoring system available to guide the decision on a biventricular versus univentricular strategy after the hybrid procedure. The available scoring systems in use are designed to guide the decision in the neonatal phase, but have not been validated in older, larger children. At present, this decision regarding univentricular versus biventricular strategy is therefore based on scoring systems combined with the experience and clinical assessment of the multidisciplinary cardiac team. Factors that should be taken into account are mitral valve size and function, estimated risk of retrograde pulmonary hypertension after repair, left ventricular size and function, left ventricular outflow tract size and obstruction, aortic valve size and function, degree of endocardial fibroelastosis, degree of tricuspid valve regurgitation, and presence of other associated heart defects.

On a practical note, we have found echocardiographic demonstration of good antegrade flow in the distal aortic arch helpful when choosing between univentricular and biventricular repair. In doubtful cases, a cardiac catheterization with test occlusion of the stented ductus and atrial septal defect can be performed to assess suitability for a specific strategy provided that the pulmonary artery bands are not too tight.

Important questions still need to be addressed, for example: is a high risk biventricular repair always preferable to univentricular repair? In our institution, whenever possible, biventricular repair is favoured, but when findings are not convincingly in favour of biventricular repair, we tend to go the hybrid route. One should take into consideration that a direct univentricular strategy has a more favourable outcome compared to univentricular repair after failed biventricular attempt. It is important to recognize that embarking on an initial hybrid strategy allows time for left heart growth and also keeps the options of either single or biventricular repair open. With increasing number of hybrid procedures performed, more data providing tools for decision making will become available.

9. Prenatal intervention

Currently, many patients with borderline left heart are diagnosed antenatally when an asymmetric four chamber view is observed on foetal echocardiography. In some institutions, intra-uterine balloon dilation of the aortic valve is offered, although success rates are variable. Improvements in technique may further allow physicians to manipulate left heart flows and growth.

10. Conclusion

In the neonate with aortic stenosis and borderline left heart, the choice between a univentricular versus biventricular strategy can be very difficult. Application of the hybrid procedure not only buys time for left heart growth, but also does not preclude a patient from either single or biventricular repair whilst simultaneously keeping future therapeutic options open.

11. Acknowledgements

The authors recognize the support of the Eddy Merckx research grant.

12. References

Akinturk, H.; Michel-Behnke, I.; Valeske, K.; Mueller, M.; Thul, J.; Bauer, J.; Hagel, K.J.; Kreuder, J.; Vogt, P. & Schranz, D. (2002). Stenting of the arterial duct and banding of the pulmonary arteries: basis for combined Norwood stage I and II repair in hypoplastic left heart. *Circulation*, 105, 9, (Mar 5 2002), pp. 1099-103

Akinturk, H.; Michel-Behnke, I.; Valeske, K.; Mueller, M.; Thul, J.; Bauer, J.; Hagel, K.J. & Schranz, D. (2007). Hybrid transcatheter-surgical palliation: basis for univentricular or biventricular repair: the Giessen experience. *Pediatr Cardiol,* 28, 2, (Mar-Apr 2007), pp. 79-87

Bacha, E. (2006). The hybrid stage I operation in hypoplastic left heart syndrome: a new alternative. *Heart Views,* 7, 3, (Sep-Nov 2006), pp. 105-110

Bacha, E.A.; Daves, S.; Hardin, J.; Abdulla, R.I.; Anderson, J.; Kahana, M.; Koenig,P.; Mora, B.N.; Gulecyuz, M.; Starr, J.P.; Alboliras, E.; Sandhu, S. & Hijazi, Z.M. (2006). Single-ventricle palliation for high-risk neonates: the emergence of an alternative hybrid stage I strategy. *J Thorac Cardiovasc Surg,* 131, 1, (Jan 2006), pp. 163-171 e2

Ballard, G.; Tibby, S.; Miller, O.; Krasemann, T.; Rosenthal, E.; Anderson, D.; Austin, C.; Qureshi, S. & Simpson, J. (2010). Growth of left heart structures following the hybrid procedure for borderline hypoplastic left heart. *Eur J Echocardiogr,* 11, 10, (Dec 2010), pp. 870-4

Brown, S.; Boshoff, D.; Eyskens, B. & Gewillig, M. (2009). Hybrid approach as a bridge to biventricular repair in a neonate with critical aortic stenosis and borderline left ventricle. *Eur J Cardiothorac Surg,* 35, 2, (Feb 2009), pp. 1080-1082

Brown, S.; Boshoff, D.; Rega, F.; Eyskens, B.; Meyns, B. & Gewillig, M. (2010). Dilatable pulmonary artery banding in infants with low birth weight or complex congenital heart disease allows avoidance or postponement of subsequent surgery. *Eur J Cardiothorac Surg,* 37, 2, (Feb 2010), pp. 296-301

Colan, S.D.; McElhinney, D.B.; Crawford, E.C.; Keane, J.F. & Lock, J.E. (2006). Validation and re-evaluation of a discriminant model predicting anatomic suitability for biventricular repair in neonates with aortic stenosis. *J Am Coll Cardiol,* 47, 9, (May 2 2006), pp. 1858-65

Corno, AF. (2005). Borderline left ventricle. *European Journal of Cardio-thoracic surgery,* Vol. 27, No. 1, (January 2005), pp. 67-73

Corsini, C.; Cosentino, D.; Pennati, G.; Dubini, G.; Hsia, T.Y. & Migliavacca, F. (2011). Multiscale models of the hybrid palliation for hypoplastic left heart syndrome. *J Biomech,* 44, 4, (Feb 24 2011), pp. 767-70

Davis, C.K.; Pastuszko, P.; Lamberti, J.; Moore, J.; Hanley, F. & El Said, H. (2011). The hybrid procedure for the borderline left ventricle. *Cardiol Young,* 21, 1, (Feb 2011), pp. 26-30

deAlmeida, A.; McQuinn, T. & Sedmera, D. (2007). Increased ventricular preload is compensated by myocyte proliferation in normal and hypoplastic fetal chick left ventricle. *Circ Res,* 100, 9, (May 11 2007), pp. 1363-70

Emani, S.M; Bacha, E.A; McElhinney, D.B; Marx, G.R; Tworetzky, W; Pigula, F.A & del Nido, P.J. (2009). Primary left ventricular rehabilitation is effective in maintaining two-ventricle physiology in the borderline left heart. *J Thorac Cardiovasc Surg,* Vol.138, No.6(December 2009), pp.1276-1282, ISSN 0022-5223

Galantowicz, M.; Cheatham, J.P.; Phillips, A.; Cua, C.L.; Hoffman, T.M.; Hill, S.L. & Rodeman, R. (2008). Hybrid approach for hypoplastic left heart syndrome: intermediate results after the learning curve. *Ann Thorac Surg,* 85, 6, (Jun 2008), pp. 2063-70; discussion 2070-1

Han, R.K.; Gurofsky, R.C.; Lee, K.J.; Dipchand, A.I.; Williams, W.G.; Smallhorn, J.F. & McCrindle, B.W. (2007). Outcome and growth potential of left heart structures after neonatal intervention for aortic valve stenosis. *J Am Coll Cardiol,* 50, 25, (Dec 18 2007), pp. 2406-14

Hayati, A.R.; Cheah, F.C.; Yong, J.F.; Tan, A.E. & Norizah, W.M. (2004). The role of serum insulin-like growth factor I (IGF-I) in neonatal outcome. *J Clin Pathol,* 57, 12, (Dec 2004), pp. 1299-301

Hickey, E.J.; Caldarone, C.A.; Blackstone, E.H.; Lofland, G.K.; Yeh, T., Jr.; Pizarro, C.; Tchervenkov, C.I.; Pigula, F.; Overman, D.M.; Jacobs, M.L. & McCrindle, B.W. (2007). Critical left ventricular outflow tract obstruction: The disproportionate impact of biventricular repair in borderline cases. *J Thorac Cardiovasc Surg,* 134, 6, (Dec 2007), pp. 1429-36; discussion 1436-7

Holzer, R.; Marshall, A.; Kreutzer, J.; Hirsch, R.; Chisolm, J.; Hill, S.; Galantowicz, M.; Phillips, A.; Cheatham, J. & Bergerson, L. (2010). Hybrid procedures: adverse events and procedural characteristics--results of a multi-institutional registry. *Congenit Heart Dis,* 5, 3, (May-Jun 2010), pp. 233-42

Holzer, R.J.; Wood, A.; Chisolm, J.L.; Hill, S.L.; Phillips, A.; Galantowicz, M. & Cheatham, J.P. (2008). Atrial septal interventions in patients with hypoplastic left heart syndrome. *Catheter Cardiovasc Interv,* 72, 5, (Nov 1 2008), pp. 696-704

Honjo, O.; Benson, L.N.; Mewhort, H.E.; Predescu, D.; Holtby, H.; Van Arsdell, G.S. & Caldarone, C.A. (2009). Clinical outcomes, program evolution, and pulmonary artery growth in single ventricle palliation using hybrid and Norwood palliative strategies. *Ann Thorac Surg,* 87, 6, (Jun 2009), pp. 1885-92; discussion 1892-3

Kasten-Sportes, C.H.; Piechaud, J.F.; Sidi, D. & Kachaner, J.(1989); Percutaneous balloon valvuloplasty in neonates with critical aortic stenosis. *J Am Coll Cardiol,* Vol.13, No.5, pp 1101-1105

McElhinney, D.B.; Lock, J.E.; Keane, J.F.; Moran, A.M. & Colan, S.D. (2005). Left heart growth, function, and reintervention after balloon aortic valvuloplasty for neonatal aortic stenosis. *Circulation,* 111, 4, (Feb 1 2005), pp. 451-8

Pizarro, C.; Bhat, M.A.; Derby, C.D. & Radtke, W.A. (2009). Bailout after failed biventricular management of critical aortic stenosis: another application of the hybrid approach. *Ann Thorac Surg,* 87, 5, (May 2009), pp. e40-2

Reini, S.A.; Dutta, G.; Wood, C.E. & Keller-Wood, M. (2008). Cardiac corticosteroid receptors mediate the enlargement of the ovine fetal heart induced by chronic increases in maternal cortisol. *J Endocrinol,* 198, 2, (Aug 2008), pp. 419-27

Rhodes, L.A.; Colan, S.D.; Perry, S.B.; Jonas, R.A. & Sanders, S.P. (1991). Predictors of survival in neonates with critical aortic stenosis. *Circulation,* 84, 6, (Dec 1991), pp. 2325-35

Roth, S. (2008). Vasodilators, In: *Handbook of Pediatric Cardiovascular Drugs,* Munoz, p 115-117, Springer-Verlag, 978-1-84628-952-1, London, UK

Rychik, J.; Szwast, A.; Natarajan, S.; Quartermain, M.; Donaghue, D.D.; Combs, J.; Gaynor, J.W.; Gruber, P.J.; Spray, T.L.; Bebbington, M. & Johnson, M.P. (2010). Perinatal and early surgical outcome for the fetus with hypoplastic left heart syndrome: a 5-year single institutional experience. *Ultrasound Obstet Gynecol,* 36, 4, (Oct 2010), pp. 465-70

Smallhorn, JF. (2009) Congenital anomalies of the aortic valve and left ventricular outflow tract, In: *Paediatric Cardiology,* Anderson, Baker, Penny, Redington, Rigby &

Wernovsky, 917-932, Churchill Livingstone/Elsevier, 978-0-7020-3064-2, Philadelphia, USA

Stasik, C.N.; Gelehrter, S.; Goldberg, C.S.; Bove, E.L.; Devaney, E.J. & Ohye, R.G. (2006). Current outcomes and risk factors for the Norwood procedure. *J Thorac Cardiovasc Surg,* 131, 2, (Feb 2006), pp. 412-7

Venugopal, P.S.; Luna, K.P.; Anderson, D.R.; Austin, C.B.; Rosenthal, E.; Krasemann, T. & Qureshi, S.A. (2010). Hybrid procedure as an alternative to surgical palliation of high-risk infants with hypoplastic left heart syndrome and its variants. *J Thorac Cardiovasc Surg,* 139, 5, (May 2010), pp. 1211-5

Vogel, M.; McElhinney, D.B.; Marcus, E.; Morash, D.; Jennings, R.W. & Tworetzky, W. (2010). Significance and outcome of left heart hypoplasia in fetal congenital diaphragmatic hernia. *Ultrasound Obstet Gynecol,* 35, 3, (Mar 2010), pp. 310-7